# *Principles & Foundations of Health Promotion and Education*

## FIFTH EDITION

Randall R. Cottrell, D.Ed., CHES
**University of Cincinnati**

James T. Girvan, Ph.D., M.P.H.
**Boise State University**

James F. McKenzie, Ph.D., M.P.H., CHES
**Professor Emeritus, Ball State University**

**Benjamin Cummings**

Boston  Columbus  Indianapolis  New York  San Francisco  Upper Saddle River
Amsterdam  Cape Town  Dubai  London  Madrid  Milan  Munich  Paris  Montréal  Toronto
Delhi  Mexico City  São Paulo  Sydney  Hong Kong  Seoul  Singapore  Taipei  Tokyo

Executive Editor: Sandra Lindelof
Director of Development: Barbara Yien
Project Manager: Carol Traver/Azimuth
  Publisher Services
Editorial Assistants: Meghan Zolnay and
  Brianna Paulson
Managing Editor: Deborah Cogan
Production Manager: Kathy Sleys

Project Management and Composition:
  Niraj Bhatt/Aptara®, Inc.
Interior and Cover Designer: Hespenheide Design
Photo Researcher: Laura Murray
Photo Editor: Donna Kalal
Manufacturing Buyer: Kathy Sleys
Executive Marketing Manager: Neena Bali
Cover Photo Credit: Image Source Ltd.

Credits and acknowledgments borrowed from other sources and reproduced, with permission, in this text-book appear on the appropriate page within the text.

Library of Congress Cataloging-in-Publication Data
Cottrell, Randall R.
  Principles & foundations of health promotion and education / Randall R. Cottrell, James T.
Girvan, James F. McKenzie.—5th ed.
    p. cm.
  Includes bibliographical references and index.
  ISBN-13: 978-0-321-73495-2
  ISBN-10: 0-321-73495-5
  1. Health education.   2. Health promotion.   I. Girvan, James T., 1946-  II. McKenzie, James F.,
1948-  III. Title.   IV. Title: Principles and foundations of health promotion and education.
  RA440.5.C685 2012
  613—dc22

                                                                              2010054547

1 2 3 4 5 6 7 8 9 10—COS—15 14 13 12 11
**Benjamin Cummings**
  is an imprint of

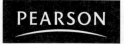

www.pearsonhighered.com

ISBN 10:    0-321-73495-5
ISBN 13: 978-0-321-73495-2

# Contents

# Foreword

In all likelihood you are reading this text as a part of an entry-level course to the field of health education/promotion. This may be your first exposure to the field, and you are probably filled with questions about what health education/promotion is all about and what you can do with a degree in this area.

If this is where you find yourself, this text is designed especially for you. If you enjoy history and want to see how health education/promotion has emerged as a profession from other health and behavioral fields, then the chapter on history will be extremely informative. In addition, the chapters on philosophy and theory will connect you to frameworks that provide a foundation for practice, research, and discovery in health education and promotion. The chapter on ethics will challenge you to think clearly about what you are doing and help you connect your practice with what you believe to be true and ethical. If you want to know what a health education specialist does, the chapter on roles and responsibilities will fully describe the competencies and skills that a practicing health education specialist should endeavor to fulfill. If you are interested in finding out what you can do with a health education/promotion degree, then the chapter describing the various settings for practice will be helpful to you. If you enjoy research, the chapter on literature in health education/promotion will prepare you for a wide range of research projects and activities. Finally, if you enjoy thinking outside the box, the chapter on future trends in health education/promotion will get you to thinking about challenges and opportunities the future will bring to the field.

This updated fifth edition of the text has several new features that you will find helpful. For example, this edition contains the latest information on the impact of health care reform on health education/promotion. This edition also includes information from the National Commission for Health Education Credentialing including the updated responsibilities, competencies and sub-competencies of a health education specialist. In addition, there is expanded information on ethical decision making, quality assurance in health education/promotion, and new information on social networking sites. Finally, this edition provides the latest information on the Health Educator Job Analysis 2010 and preliminary information on Healthy People 2020. Of course, you will enjoy the case studies and practitioner perspectives from previous editions, and the expanded Weblinks will continue to bring the text to life as you interact and connect with various organizations and entities that you are reading about in the text and learning about in class.

When I read a book or suggest a text for others to read, I want to know a bit about the author(s). It is important to me that an author actually knows something about what he/she is writing. Rest assured, the authors of this text are outstanding professors in the field of health education/promotion. Each of them has assumed significant leadership roles in the profession of health education/promotion. So, each of them has extensive experience and background about the things they are writing.

As you read this text and study for your course, let me encourage you to take time to find ways to put into practice what you are learning in class. Ask your faculty advisor if there is a health education/promotion project you can do around your academic department. Join a professional society or your student majors club. Ask one of your professors if he/she is working on a research project that you can assist with. Volunteer to assist a health education specialist at a local health department, voluntary agency, or public school. Find a service project to do with a local health or social service agency.

Welcome to the profession of health education/promotion! This text will be a first step to connect you to research, resources, and practitioners in the field. Through the years you will refer back to the basics that you will learn here—and this text will continue to be a resource for you. As you grow in your professional development, remember to take advantage of the resources and associations presented in this text. They will enrich your life and add value to your professional experience.

Once again, welcome to health education/promotion!

Steve M. Dorman, MPH, Ph.D.
*Professor and Dean*
*College of Health and Human Performance*
*University of Florida*

# Preface

Many students enter the field of health education/promotion knowing only that they are interested in health and wish to help others improve their health status. Typically, students' interest in health education/promotion is derived from their own desire to live a healthy lifestyle and not from an in-depth understanding of the historical, theoretical, and philosophical foundations of this profession. Other than perhaps a high school health education teacher, many students do not know any health education/promotion practitioners. In fact, most beginning students are unaware of employment opportunities, the skills needed to practice health education/promotion, and what it would be like to work in a given health education/promotion setting.

This text is written for such students. The contents will be of value to students who are undecided as to whether health education/promotion is the major they want to pursue, as well as for new health education/promotion majors who need information about what health education/promotion is and where health education specialists can be employed. The text is designed for use in an entry-level health education/promotion course in which the major goal is to introduce students to health education/promotion. In addition, it may have value in introducing new health education graduate students, who have undergraduate degrees in fields other than health education/promotion, to the health education/promotion profession.

## NEW TO THE FIFTH EDITION

- All chapters have been updated for currency including tables, figures, references, terminology, end-of-chapter materials, Weblinks, and appendices.
- Many of the Practitioner's Perspective boxes have been replaced, offering fresh insights from practitioners in such diverse fields as community health education/promotion; health and wellness center education/promotion; wellness peer education/promotion in a higher education setting; health education/promotion for a governmental agency; and local school and community-based injury prevention programs, among others. One new Practitioner's Perspective box details a student internship in Uganda.
- Important new issues and trends covered include
  - the impact of health care reform on health education/promotion;
  - Health Educator Job Analysis 2010;
  - Healthy People 2020;
  - updated responsibilities, competencies, and sub-competencies of a health education specialist;

- NCHEC's new MCHES certification;
- quality assurance in health education/promotion; and
- ethical issues related to community interventions.

## CHAPTER OVERVIEW

Chapter 1, "A Background for the Profession," provides an overview of health education/promotion and sets the stage for the remaining chapters. Chapter 2, "The History of Health and Health Education/Promotion," examines the history of health and health care, as well as the history of health education/promotion. This chapter was written to help students understand the tremendous advances that have been made in keeping people healthy, and it provides perspective on the role of health education/promotion in that effort. One cannot appreciate the present without understanding the past. The chapter will bring students up-to-date with the most recent happenings in the profession, such as the new Patient Protection and Affordable Care Act. Chapters 3, 4, and 5 provide what might best be called the basic foundations. All professions, such as law, medicine, business, and teacher education, must provide students with information related to the philosophy, theory, and ethics inherent in the field.

Chapter 6, "The Health Education Specialist: Roles, Responsibilities, Certifications, Advanced Study," is designed to acquaint new students with the skills that are needed to practice in the field of health education/promotion. It also explains the certification process to students and encourages them to begin thinking of graduate study very early in their undergraduate programs. New information related to changes in the competencies and sub-competencies of a health education specialist based on the Health Education Job Analysis Study is incorporated into this chapter. Chapter 7, "The Settings for Health Education/Promotion," introduces students to the job responsibilities inherent in different types of health education/promotion positions and provides a discussion of the pros and cons of working in various health education/promotion settings. With its "A Day in the Career of . . ." sections and the "Practitioner's Perspective" boxes, this chapter is unique among introductory texts. A new section has been added, warning students to be careful about what they post to social networking websites, and information is included on landing one's first job and how to excel in a health education/promotion career. This chapter truly provides students with important insights into the various health education/promotion settings and the overall profession of health education/promotion.

Chapter 8, "Agencies/Associations/Organizations Associated with Health Education/Promotion," introduces students to the many professional agencies, associations, and organizations that support health education/promotion. This is an extremely important chapter, since all health education specialists need to know of these resources and allies. We believe that all introductory students should be encouraged to join one or more of the professional associations described in this chapter. For that reason, contact information for all of the professional associations discussed is included in the chapter. Chapter 9, "The Literature of Health Education/Promotion," directs students to the information and resources necessary to work in the field. Included in this chapter is basic information related to the Internet and the World Wide Web that should be especially helpful to new students. With the explosion of knowledge related to health, being able to locate needed resources is a critical skill for health education specialists. Finally, health education/promotion students need to consider what future changes in health knowledge, policy, and funding may mean to those working in health education/promotion. They must learn to project into the future and prepare themselves to meet these challenges. Chapter 10, "Future Trends in Health Education/Promotion," is an attempt to provide a window into the future for today's health education/promotion students.

As one reads the text, it will be apparent that certain standard features exist in all chapters. These are designed to help the student identify important information, guide the student's learning, and extend the student's understanding beyond the basic content information. Each chapter begins by identifying objectives. Prior to reading a chapter, students should carefully read the objectives, as they will guide the student's learning of the information contained in that chapter. After reading a chapter, it may also be helpful to review the objectives to make certain major points were understood. Being able to respond to each objective and define each highlighted term in a chapter is typically of great value in understanding the material and preparing for examinations.

Throughout the book take note of the "Practitioner's Perspective" boxes. These are boxes by young health education/promotion professionals who are currently working in the field. Some of the boxes relate to working in a particular setting, while others focus on such areas as ethics, certification, internships, hiring, and graduate study. There are 13 new and informative "Practitioner's Perspectives" in this edition.

At the end of each chapter, the student will find a brief summary of the information contained in that chapter. Following the summary are review questions. Students are encouraged to answer these questions, as they provide an additional method for targeting learning and reviewing the chapter's contents. A case study follows the review questions. Case studies allow readers to project themselves into realistic health education situations and problem-solve how to handle such situations. Next, readers will find critical thinking questions designed to extend readers' learning beyond what is presented in the chapter. They require readers to apply what they have learned, contemplate major events, and project their learning into the future. A list of activities, designed to extend readers' knowledge beyond what can be obtained by reading the chapter, is also included. In some activities students are asked to apply or synthesize the chapter's information. In others, students are encouraged to get actively involved with experiences that will help integrate learning from the text with a practical, real-world setting. By completing these activities, students should have a better understanding of health education/promotion. The activities are followed by Weblinks, which have been updated and expanded for this edition. Weblinks are sites that students can access to read more about a topic, extend their learning, or obtain interesting resource materials. Each chapter ends with a list of references the authors used to develop the chapter. All references are cited in the chapter, and students can use the references to obtain more detailed information on a topic from an original source when they desire to do so.

## SUPPLEMENTS

The following instructor supplements are available with the fifth edition:

- An Instructor's Manual that includes a synopsis, an outline, teaching ideas, website activities, and video resources for each chapter.
- A Test Bank that includes multiple-choice, true/false, and essay questions for each chapter.  A computerized Test Bank is also available.
- PowerPoint presentations that feature chapter outlines and key points from the text.

All of the supplements can be downloaded from Pearson's Instructor Resource Center at http://www.pearsonhighered.com/educator.

This text is also available as a CourseSmart eTextbook (ISBN: 0-321-70975-6). CourseSmart eTextbooks are an exciting new choice for students looking to save money. As an alternative to purchasing the printed textbook, students can subscribe to the same content online and save 40 percent off the suggested list price of the printed text. Access the CourseSmart eText at www.coursesmart.com.

We readily acknowledge that the information contained in this text represents our bias regarding what material should be taught in an introductory course. There may be important introductory information we have not included, or we may have included information that may not be considered introductory by all users. We welcome and encourage comments and feedback, both positive and negative, from all users of this text. Only with such feedback can we make improvements and include the most appropriate information in future editions.

Randall R. Cottrell
James T. Girvan
James F. McKenzie

# Acknowledgments

First, we would like to thank all of the health education faculty who have adopted our text and all of the students who have used the text with each new edition. The response we have received has been truly gratifying. Without you, we would not be writing the fifth edition.

We would also like to thank Pearson/Benjamin Cummings for producing the book. We would especially like to thank Sandy Lindelof for her editorial guidance as well as Megan Power and Dorothy Cox for their hard work on this project. In addition, we would like to thank Carol Traver and Azimuth Publisher Services for their diligent work on our behalf and their outstanding administrative and organization skills.

We would like to express our sincere appreciation to those health education/promotion professionals who served as reviewers for the fifth edition. They had many good ideas that we tried to incorporate whenever possible. The reviewers were John Batacan, Idaho State University; Holly Harring, University of South Carolina; Joanna Hayden, William Paterson University; Adriana Rascon-Lopez, University of Texas at El Paso; Manoj Sharma, University of Cincinnati; and Erica Sosa, University of Texas at San Antonio. We would also like to thank the reviewers of previous editions: Georgia Polacek of the University of Texas, San Antonio; Kathleen Allison of Lock Haven University; Gregg Kirchofer of Canisius College; Dawn Larsen of Minnesota State University, Mankato; Sharon Thompson of The University of Texas, El Paso; M. Allison Ford of Florida Atlantic University; Mike Perko of the University of Alabama; Georgia Johnston of the University of Texas, San Antonio; Craig Huddy of Concord College; Whitney Boling of the University of Houston; Virginia Noland of the University of Florida; R. Morgan Pigg, Jr. of the University of Florida; Marilyn Morrow of Illinois State University; Steve Nagy of Western Kentucky University; Emily Tyler of the University of North Carolina at Greensboro (with additional helpful feedback from Julie Orta, MPH student); and Marianne Frauenknecht of Western Michigan University.

We are lucky to have had excellent secretarial assistance with this project. A big thanks goes to Billie Kennedy, Debbie Morris, Carol Carroll, Linda Miller, Lennell Wade, and Pat Borusiewicz.

Finally, we would like to dedicate this book to the people in our lives who mean the most to us: our wives, Karen, Georgia, and Bonnie; our children, Kyle, Lisa, Kory, Jennifer, Erik, Becky, Erik, Anne, and Greg; our grandchildren, Kaylee, Anna, Mitchell, Julia, Jonah, Rose, and Aevan; and our parents, Russell and Edith Cottrell, Terry and Margaret Girvan, and Gordon and Betty McKenzie.

## CHAPTER 1

# A Background for the Profession

After reading this chapter and answering the questions at the end, you should be able to:

- Define the terms *health, health education, health promotion, disease prevention, public health, community health, global health, population health, coordinated school health program,* and *wellness.*
- Explain why health education/promotion should be considered an emerging profession.
- Describe the current status of health education/promotion.
- Define *epidemiology.*
- Explain the means by which health or health status can be measured.
- List and explain the goal and objectives of health education/promotion.
- Identify the practice of health education/promotion.
- Explain the following concepts and principles:
  a. Health Field Concept
  b. levels of prevention
  c. risk factors
  d. health risk reduction
  e. chain of infection
  f. communicable disease model
  g. multicausation disease model
  h. Selected principles of health education/promotion—*participation, empowerment,* and *culturally competent*

Health education/promotion has come a long way since its early beginnings. Health education/promotion as we know it today dates back only about eighty years, but the progress in development has accelerated most rapidly in the past thirty years (Glanz & Rimer, 2008). As the profession has grown and changed, so have the role and

1

responsibilities of health education specialists. The purpose of this book is to provide those new to this profession with a sense of the past—how the profession was born and on what principles it was developed; a complete understanding of the present—what it is that health education specialists are expected to do, how they should do it, and what guides their work; and a look at the future—where the profession is headed, and how health education specialists can keep pace with the changes in order to be responsive to those whom they serve.

This first chapter provides a common background in the terminology, concepts, and principles of the profession. It defines many of the key words and terms used in the profession, briefly discusses why health education/promotion is referred to as an emerging profession, looks at the current state of the profession, shows how health and health status have been measured, outlines the goals and objectives of the profession, identifies the practice of health education/promotion, and discusses some of the basic, underlying concepts and principles of the profession.

## Key Words, Terms, and Definitions

Each chapter introduces new terminology that is either important to the specific content presented in the chapter or used frequently in the profession. This chapter discusses the more common terms that will be used throughout this text. Like the profession, these words and definitions have evolved over the years. Over the past seventy plus years there have been several efforts to standardize the terms used in the profession. The most recent effort occurred in 2000 (Joint Committee, 2001). (Note: At the time this book was going to press, the American Association [AAHE] for Health Education was in the process of convening the "Joint Committee." Readers should check the AAHE Web site for changes in terminology that may have occurred.) Every ten years the American Association for Health Education forms a task force, called the Joint Committee on Health Education and Health Promotion Terminology, to review and update the terminology of the profession (see Chapter 8 for information on this and other professional associations). The members of the 2000 Committee represented all of the professional associations within the Coalition of National Health Education Organizations (see Chapter 8), as well as key federal agencies (Joint Committee, 2001). Prior to this meeting, there have been six major terminology reports developed for the profession with the first dating back to 1927 (Johns, 1973; Joint Committee on Health Education Terminology, 1991a, 1991b; Moss, 1950; Rugen, 1972; Williams, 1934; Yoho, 1962).

Prior to presenting some of the key terms used in the profession, an in-depth discussion of the word *health* may be helpful. Health is a difficult concept to put into words, but it is one that most people intuitively understand. The World Health Organization has defined health as "the state of complete mental, physical and social well being not merely the absence of disease or infirmity" (WHO, 1947, p. 1). This classic definition is important as it identifies the vital components of health. It further implies that health is a holistic concept involving an interaction and interdependence among these various components. A number of years after the writing of the WHO definition, Hanlon (1974) defined health as "a functional state which makes possible the achievement of other goals and activities. Comfort, well-being, and the distinction between physical and mental health differ in social classes, cultures, and religious groups" (p. 73). And more recently, the WHO (1986) has stated that "To reach a state of complete physical, mental, and social well-being, an individual or group must be able to identify and to realize aspirations, to satisfy needs, and to change or cope with the environment. Health is, therefore, seen as a resource for everyday life, not the object of living. Health is a positive concept emphasizing social and personal resources, as well as physical capacities" (p. 5). In other words, good health should not be the goal of life, but rather a vehicle to reaching one's goals of life. We feel that these major concepts of health are captured in the definition that states that **health** "is a *dynamic* state or condition of the human organism that is multidimensional (i.e., physical, emotional, social, intellectual, spiritual, and occupational) in nature, a resource for living, and results from a person's interactions with and adaptations to his or her environment" (McKenzie, Pinger, & Kotecki, 2012, p. 6). As such, health can exist in varying degrees—ranging from good to poor and everywhere in between—and depends on each person's individual circumstances. "For example, a person can be healthy while dying, or a person who is quadriplegic can be healthy in the sense that his or her mental and social well-being is high and physical health is as good as it can be" (Hancock & Minkler, 2005, p. 144).

In addition to the word *health*, it is also important to have an understanding of the following key terms and definitions:

**community health**—"the health status of a defined group of people and the actions and conditions to protect and improve the health of the community" (Green & McKenzie, 2002, p. 247)

**health education**—"any combination of planned learning experiences based on sound theories that provide individuals, groups, and communities the opportunity to acquire information and the skills needed to make quality health decisions" (Joint Committee, 2001, p. 99)

**health promotion**—"any planned combination of educational, political, environmental, regulatory, or organizational mechanisms that support actions and conditions of living conducive to the health of individuals, groups, and communities" (Joint Committee, 2001, p. 101) (See **Figure 1.1** for the relationship between health education and health promotion.)

**disease prevention**—"the process of reducing risks and alleviating disease to promote, preserve, and restore health and minimize suffering and distress" (Joint Committee, 2001, p. 99)

**public health**—"is the science and the art of protecting and improving the health of communities through education, promotion of healthy lifestyles, and research for disease and injury prevention" (Association of Schools of Public Health, n. d., ¶ 1)

**global health**—"health problems, issues, and concerns that transcend national boundaries, may be influenced by circumstances or experiences in other countries, and are best addressed by cooperative actions and solutions" (IOM, 1997, p. 3)

**population health**—"the health status of people who are not organized and have no identity as a group or locality and the actions and conditions to promote, protect, and preserve their health" (McKenzie et al., 2012, p. 7)

**coordinated school health program**—"an organized set of policies, procedures, and activities designed to protect, promote, and improve the health and well-being of students and staff, thus improving a student's ability to learn. It includes, but is not limited to, comprehensive school health education; school health services; a healthy

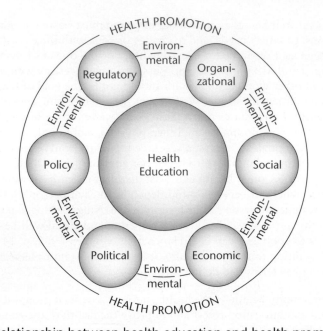

**Figure 1.1** Relationship between health education and health promotion

*Source:* From J. F. Mckenzie, B. L. Neiger, and R. Thackeray, *Planning, Implementing and Evaluating Health Promotion Programs: A Primer.* 5th ed., p. 4, Fig 1.1 © 2009 Reproduced by permission of Pearson Education, Inc., Upper Saddle River, NJ.

school environment; school counseling; psychological and social services; physical education; school nutrition services; family and community involvement in school health; and school-site health promotion for staff" (Joint Committee, 2001, p. 99)

**wellness**—"an approach to health that focuses on balancing the many aspects, or dimensions, of a person's life through increasing the adoption of health-enhancing conditions and behaviors rather than attempting to minimize conditions of illness" (Joint Committee, 2001, p. 103)

Before we leave the discussion about key words and terms of the profession, it should be noted that there is not complete agreement on terminology. We could easily have found another definition for each of the terms presented above written by either a respected scholar in health education/promotion or a legitimate professional or governmental health agency.

## An Emerging Profession

Health education/promotion "is eclectic in nature. As an applied science, it derives its body of knowledge from a variety of disciplines" (Galli, 1976, p. 158). More specifically, health education/promotion's body of knowledge represents a synthesis of facts, principles, and concepts drawn from biological, behavioral, sociological, and health sciences, but interpreted in terms of human needs, human values, and human potential" (Cleary & Neiger, 1998, p. 11). As the applied science of health education/promotion has developed over the years, it has been labeled in a variety of ways as a process, a field, a discipline, and/or a profession. Most would agree health education/promotion is a process or several processes, but to label it as only a process would not be accurate. The words *field* and *discipline* have been used interchangeably, so for the purposes of this discussion, we will use the term *discipline*. Thus, the real question becomes, Is health education/promotion a discipline or a profession? Health education/promotion is neither but is somewhere between the two; in other words, an **emerging profession.** Though the debate may seem trivial, more technical than significant, or just a question of semantics, it is important that those studying to be health education specialists have an understanding of this discussion and be able to see how health education/promotion fits into the bigger picture.

One reason health education/promotion has been described in so many ways is that health education specialists have not been consistent in their use of labels. In the past, health education specialists either did not think it important to make a distinction in terminology or did not give much thought as to what the individual labels meant.

A **discipline** has been defined as "a field of study" (Merriam-Webster, 2010a, ¶ 3). Health education/promotion fits this definition, and then some. We see a discipline as something smaller than a **profession,** which has been defined as "a calling requiring specialized knowledge and often long and intensive academic preparation" (Merriam-Webster, 2010b, ¶ 4). Or, as Livingood (1996, p. 421) has stated, a profession is "the sociological construct for an occupation that has special status." Using these definitions, we see health education/promotion as fitting somewhere between a discipline and a profession, thus the term *emerging profession.*

To further support our claim that health education/promotion is an emerging profession, it might be helpful to present a list of characteristics of a profession. Feeney and Freeman (1999) felt that the following functions distinguish a profession. The words in brackets are our opinions on how health education/promotion stacks up with each of these characteristics.

- A profession requires practitioners to participate in *prolonged training* based on principles that involve judgment for their application, not a precise set of behaviors that apply in all cases. [Health education specialists are not in agreement over what constitutes an extensive period of preparation. Some say a bachelor's degree is necessary; others say a master's degree.]

- Professional training is delivered in accredited institutions. Rigorous *requirements for entry* to the training are controlled by members of the profession. [Health education/promotion has no requirement that training must take place in accredited institutions, nor does health education/promotion have requirements for entry into training.]

- A profession bases its work on a *specialized body of knowledge and expertise,* which is applied according to the particular needs of each case. [As noted earlier, health education/promotion's body of knowledge represents a synthesis of facts, principles, and concepts from several disciplines.]

- Members of the profession have agreed on *standards of practice*—procedures that are appropriate to the solution of ordinary predicaments that practitioners expect to encounter in their work. [Health education/promotion has identified the

responsibilities and competencies for those who practice health education/
promotion (See Appendix B).]

- A profession is characterized by *autonomy*—it makes its own decisions regarding
  entry to the field, training, licensing, and standards. The profession exercises internal
  control over the quality of the services offered and regulates itself. [This is emerging,
  because not all of these aspects are clearly defined by health education/promotion.
  Currently, there is only informal control of the quality of services offered.]

- A profession has a *commitment to serving a significant social value*. It is altruistic
  and service oriented rather than profit oriented. Its primary goal is to meet the
  needs of clients. Society recognizes a profession as the only group from within the
  community that can perform this specialized function. [Health education/promotion
  has a commitment to serving a significant social value. With the acknowledgment
  in 1998 of the U.S. Department of Commerce and Labor formally recognizing
  "health educator" as a distinct occupation, health education/promotion is moving
  in the right direction, but there are still many, including some health professionals,
  who do not recognize the work of health education specialists.]

- A profession has a *code of ethics* that spells out its obligations to society. [Health
  Education has a code of ethics (see Appendix A).]

Though many of the characteristics on Feeney and Freeman's list can be met by health
education/promotion, not all can be.

Further, Barber (1988) states that an emerging profession is an occupation that
does not rank so clearly high or so clearly low on those attributes that distinguish an
occupation from a profession. In other words, Barber indicates that an emerging profession has not been clearly defined by itself or others. We feel Feeney and Freeman's
list and our comments on his list show that health education/promotion is an emerging profession.

Stating that health education/promotion is not at full profession status is not to
say that those who engage in the work—health education specialists—are not professionals. A professional is "one that is professional; *especially* one that engages in a
pursuit or activity professionally" (Merriam-Webster, 2010c, ¶ 1). Professionals must
exercise discretion, judgment, and personal responsibility when applying the knowledge (Turnock, 2006) and skills of their profession in order to enhance, not only the
lives of those whom they are helping, but also the profession. When professionals do
such work throughout their career while maintaining high standards of excellence it is
called *professionalism* (Young & Perko, 2009). It is our belief that health education
specialists do this type of work. When applying the characteristics of a professional,
the Joint Committee (2001) has defined a **health educator** as "a professionally prepared individual who serves in a variety of roles and is specifically trained to use
appropriate educational strategies and methods to facilitate the development of policies,
procedures, interventions, and systems conducive to the health of individuals, groups,
and communities" (p. 99). [Note: Based upon a study titled "Marketing the Health
Education Profession: Knowledge, Attitudes, and Hiring Practices of Employers" conducted by Hezel Associates (2007), the term *health education specialist* has gained
favor over the use of the term health educator. A **health education specialist** has been
defined as "someone having completed the education and/or training requirements
currently associated with professionally prepared" (Hezel Associates, 2007, p. 8).

Thus the term health education specialist will be used throughout the remainder of this book.]

Have we convinced you that health education/promotion is an emerging profession? Maybe we have and maybe we have not; however, throughout the remainder of this book we use the term *profession* to represent *emerging profession*. We are also sure the debate (discipline vs. emerging profession vs. profession) will continue.

## Current Status of Health Education/Promotion

In looking back through history, there have been a number of occasions that can be pointed to as "critical" to the development of health education/promotion. (See Chapter 2 for an in-depth presentation of the history.) But there has been no time in history in which the status of the profession has been more visible to the average person or as widely accepted by other health professionals as it is today. Much of this notoriety can be attributed to the health promotion era of public health history that began about 1974 in the United States.

The United States' first public health revolution spanned the late nineteenth century through the mid-twentieth century and was aimed at controlling the harm (morbidity and mortality) that came from infectious diseases. By the mid-1950s, many of the infectious diseases in the United States were pretty much under control (see **Figure 1.2**). This was evidenced by the improved infant mortality rates, the reduction in the number of children who were contracting childhood diseases, the reduction in the overall death rates in the country, and the increase in life expectancy (see **Table 1.1**). With the control of many communicable diseases, the focus moved to the major chronic diseases

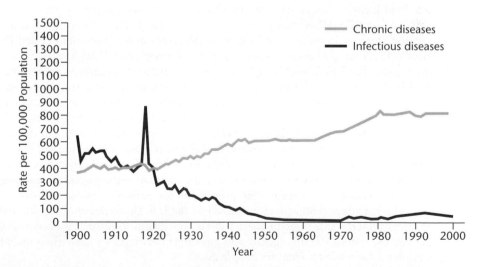

**Figure 1.2** Infectious and chronic disease death rates in the United States, 1900–2000

*Source:* Adapted from G. L. Armstrong, L. A. Conn, and R. W. Pinner, "Trends in Infectious Disease Mortality in the United States During the 20th Century," *Journal of the American Medical Association 281*, 1 (1999): 61–66.

**Table 1.1**    Life expectancy at birth, at sixty-five years of age, and at seventy-five years of age, according to sex: United States, selected years 1900–2008

| | At Birth | | | At 65 Years | | | At 75 Years | | |
|---|---|---|---|---|---|---|---|---|---|
| Year | Both Sexes | Male | Female | Both Sexes | Male | Female | Both Sexes | Male | Female |
| 1900 | 47.3 | 46.3 | 48.3 | 11.9 | 11.5 | 12.2 | * | * | * |
| 1950 | 68.2 | 65.6 | 71.1 | 13.9 | 12.8 | 15.0 | * | * | * |
| 1960 | 69.7 | 66.6 | 73.1 | 14.3 | 12.8 | 15.8 | * | * | * |
| 1970 | 70.8 | 67.1 | 74.7 | 15.2 | 13.1 | 17.0 | * | * | * |
| 1980 | 73.7 | 70.7 | 77.4 | 16.4 | 14.1 | 18.3 | 10.4 | 8.8 | 11.5 |
| 1990 | 75.4 | 71.8 | 78.8 | 17.2 | 15.1 | 18.9 | 10.9 | 9.4 | 12.0 |
| 1995 | 75.8 | 72.5 | 78.9 | 17.4 | 15.6 | 18.9 | 11.0 | 9.7 | 11.9 |
| 2000 | 77.0 | 74.3 | 79.7 | 18.0 | 16.2 | 19.3 | 11.4 | 10.1 | 12.3 |
| 2008 | 77.8 | 75.3 | 80.3 | 18.6 | 17.1 | 19.8 | 11.6 | 10.5 | 12.4 |

* = Data not available
*Source:* Data from U.S. Department of Health and Human Services, National Center for Health Statistics. (2010). *Health, United States, 2009: With Special Feature on Medical Technology.* Hyattsville, MD: Author; and Miniño, A .M., Xu, J., & Kochanek, K. D. (2010). Deaths: Preliminary Data for 2008. *National Vital Statistics Reports, 59* (2), 1–72.

such as heart disease, cancer, and strokes—diseases that were, in large part, the result of the way people lived.

By the mid-1970s, it had become apparent that the greatest potential for reducing morbidity, saving lives, and reducing health care costs in the United States was to be achieved through health promotion and disease prevention. At the core of this approach was health education/promotion. In 1980, the U.S. Department of Health, Education, and Welfare (USDHEW) presented a blueprint of the health promotion and disease prevention strategy in its first set of health objectives in the document called *Promoting Health/Preventing Disease: Objectives for a Nation* (USDHEW, 1980). This document proposed a total of 226 objectives divided into three main areas—preventive services, health protection, and health promotion. This was the first time a comprehensive national agenda for prevention had been developed, with specific goals and objectives for anticipated gains (McGinnis, 1985). In 1985, it was apparent that only about one-half of the objectives established in 1980 would be reached by 1990, another one-fourth would not be reached, and progress on the others could not be judged because of the lack of data (Mason & McGinnis, 1990). Even though not all objectives were reached, the 1980 planning process demonstrated the value of setting goals and listing specific objectives as a means of measuring progress in the nation's health and health care services. These goals and objectives published by the U.S. Department of Health and Human Services (USDHHS), now in their fourth generation as *Healthy People 2020*, have defined the nation's health agenda and guided its health policy since their inception. (See Chapter 2 for more on *Healthy People 2020*).

Now ten plus years into the twenty-first century, the health of the people in the United States is better than any time in the past. "By every measure, we are healthier, live longer, and enjoy lives that are less likely to be marked by injuries, ill health, or premature death" (Institute of Medicine [IOM], 2002, p. 2). Yet, we could do better.

"Four modifiable health risk behaviors—lack of physical activity, poor nutrition, tobacco use, and excessive alcohol consumption—are responsible for much of the illness, suffering, and early death related to chronic diseases" (CDC, 2010b, ¶ 3). Thus, "behavior patterns represent the single most prominent domain of influence over health prospects in the United States" (McGinnis, Williams-Russo, & Knickman, 2002, p. 82).

Clearly, there is a greater need for health education/promotion interventions in the United States both today and in the future.

## Measuring Health or Health Status

Though the definition of health is easy to state, trying to quantify the amount of health an individual or a population possesses is not easy. Therefore, most measures of health are expressed using health statistics based on the traditional medical model of describing ill health (injury, disease, and death) instead of well health. Thus, the higher the presence of injury, disease, and death indicators, the lower the level of health; the lower the presence of injury, disease, and death indicators, the higher the level of health. Out of necessity we have defined the level of health with just the opposite—ill health (McKenzie et al., 2012).

The information gathered when measuring health is referred to as **epidemiological data.** These data are gathered at the local, state, and national levels to assist with the prevention of disease outbreaks or control those in progress and to plan and assess health education/promotion programs. Epidemiology is one of those disciplines noted earlier in the chapter that helps provide the foundation for the health education/promotion profession (see **Box 1.1**). Epidemiology is defined as "the study of the distribution and determinants of health-related states or events in specific populations, and the application of this study to control health problems" (*Dictionary of Epidemiology* as cited in Last, 2007, p. 111). In the following sections, several of the more common epidemiological means by which health, or lack thereof, are described and quantified.

---

**Box 1.1** Practitioner's Perspective    **Epidemiology**

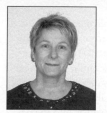

(Reprinted by permission of Jean Woodward)

NAME: Jean Woodward, B.S., M.H.S. CHES

CURRENT POSITION: Project Director, Access to Recovery Program, Division of Behavioral Health

EMPLOYER: Idaho Department of Health and Welfare

DEGREE/INSTITUTION/YEAR: Bachelor of Science, Boise State University, 2001; Master of Health Science, Boise State University, 2005

MAJOR: B.S. HEALTH PROMOTION; M.H.S. HEALTH PROMOTION

**How I obtained my job:** I think that my diverse employment background prepared me well to be a public health educator. Prior to my public health service, I was a teacher (grades 1–12) for 10 years and an acute care nurse for 18 years. In addition, I was involved in several community-level programs, many of which I was the initiator. My background in health and education along with my community mobilization experience made public health educator a natural choice for me. I started at the local health district level, and after four years moved to the state level. My public

**Box 1.1 Practitioner's Perspective**   Continued

health background includes environmental health, chronic disease prevention, and currently I manage a substance abuse treatment program.

**How I utilize an understanding of epidemiology in my job:** Public health is a population-based practice that includes assessing health status, diagnosing and investigating health problems and health hazards, designing solutions for health problems, and evaluating the efficacy of those solutions. Epidemiology is the tool that I use to perform each of these functions. Epidemiology tells me if there is a health problem, who has the problem, how much of the problem there is, and how severe the problem is. It can also guide me to an effective intervention point and solution to the problem. Epidemiology provides the science-base for my public health interventions.

**What I like most about my job:** Health promotion is always challenging; no two days are ever the same. Because of its prevention focus, I feel as though I can truly make a difference in peoples' lives. I also enjoy the synergy of a team effort. Public health is collaborative by nature; and through engaging community partners, I am able to provide more comprehensive, effective, and efficient health promotion programs.

**What I like least about my job:** Funding for public health tends to be categorical. There are separate pots of money for each health issue, no matter that most health issues are related at some level. This compartmentalization leads to inefficiency through duplication of efforts and wasting of resources. Health doesn't occur in a vacuum. I feel that only through utilizing an integrated, systems approach to health that we can effectively support the health behavior changes that result in improved public health.

**Recommendations for those preparing to be health education specialists:** There are four recommendations that I would make to those preparing to be health education specialists: 1) You cannot get too much education so stay in school; 2) Get broad experience through graduate assistantships/internships/work; 3) Apply

what you learn as quickly as possible; and 4) Learn to write succinctly.

**What role do you see for health education specialists in the future?** The future holds many challenges for health education specialists: the aging of the population; changes in ethnic/racial composition; changes in family structure; changes in the health care delivery system; an explosion of information technologies; the changing needs in the public health workforce; credentialing; and growth in health-related partnerships. Each of these will require high-level health education specialist competency.

Two competency areas of recent focus are health literacy and cultural competency. The USDHHS's Office of Disease Prevention and Health Promotion defined health literacy as "the capacity to obtain, process, and understand basic health information and services needed to make appropriate health decisions." A recent Institute of Medicine study found that many Americans lack the literacy to obtain basic health information and services. Designing health education/promotion interventions to address low literacy currently challenges and will continue to challenge public health professionals in the future.

Changing demographics will drive the need for cultural competency in health education/promotion. Cultural competency will allow health education specialists to design effective interventions to meet the needs of America's increasingly racial and ethnic diversity.

While there are many challenges for health education specialists in the future, there will be increasing opportunities, as well. Health education/promotion is an essential public health service. Through its focus on prevention, it reduces the costs that individuals, employers, medical facilities, insurance companies, and the nation would spend on medical treatment. As a result, there will be increasing demand for health education specialists in schools, colleges, worksites, medical care, public health, community-based agencies and organizations, and other settings, such as nursing, social work, mental health, substance abuse/HIV counselors, etc.

**Table 1.2** Crude death rates for all causes and selected causes of death: United States, 2008

| Cause | Deaths per 100,000 Population |
|---|---|
| All causes | 813.2 |
| Diseases of the heart | 203.1 |
| Malignant neoplasms (cancer) | 186.2 |
| Chronic lower respiratory diseases | 46.4 |
| Cerebrovascular diseases (stroke) | 44.0 |
| Intentional self-harm (suicide) | 11.8 |
| Parkinson's disease | 6.7 |
| Assault (homicide) | 5.9 |

*Source:* Data from U.S. Department of Health and Human Services, National Center for Health Statistics. (2010). *Health, United States, 2009: With Special Feature on Medical Technology.* Hyattsville, MD: Author. Miniño, A. M., Xu, J., & Kochanek, K. D. (2010). Deaths: Preliminary Data for 2008. *National Vital Statistics Reports, 59* (2), 1–72.

## Rates

A **rate** "is a measure of some event, disease, or condition in relation to a unit of population, along with some specification of time" (NCHS, 2010, p. 544). Rates are important because they provide an opportunity for comparison of events, diseases, or conditions that occur at different times or places. Some of the more commonly used rates are death rates, birth rates, and morbidity rates. **Death rates** (the number of deaths per 100,000 resident population), sometimes referred to as *mortality* or *fatality rates*, are probably the most frequently used means of quantifying the seriousness of injury or disease. (See **Table 1.2** for death rates and **Table 1.3** for an example of a formula used to tabulate rates.) "The transition from wellness to ill health is often gradual and poorly defined. Because death, in contrast, is a clearly defined event, it has continued to be the most reliable single indicator of health status of a population. Mortality statistics, however, describe only a part of the health status of a population, and often only the endpoint of an illness process" (USDHHS, 1991, p. 15). Rates can be expressed in three forms—(1) crude, (2) adjusted, and (3) specific. A **crude rate** is the rate expressed for a total population. An **adjusted rate** is

**Table 1.3** Selected mortality rates and their formulas

| Rate | Definition | Example (U.S. 2008) |
|---|---|---|
| Crude death rate $= \dfrac{\text{Number of deaths (all causes)}}{\text{Estimated midyear population}} \times 100{,}000$ | | 813.2/100,000 |
| Age-specific death rate $= \dfrac{\text{Number of deaths, } 45 - 54}{\text{Estimated midyear population, } 45 - 54} \times 100{,}000$ | | 420.6/100,000 |
| Cause-specific mortality rate $= \dfrac{\text{Number of deaths (HIV)}}{\text{Estimated midyear population}} \times 100{,}000$ | | 3.4/100,000 |

*Source:* Data from U.S. Department of Health and Human Services, National Center for Health Statistics. (2010). *Health, United States, 2009: With Special Feature on Medical Technology.* Hyattsville, MD: Author. Miniño, A. M., Xu, J., & Kochanek, K. D. (2010). Deaths: Preliminary Data for 2008. *National Vital Statistics Reports, 59* (2), 1–72.

also expressed for a total population but is statistically adjusted for a certain characteristic, such as age. A **specific rate** is a rate for a particular population subgroup such as for a particular disease (i.e., disease-specific) or for a particular age of people (i.e., age-specific). Examples include calculating the death rate for heart disease in the United States, or the age-specific death rate for forty-five- to fifty-four-year-olds.

There are three other epidemiological terms that are used to describe the magnitude of a rate of some event, disease, or condition in a unit of population. They are: (1) **endemic**—occurs regularly in a population as a matter of course; (2) **epidemic**—an unexpectedly large number of cases of an illness, specific health-related behavior, or other health-related event in a population; and (3) **pandemic**—an outbreak over a wide geographical area, such as a continent. As you continue your preparation to become a health education specialist, you will be introduced to more and more epidemiological principles and terms.

## Life Expectancy

Life expectancy is another means by which health or health status has been measured. It, too, however, is based on mortality. Even with this limitation, though, life expectancy has been described as "the most comprehensive indicator of patterns of health and disease, as well as living standards and social development" (Centers for Disease Control and Prevention [CDC], 1994, pp. 2–8). **Life expectancy** "is the average number of years of life remaining to a person at a particular age and is based on a given set of age-specific death rates, generally the mortality conditions existing in the period mentioned. Life expectancy may be determined by race, sex, or other characteristics using age-specific death rates for the population with that characteristic" (NCHS, 2010, p. 525). The most frequently used times to state life expectancy are at birth, at the age of sixty-five, and more recently at age seventy-five (see Table 1.1). It must be remembered that life expectancy is an average for an entire cohort (usually a single birth year) and is not necessarily a useful predictor for any one individual. In terms of evaluating the effect of chronic disease on a population, life expectancies calculated *after* birth have been found to be more useful measures than life expectancy *at* birth, because life expectancy at birth reflects infant mortality rates.

## Years of Potential Life Lost

A third means by which health or health status has been measured is **years of potential life lost (YPLL)**. YPLL "is a measure of premature mortality" (NCHS, 2010, p. 549). (see **Table 1.4**). It is calculated by subtracting a person's age at death from seventy-five years. For example, for a person who dies at age thirty, the YPLL are forty-five. Until 1996, the U.S. government used age sixty-five in calculating YPLL, but because life expectancy in the United States has continued to increase and is greater than seventy-five years that age is now used (NCHS, 2010).

## Disability-Adjusted Life Years

The three measures of health and health status noted previously are commonly used in the United States and other developed countries. However, because mortality does not express the burden of living with disability (for example, the resulting paralysis from an

**Table 1.4**   Age-adjusted years of potential life lost (per 100,000 population) before age 75 for selected leading causes of death: United States, 1990 and 2006

| Cause | 1990 | 2006 |
|---|---|---|
| Malignant neoplasms | 2,003.8 | 1585.7 |
| Diseases of the heart | 1,617.7 | 1138.0 |
| Accidents (unintentional injuries) | 1,162.1 | 1165.4 |
| Intentional self-harm (suicide) | 393.1 | 349.2 |
| Assault (homicide) | 417.4 | 281.0 |
| Cerebrovascular diseases (stroke) | 259.6 | 199.3 |
| Chronic lower respiratory diseases | 187.4 | 181.4 |
| Diabetes mellitus | 155.9 | 157.4 |
| HIV | 383.8 | 124.5 |
| Chronic liver disease and cirrhosis | 196.9 | 157.4 |
| Influenza and pneumonia | 141.5 | 78.8 |

*Source:* Data from U.S. Department of Health and Human Services, National Center for Health Statistics. (2010). *Health, United States, 2009 with Special Feature on Medical Technology.* Hyattsville, MD: Author, p. 194.

automobile crash or the depression that often follows a stroke), the WHO and the World Bank developed a measure called **disability-adjusted life years (DALYs)**. One DALY can be thought of as one lost year of "healthy" life due to being in states of poor health or disability (Murray & Lopez, 1996; WHO, 2008).

To calculate total DALYs for a given condition in a population, years of life lost (YLL) and years lived with disability of known severity and duration (YLDs) for that condition must each be estimated, then the total summed. For example, to calculate DALYs incurred through road accidents in India in 1990, add the total years of life lost in fatal road accidents and the total years of life lived with disabilities by survivors of such accidents (Murray & Lopez, 1996, p. 7).

**Figure 1.3** presents the DALYs for selected regions of the world. As noted, "DALYs in Africa are at least two times higher than in any other region" (WHO, 2008, p. 40).

## Health-Adjusted Life Expectancy

One other measurement of health, which is used by the WHO and is based on disability and life expectancy rather than mortality, is **health-adjusted life expectancy (HALE)**. Sometimes referred to as healthy life expectancy, HALE is the number of years of healthy life expected, on average, in a given population. Like life expectancy, HALE can be calculated at birth and at other ages. The methods used to calculate HALE are beyond the scope of this textbook, but have been described else (Mathers, Sdana, Salmon, Murray, & Lopez, 2001).

## Health-Related Quality of Life

Even though DALYs and HALE go beyond measuring health in terms of just mortality, they really do not get at the quality of life (QOL). While QOL refers to a person or group's general well-being, **health-related quality of life (HRQOL)** "refers to a person or group's perceived physical and mental health over time" (CDC, 2010c, ¶ 1). Health

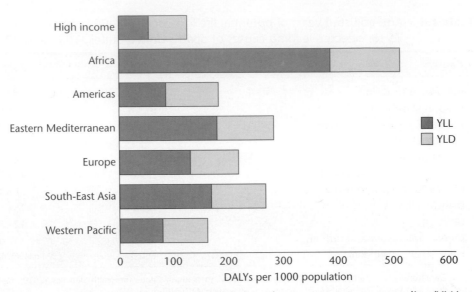

**Figure 1.3** Burden of disease: years of life lost due to premature mortality (YLL) and years of life lived with a disability (YLD) per thousand by region, 2004. DALYs, disability-adjusted life years

*Source:* From "Burden of Disease: DALYs" in *The Global Burden of Disease: 2004 Update.* © World Health Organization, 2008. Reproduced by permission of the World Health Organization. http://www.who.int/healthinfo/global_burden_disease/GBD_report_2004update_part4.pdf

care providers have often used HRQOL to measure the effects of chronic disease in their patients to better understand how a disease interferes with a person's daily life. Similarly, public health professionals have used HRQOL to measure the effects of numerous disorders, short- and long-term disabilities, and diseases in different populations. Tracking HRQOL in different populations can identify subgroups with poor physical or mental health and can help guide policies or other interventions to improve their health (CDC, 2010c).

In recent years, more and more health professionals have been using the concept of HRQOL to quantify and track the health status of people. Measures of HRQOL are now included on a number of different health surveys, including the Behavioral Risk Factor Surveillance Survey (BRFSS) and the National Health and Examination Survey (NHANES) (see next section for discussion of these surveys). Both the BRFSS and the NHANES use the standard 4-item "Healthy" Days core questions (CDC HRQOL-4) created by the Centers for Disease Control and Prevention and presented in **Box 1.2**.

## Health Surveys

Data collected through surveys conducted by governmental agencies are other means by which health or health status has been measured in the United States. Six examples are presented here. The first two, the National Health Interview Survey (NHIS) and the National Health and Nutrition Examination Survey (NHANES), are conducted by the National Center for Health Statistics. The NHIS, which has been used for over fifty years, is a telephone interview in which respondents are asked a number of questions about

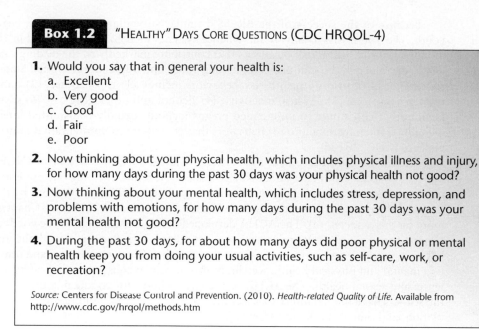

**Box 1.2** "HEALTHY" DAYS CORE QUESTIONS (CDC HRQOL-4)

**1.** Would you say that in general your health is:
   a. Excellent
   b. Very good
   c. Good
   d. Fair
   e. Poor

**2.** Now thinking about your physical health, which includes physical illness and injury, for how many days during the past 30 days was your physical health not good?

**3.** Now thinking about your mental health, which includes stress, depression, and problems with emotions, for how many days during the past 30 days was your mental health not good?

**4.** During the past 30 days, for about how many days did poor physical or mental health keep you from doing your usual activities, such as self-care, work, or recreation?

*Source:* Centers for Disease Control and Prevention. (2010). *Health-related Quality of Life.* Available from http://www.cdc.gov/hrqol/methods.htm

their health and health behavior. One of the questions, for example, asks the respondents to describe their health status using one of five categories: excellent, very good, good, fair, or poor.

The NHANES data are collected using a mobile examination center. Through direct physical examinations, clinical and laboratory testing, and related procedures, data are collected on a representative group of Americans. These examinations result in the most authoritative source of standardized clinical, physical, and physiological data on the U.S. population. Included in the data are the prevalence of specific conditions and diseases and data on blood pressure, blood cholesterol, body mass index, nutritional status and deficiencies, and exposure to environmental toxins (McKenzie et al., 2012).

The third example of data collected from surveys actually comes from a family of surveys called the National Health Care Surveys (NHCS). At the time this book was written, this group of surveys was comprised of six different surveys that are designed to answer key questions about health care providers (i.e., outpatient care, hospitals, and long-term care). A seventh survey will be added soon to survey residential care facilities. All surveys yield objective, reliable information about the organizations and providers that supply health care, the services rendered, and the patients they serve (NCHS, 2009).

The fourth example of data collected through a survey is the data collected through the Behavioral Risk Factor Surveillance System (BRFSS). These data are collected by individual states, territories, and the District of Columbia through cooperative agreements with the Centers for Disease Control and Prevention (CDC). Through the use of telephone survey techniques, each state selects a probability sample from the civilian, noninstitutionalized adult population (over eighteen years of age). Those selected are asked a set of standard core questions, developed by the CDC in order to produce data about health behaviors that can be compared across states (CDC, 2010a). In addition, states may include other questions that would be useful in monitoring health in that particular state.

Because of the success of the BRFSS a similar surveillance system was begun for youth. The Youth Risk Behavior Surveillance System (YRBSS) was developed in 1990 to monitor priority health risk behaviors that contribute markedly to the leading causes of death, disability, and social problems among youth and adults in the United States. The six categories of priority health-risk behaviors include (1) tobacco use; (2) unhealthy dietary behaviors; (3) physical inactivity; (4) alcohol and other drug use; (5) sexual behaviors that contribute to unintended pregnancy and sexually transmitted infections, including HIV infection; and (6) behaviors that contribute to unintentional injuries and violence (CDC, 2010d).

The final survey presented, the National College Health Assessment (NCHA), is one that collects health data about college students. It is also the only one presented here that is not conducted by a governmental agency. The NCHA is carried out by the professional organization American College Health Association (ACHA) (see Chapter 8 for more on this association). The ACHA developed the NCHA, which can be conducted as either a paper-pencil or online survey, to assist schools in collecting data about students' habits, behaviors, and perceptions about topics such as alcohol, tobacco, and other drug use; mental and physical health; weight, nutrition, and exercise; personal safety and violence; and sexual health. The ACHA does charge schools for conducting the NCHA but the schools have the flexibility to select the surveying method, sample size, priority population, and time it is offered (ACHA, 2009).

## Using Health Data in Health Education/Promotion

In the previous sections of this chapter we presented information on measuring health and health status, as well as where health education specialists may find health-related data that are collected by governmental and other organizations. Now we would like to give you an example of how health education specialists may use data. As you will soon learn, a major task of health education specialists is to assist those in the priority population (individuals, groups, and communities) in obtaining, maintaining and improving their health. Often this means planning some type of health education/promotion program that can be used by those in the priority population. These programs should be based on the needs of the priority population, and the needs are often described using data.

For example, let's say a health education specialist is working for a local (county) health department at a time when the state health department has just made funds available through a competitive grant process to deal with the high rates of cancer in the state. Because of some past concerns about cancer in the county, her supervisor has suggested she seek funding. Though she has heard some residents express concern about possible higher rates of cancer, she is really not sure about the type of cancer or whether there is a specific group of people affected. Therefore she needs to be able to describe the potential problem and identify a priority population. One approach would be to determine if there are any health disparities associated with cancer in her county. It has long been "recognized that some individuals are healthier than others and that some live longer than others do, and that often these differences are closely associated with social characteristics such as race, ethnicity, gender, location, and socioeconomic status" (King, 2009, p. 339). These gaps between groups have been referred to as *health disparities* (also called health inequalities in some countries). More formally, **health disparity** has been defined as the difference in health between populations often caused by two health inequities—lack of access to care and lack of quality care (McKenzie et al., 2012).

One place to start looking for cancer health disparities would be the cancer mortality rates (i.e., crude and age-adjusted) for the state as a whole compared with the county where the health education specialist works. These data may be available from the National Center for Health Statistics or another center within the Centers for Disease Control and Prevention, from the state department of health, or from a university research center. Similar comparisons could also be made based upon the mortality rates for various types of cancer. If the health education specialist knew what types of cancers were of greatest concern in the county, she could then examine the data for the county on the basis of certain demographic characteristics that have been associated with certain cancers. So the health education specialist may be using sex-, age-, or race/ethnicity-specific rates to compare various subgroups while looking for disparities. Once the health education specialist identifies a subgroup problem with a type of cancer, she may turn to data from the Behavioral Risk Factor Surveillance System to look for risk behaviors that are known to contribute to or cause the type of cancer identified. Again, the health education specialist may find the needed data in a state or local agency or university as well. Using all of these different sources of data should help the health education specialist find the focus of her program for the priority population and put her in a position to compete for the grant money from the state department of health. Examples of what the health education specialist may have found through this process are higher rates of prostate cancer in African-American men between the ages of 45 and 64 years, or a higher prevalence of certain types of leukemia in children under 15 years of age.

In summary, to get to the point of being able to identify a priority population (i.e., a certain subgroup of people) and program focus (i.e., risk factors associated with a certain type of cancer) several different types of data were used. Initially, the health education specialist used cancer mortality data, then prevalence rates for various types of cancer and different subgroups, and finally risk factor data for various types of cancer.

## The Goal and Purpose of the Profession

The ultimate goal of all service professions, including health education/promotion, is to improve the quality of life, even though the quality of life is difficult to quantify (Raphael, Brown, Renwick, & Rootman, 1997). However, many professionals feel that there is a direct relationship between quality of life and health status. Quality of life is usually improved when health status is improved, or, as Ashley Montagu (1968, p. 206) has stated, "The highest goal in life is to die young, at as old an age as possible." To that end, "the goal of health education is to promote, maintain, and improve individual and community health. The teaching-learning process is the hallmark and social agenda that differentiates the practice of health education from that of other helping professions in achieving this goal" (NCHEC, 1996, pp. 2–3).

Because quality of life and health status are complex variables, they are not usually changed in a short period of time. In order to reach these goals, people usually, over a period of time, work their way through a number of small steps that equip them with all that is necessary to impact both their health status and, in turn, their quality of life.

Thus, it is the work of health education/promotion specialists to create interventions (programs) that can assist people in working toward better health. This work is reflected in the purpose of health education that "is to positively influence the health behavior of individuals and communities as well as the living and working conditions that influence their health" (New York State as presented at CNHEO, 2007, p. 1).

## The Practice of Health Education/Promotion

Although the specific practice of health education specialists is outlined in the responsibilities and competencies presented in Chapter 6, as noted in our discussion of the use of data earlier, the primary role of health education specialists is to develop appropriate health education/promotion programs for the people they serve. The practice of health education/promotion is based on the assumption "that beneficial health behavior will result from a combination of planned, consistent, integrated learning opportunities. This assumption rests on the scientific evaluations of health education programs in schools, at worksites, in medical settings, and through mass media" (Green & Ottoson, 1999, pp. 93–94). The results of these *scientific evaluations,* referred to by Green and Ottoson, are one source of data that contribute to a body of data known as evidence. **Evidence** is data that can be used to make decisions about planning. When health education specialists practice in such a way that they systematically find, appraise, and use evidence as the basis for decision-making when planning health education/promotion programs it is referred to as **evidence-based practice** (Cottrell & McKenzie, 2011).

While the practice of health education specialists is easily stated, it is by no means easy to carry out. Much time, effort, practice, and on-the-job training are required to be successful. Even the most experienced health education specialists find program development challenging because of the constant changes in settings, resources, and priority populations (McKenzie, Neiger, & Thackeray, 2009).

The specific steps taken to develop a health education/promotion program vary depending on the planning model used (see Chapter 4); most models include the following steps (McKenzie et al., 2009) (see Figure 4.18):

1. Assessing the needs of the priority population

2. Setting goals and objectives

3. Developing an intervention that considers the peculiarities of the setting

4. Implementing the intervention

5. Evaluating the results

Therefore, it becomes the practice of health education specialists to be able to carry out all that is associated with these tasks.

## Basic Underlying Concepts of the Profession

As is noted earlier in this chapter and discussed in greater detail in Chapter 2, the profession of health education/promotion is one that has been built on the principles and concepts of a number of disciplines and professions. Within health education/promotion can be found pieces of community development and organizing, education, epidemiology, medicine, psychology, and sociology. In the sections that follow, we present some of the basic underlying concepts of the profession. Please note that we have not exhausted the discussion of each of these topics but, rather, present sufficient information to allow a basic understanding of each.

## The Health Field Concept and the Determinants of Health

Shortly after the Canadian government implemented its national health plan that insured health care for all Canadians, it began to look more closely at the health field as a way of improving Canadians' health. The **health field** is a term the government described as being far more encompassing than the "health care system." This term was much broader and included all matters that affected health (Lalonde, 1974). Because the health field was such a broad concept, it was felt that there was a need to develop a framework that would subdivide the concept into principal elements so that the elements could be studied. Such a framework was developed and called the **Health Field Concept** (Laframboise, 1973).

The Health Field Concept divided the health field into four elements: (1) human biology, (2) environment, (3) lifestyle, and (4) health care organization. "These four elements were identified through an examination of the causes and underlying factors of sickness and death in Canada, and from an assessment of the parts the elements play in affecting the level of health in Canada" (Lalonde, 1974, p. 31). **Human biology** "includes all those aspects of health, both physical and mental, which are developed within the human body as a consequence of the basic biology of man [sic] and the organic make-up of an individual" (Lalonde, 1974, p. 31). This includes not only the genetic inheritance of an individual but also the processes of maturation and aging and the complex interaction of the various systems of the human body (Lalonde, 1974). The element of **environment** "includes all those matters related to health which are external to the human body and over which the individual has little or no control" (Lalonde, 1974, p. 32). Some examples of things often included in the element of environment are geography, climate, community size, industrial development, economy, and social norms.

The element of **lifestyle** comprises the "aggregation of decisions by individuals which affect their health and over which they more or less have control" (Lalonde, 1974, p. 32). In more recent times, lifestyle has been more commonly referred to as **health behavior** (those behaviors that impact a person's health). The fourth element in the Health Field Concept is health care organization. **Health care organization** "consists of the quantity, quality, arrangement, nature and relationships of people and resources in the provision of health care" (Lalonde, 1974, p. 32). This fourth element is often referred to as the health care system.

The utility of the Health Field Concept has proved to be very helpful over the years, both in Canada and the United States. Its greatest importance may have been to bring attention to the concept of health promotion and disease prevention. Prior to this point in history, the primary focus of health care had been on the cure of disease, not the prevention of disease. In fact, it was stated that the Health Field Concept put human biology, environment, and lifestyle on equal footing with health care organization (Lalonde, 1974). Since its development, studies using this concept in both Canada and the United States have provided a greater understanding of what contributes to morbidity and mortality, and what health professionals can do to help improve the health of those whom they serve.

Using a similar framework as that of the elements of the Health Field Concept, it is now believed that the health of populations is shaped by five intersecting domains (i.e., the **Determinants of Health**): (1) gestational endowment (i.e., genetic makeup), (2) social circumstances (e.g., education, socio-economic status, housing, crime), (3) environmental conditions (e.g., toxic agents, microbial agents, natural and humanmade hazards), (4) health behavior (i.e., diet, physical activity), and (5) access to quality medical care (IOM, 2001; McGinnis, 2001; USDHHS, 2000) (see the discussion of Multicausation Disease Model later in the chapter). Further, these domains are dynamic and vary in impact depending on where one is in the life cycle (IOM, 2001). For example, we know that genetics play a big part in late onset diseases such as diabetes, cancer, and cardiovascular disease, while employment and income (social circumstances) have a significant influence on health and health care throughout life.

On a population basis, using the best available estimates, the impacts of various domains on early deaths in the United States distribute roughly as follows: genetic predispositions, about 30%, social circumstances, 15%, environmental exposures, 5%, behavioral patterns, 40%; and shortfalls in medical care about 10%. But more important than these proportions is the nature of the influences in play where the domains intersect. Ultimately, the health fate of each of us is determined by factors acting not mostly in isolation but by our experience where domains interconnect. Whether a gene is expressed can be determined by environmental exposures or behavioral patterns. The nature and consequences of behavioral choices are affected by our social circumstances. Our genetic predispositions affect the health care we need, and our social circumstances affect the health care we receive. (McGinnis et al., 2002, p. 83)

## The Levels and Limitations of Prevention

The word *prevention* has already been used several times in this chapter. We now want to formally define the term, present the different levels of prevention, and briefly discuss the limitations of prevention. **Prevention,** as it relates to health, has been defined as the planning for and the measures taken to forestall the onset of a disease or other health problem before the occurrence of undesirable health events. This definition presents three distinct levels of prevention: primary, secondary, and tertiary prevention. **Primary prevention** comprises those preventive measures that forestall the onset of illness or injury during the prepathogenesis period (before the disease process begins) (McKenzie et al., 2012). Examples of primary prevention measures include wearing a safety belt, using rubber gloves when there is potential for the spread of disease, immunizing against specific diseases (see **Figure 1.4**), exercising, and brushing one's teeth. And any health education/promotion program aimed specifically at forestalling the onset of illness or injury is also an example of primary prevention.

Illness and injury cannot always be prevented. In fact, many diseases, such as cancer and heart disease, can establish themselves in humans and cause considerable damage before they are detected and treated. In such cases, the sooner a condition is detected and medical personnel intervene, the greater the chances of limiting disability and preventing death. Such identification and intervention are known as secondary prevention. More specifically, **secondary prevention** includes the preventive measures that lead to an early diagnosis and prompt treatment of a disease or an injury to limit disability and prevent more serious pathogenesis. Good examples of secondary prevention include personal and clinical screenings and exams such as blood pressure, blood cholesterol, and

**Figure 1.4** Vaccination is an example of primary prevention.

(F. Hoffman/The Image Works)

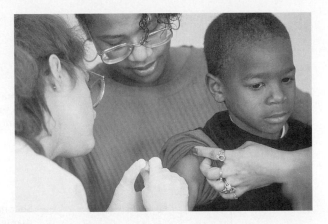

hemocult (hidden blood) screenings; breast self-exams (BSE); and testicle self-exams (TSE). The goal of such screenings and exams is not to prevent the onset of the disease but rather to detect its presence during early pathogenesis, thus permitting early treatment and limiting disability (McKenzie et al., 2012).

The final level of prevention is **tertiary prevention**. It is at this level that health education specialists work to retrain, reeducate, and rehabilitate the individual who has already incurred disability, impairment, or dependency. Examples of some tertiary measures include educating a patient after lung cancer surgery or working with an individual who has diabetes to ensure that the daily insulin injections are taken. **Figure 1.5** provides a visual representation of the levels of prevention in relation to health status.

Though health education specialists can intervene at any of the three levels of prevention, and can have a great deal of success, it should be obvious from the earlier discussion of the Health Field Concept and the Determinants of Health that prevention is not the "magic bullet" for an endless life. Prevention does have its limits. McGinnis (1985) has noted four major categories of limitations: (1) biological, (2) technological, (3) ethical, and (4) economic. Biological limitations center around life span. How long should individuals expect to live healthy lives or, for that matter, how long should they expect to live at all? Even with the very best inputs and a bit of luck, one should not expect to live longer than 80 to 110 years. Body parts will eventually wear out from use.

Technological advances also have their limitations. Today, health care workers have a vast array of technical equipment available to help them care for their patients, but technology still has not been able to eradicate AIDS or malaria, or to explain the cause of Alzheimer's disease.

Prevention is also limited by ethical concerns (see Chapter 5). Even though helmets would increase the chances of survival in automobile crashes, is it ethical to have a law that says all drivers and passengers in automobiles must wear them? Or is it ethical to penalize people via fines, taxes, or surcharges for acting in unhealthy ways, such as driving an automobile without a safety belt on, buying and using tobacco products, or for not having a smoke detector and fire extinguisher in the home?

Finally, prevention has economic limitations. Prevention is limited by the amount of money that is put into it. Though the exact figures are difficult to determine, it is commonly understood that less than 5 percent of all dollars spent on health in the United States each year is spent on prevention. Stated another way, approximately 95 percent

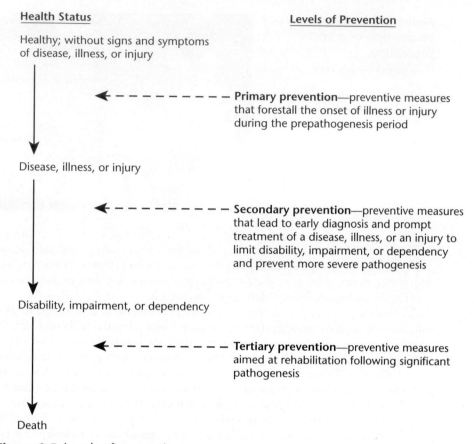

**Figure 1.5** Levels of prevention

*Source:* Adapted from *Public Health: Administration and Practice,* 9th ed., by G.E. Pickett et al., eds. Copyright © Elsevier 1990. By permission of Elsevier Ltd.

of the two trillion plus dollars spent on health in the United States each year is spent on curing ill health, not on preventing it (IOM, 2000; 2002).

## Risk Factors

The Health Field Concept and the Determinants of Health have provided those interested in health issues with a framework from which the health field can be studied. The levels of prevention and their limitations have provided this same group of people with a time frame from which to plan to help forestall the onset of, limit the spread of, and rehabilitate after pathogenesis or another health problem. What none of these concepts fully discloses is the focus at which health promotion and disease prevention programming should be aimed. The targets of such programming are **risk factors,** those inherited, environmental, and behavioral influences "which are known (or thought) to increase the likelihood of physical or mental problems" (Slee, Slee, & Schmidt, 2008, p. 510). Risk factors increase the probability of morbidity and premature mortality but do not guarantee that people with a risk factor will suffer the consequences.

Risk factors can be divided into two categories: (1) **modifiable** (changeable or controllable) and (2) **nonmodifiable** (nonchangeable or noncontrollable) **risk factors.** The former include such factors as sedentary lifestyle, smoking, and poor dietary habits—things that individuals can change or control while the latter group includes factors such as age, sex, and inherited genes—things that individuals cannot change or do not have control over. Note that these two categories of risk factors are often interrelated. In fact, the combined potential for harm from a number of risk factors is greater than the sum of their individual potentials. For example, asbestos workers have an increased risk for cancer because of their exposure to this carcinogen. Further, if they smoke, they have a thirty times greater chance of developing lung cancer than do their nonsmoking coworkers and a ninety times greater chance of getting lung cancer than do people who neither work with asbestos nor smoke. The risk increases further if they have an inherited respiratory disease.

Over the years, knowledge about the impact of risk behaviors has continued to grow. In looking back over the twentieth century, we have seen disease prevention change "from focusing on reducing environmental exposures over which the individual had little control, such as providing potable water, to emphasizing behaviors such as avoiding use of tobacco, fatty foods, and a sedentary lifestyle" (Breslow, 1999, p. 1030). As noted earlier, approximately 40 percent of the early deaths in the United States each year are caused by these behavior patterns that could be modified by preventive interventions (McGinnis et al., 2002). Therefore, much of the focus of the work of health education specialists has been to help individuals identify and control their modifiable risk factors.

## Health Risk Reduction

In order to be able to take aim at specific risk factors, health education specialists must have a basic understanding of both communicable (infectious) and noncommunicable (noninfectious) diseases. **Communicable diseases** are those diseases for which biological agents or their products are the cause and that are transmissible from one individual to another (McKenzie et al., 2012), while **noncommunicable diseases** or illnesses are those that cannot be transmitted from an infected person to a susceptible, healthy one (McKenzie et al., 2012). Our intent in this section and the ones that follow is not to present information on all possible diseases and their related risk factors that a health education specialist may have to develop programs for, but rather to provide a general understanding of the spread and cause of disease. (See **Table 1.5** for leading causes of death and their risk factors.)

Before moving on, we would like to make a special note about one of the terms presented in Table 1.5. The term *leading causes of death* is used in this table. That term refers to "the primary pathophysiological conditions identified at the time of death, as opposed to the root causes" (McGinnis & Foege, 1993, p. 2207). In 1993 McGinnis and Foege conducted a study to see if they could identify the root causes of death. What they found was that the leading *actual causes of death* were modifiable behaviors; behaviors that people could change. The behavior that was the leading actual cause of death was tobacco use, accounting for some 400,000, or 19 percent, of the mortality in 1990. A similar study to that of McGinnis and Foege (1993) was conducted by Mokdad, Marks, Stroup, and Gerberding in 2004 using 2000 mortality data. They also found tobacco to be the leading actual cause of death, but that poor diet and physical inactivity killed almost as many (see **Table 1.6**). It is now estimated that tobacco is the primary cause of 443,000 deaths per year (CDC, 2009). "These findings, along with

**Table 1.5** Leading causes of death and associated risk factors for all ages: United States, 2008

| Rank | Cause | Risk Factors |
| --- | --- | --- |
| 1 | Diseases of the heart | Tobacco use, high blood pressure, elevated serum cholesterol, diet, diabetes, obesity, lack of exercise, alcohol abuse, genetics |
| 2 | Malignant neoplasms (cancer) | Tobacco use, alcohol misuse, diet, solar radiation, ionizing radiation, worksite hazards, environmental pollution, genetics |
| 3 | Chronic lower respiratory diseases | Tobacco use diseases |
| 4 | Cerebrovascular diseases (stroke) | Tobacco use, high blood pressure, elevated serum cholesterol, diabetes, obesity, genetics |
| 5 | Accidents (unintentional injuries) | Alcohol misuse, tobacco use (fires), product design, home hazards, handgun availability, lack of safety restraints, excessive speed, automobile design, roadway design |
| 6 | Alzheimer's disease | Age, family history, genetics, head injury, heart-health, general healthy aging[a] |
| 7 | Diabetes mellitus | Obesity (for type II diabetes), diet, lack of exercise, genetics |
| 8 | Pneumonia and influenza | Tobacco use, infectious agents, biological factors |
| 9 | Nephritis, nephrotic syndrome, and nephrosis | Infectious agents, drug hypersensitivity, genetics, trauma |
| 10 | Septicemia | Infectious agents[b] |

*Sources:* [a] Alzheimer's Association. (2010). *Risk Factors.* Retrieved August 19, 2010 from http://www.alz.org/alzheimers_disease_causes_risk_factors.asp#riskfactors
[b] Society of Critical Care Medicine. (n.d.). *Sepsis: What you should know.* Retrieved August 19, 2010 from http://ssc.sccm.org/sepsis/what_you_should_know
Miniño, A. M., Xu, J., Kochanek, K. D. (2010). Deaths: Preliminary Data for 2008. *National Vital Statistics Reports, 59* (2), 1–72.

escalating health care costs and aging population, argue persuasively that the need to establish a more preventive orientation in the U.S. health care and public health systems has become more urgent" (Mokdad et al., 2004, p. 1238).

**The Chain of Infection**   The **chain of infection** (see **Figure 1.6**) is a model used to explain the spread of a communicable disease from one host to another. The basic premise represented in the chain of infection is that individuals can break the chain (reduce the risk) at any point; thus, the spread of disease can be stopped. For example, the spread of some waterborne diseases is stopped when the first link of the chain is broken with the chlorination of the water supply, thus killing the pathogens that cause a disease. The risk is reduced because the pathogen is destroyed before it is consumed. The chain can also be broken by placing a barrier between the means of transmission and the portal of

**Table 1.6**    Actual causes of death in the United States, 1990 and 2000

| | 1990 | | 2000 | |
|---|---|---|---|---|
| **Actual Cause** | **Number** | **%ᵃ** | **Number** | **%ᵃ** |
| Tobacco | 400,000 | 19 | 435,000 | 18.1 |
| Poor diet and physical inactivity | 300,000 | 14 | 365,000 | 15.2 |
| Alcohol consumption | 100,000 | 5 | 85,000 | 3.5 |
| Microbial agents | 90,000 | 4 | 75,000 | 3.1 |
| Toxic agents | 60,000 | 3 | 55,000 | 2.3 |
| Motor vehicle | 25,000 | 1 | 43,000 | 1.8 |
| Firearms | 35,000 | 2 | 29,000 | 1.2 |
| Sexual behavior | 30,000 | 1 | 20,000 | 0.8 |
| Illicit drug use | 20,000 | | 17,000 | 0.7 |
| **Total** | **1,060,000** | **50** | **1,124,000** | **46.7** |

ᵃThe percentages are for all deaths

*Sources:* The 1990 data from J. M. McGinnis and W. H. Foege, "Actual Causes of Death in the United States." *Journal of the American Medical Association 270,* 18 (1993): 2207–2212. The 2000 data from Mokdad, A. H., Marks, J. S., Stroup, D. F., and Gerberding, J. L. "Correction: Actual Causes of Death in the United States, 2000." *Journal of the American Medical Association 292,* 3 (2005): 293–294.

entry, as when health care providers protect themselves with surgical masks and rubber gloves. In this case, the risk is reduced because individuals are not exposing themselves to the pathogen. With such information, health education specialists can help create programs that are aimed at "breaking" the chain and reducing the risks.

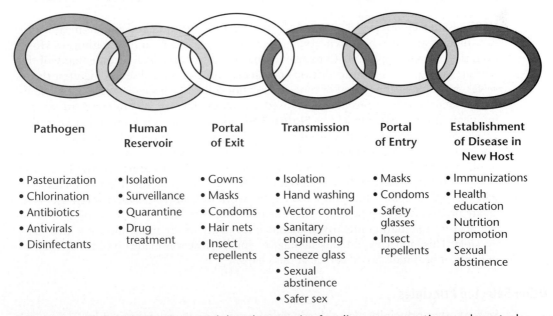

| Pathogen | Human Reservoir | Portal of Exit | Transmission | Portal of Entry | Establishment of Disease in New Host |
|---|---|---|---|---|---|
| • Pasteurization | • Isolation | • Gowns | • Isolation | • Masks | • Immunizations |
| • Chlorination | • Surveillance | • Masks | • Hand washing | • Condoms | • Health education |
| • Antibiotics | • Quarantine | • Condoms | • Vector control | • Safety glasses | • Nutrition promotion |
| • Antivirals | • Drug treatment | • Hair nets | • Sanitary engineering | • Insect repellents | • Sexual abstinence |
| • Disinfectants | | • Insect repellents | • Sneeze glass | | |
| | | | • Sexual abstinence | | |
| | | | • Safer sex | | |

**Figure 1.6** Chain of infection model and strategies for disease prevention and control

*Source:* From J. F. McKenzie, R. R. Pinger, and J. E. Kotecki. *An Introduction to Community Health.* 7th ed. © 2012 Jones and Bartlett Publishers, Sudbury, MA. www.jbpub.com. Reprinted with permission.

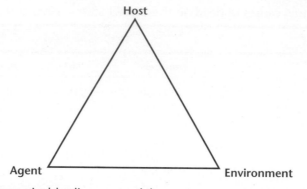

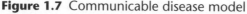

**Figure 1.7** Communicable disease model

*Source:* From J. F. McKenzie, R. R. Pinger, and J. E. Kotecki. *An Introduction to Community Health*, 7th edition. © 2012 Jones and Bartlett Publishers, Sudbury, MA. www.jbpub.com. Reprinted with permission.

**Communicable Disease Model**    A second model used to describe the spread of a communicable disease is the **communicable disease model**. **Figure 1.7** presents the elements of this model—agent, host, and environment. These three elements summarize the minimal requirements for the presence and spread of a communicable disease in a population. The agent is the element (or, using the chain of infection labels, the pathogen) that must be present for a disease to spread—for example, bacteria or a virus. The host is any susceptible organism that can be invaded by the agent. Examples include plants, animals, and humans. The environment includes all other factors that either prohibit or promote disease transmission. Thus, communicable disease transmission occurs when a susceptible host and a pathogenic agent exist in an environment conducive to disease transmission.

**Multicausation Disease Model**    Obviously, the chain of infection and communicable disease models are most helpful in trying to prevent disease caused by a pathogen. However, they are not applicable to noncommunicable diseases, which include many of the chronic diseases such as heart disease and cancer. Most of these diseases manifest themselves in people over a period of time and are not caused by a single factor but by combined factors. The concept of "caused by many factors" is referred to as the **multicausation disease model** (see **Figure 1.8**). For example, it is known that heart disease is more likely to manifest itself in individuals who are older, who smoke, who do not exercise, who are overweight, who have high blood pressure, who have high cholesterol, and who have immediate family members who have had heart disease. Note that within this list of factors there are both modifiable and nonmodifiable risk factors. As when using the chain of infection model, the work of health education specialists is to create programs to help people reduce the risk of disease and injury by helping those in the priority population identify and control as many of the multicausative factors as possible. This model should look familiar to you because it is made up of the five determinants of health discussed earlier in this chapter.

## Other Selected Principles

Several other principles of health education/promotion have been noted by Cleary and Neiger (1998). They have identified via the work of others that health education

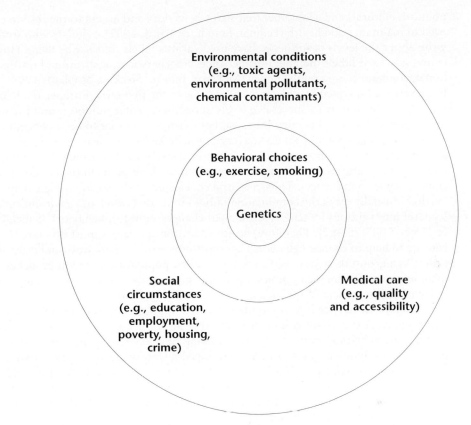

**Figure 1.8** Multicausation disease model

specialists must address the principles of participation, empowerment, and cultural competency if health education/promotion is to be successful. We would like to add two other principles to this list, socio-ecological approach and advocacy. **Participation** refers to the active involvement of those in the priority population in helping identify, plan, and implement programs to address the health problems they face. Without such participation, ethical issues associated with program development come into play, and the priority population probably will not support and feel **ownership** of (responsibility for) the program. For example, if the health education specialists for a large corporation are creating a health promotion program for all employees, they should not begin to plan without the participation of (or at least representation by) each of the segments (clerical, labor, and management) of the employee population.

In recent years, health education/promotion activities have placed more emphasis on socio-ecological approaches to improving health. The underlying concept of the **socio-ecological approach** (sometimes referred to as the *ecological perspective*) is that behavior has multiple levels of influences. This approach "emphasizes the interaction between, and the interdependence of factors within and across all levels of a health problem" (Rimer & Glanz, 2005, p. 10). That is to say, seldom does behavior change based on influence from a single level. People live in environments (i.e., physical, social, political, cultural, and economic) that shape behaviors and access to the resources they need to maintain good health (Pellmar, Brandt, & Baird, 2002). Scholars who study and write about the levels of influence have used various labels to describe them. However, commonly used labels include: intrapersonal, interpersonal, institutional or organizational, community, and public policy (McLeroy, Bibeau, Steckler, & Glanz, 1998). These five levels are presented in a hierarchical order with the first level, intrapersonal, impacting a single person, with successive levels impacting greater numbers, and the highest level—public policy—impacting the most. For example, in order to get a person to begin an exercise program it may take a conversation with his/her physician (i.e., interpersonal-level influence), a company policy (i.e., institutional- or organizational-level influence), and also the county commissioners voting to put walking paths in the community (i.e., community-level influence). Thus, a central conclusion of the socio-ecological approach "is that it usually takes the combination of both individual-level and environmental/policy-level interventions to achieve substantial changes in health behavior" (Sallis, Owen, & Fisher, 2008, p. 467). Therefore, health education specialists must do more than just educate to help to change behavior. They must now work in new ways and develop new skills. As a group these new skills are often called **population-based approaches**. They include policy development, policy advocacy, organizational change, community development, empowerment of individuals, and economic supports.

To more clearly see how a population-based approach works, consider the following example. A state-level voluntary health organization was spending most of its time and resources helping individuals quit smoking or preventing others from starting to smoke. Recently the organization has developed a state-wide advocacy network to respond to tobacco-related legislation. They are using a population-based approach to influence legislation and policy that will ultimately impact individual smoking behaviors. They still maintain the more individual approaches to dealing with the tobacco issue but have added the population-based approach.

Advocacy is another principle in which health education specialists have become more involved. **Advocacy** is defined "as the actions or endeavors individuals or groups engage in order to alter public opinion in favor or in opposition to a certain policy" (Pinzon-Perez & Perez, 1999, p. 29). Whereas, **health advocacy** has been defined as "the processes by which the actions of individuals or groups attempt to bring about social and/or organizational change on behalf of a particular health goal, program, interest, or population" (Joint Committee, 2001, p. 99). Professional associations encourage health education specialists to get more involved in advocacy for the profession and for health-related issues (Auld & Dixon-Terry, 2010). As an example, the Coalition of National Health Education Organizations (CNHEO) (see Chapter 8 for more on this organization) sponsors the Health Education Advocate Web site (see the Weblink at the end of this chapter for the URL for this site). This site provides health education specialists with an easy link to contact their legislators whenever health education/promotion–related bills or concerns are considered by Congress.

If health education/promotion is going to create lasting change, then those in the priority population must be empowered as a result of the health education/promotion programming. **Empowerment** is a "social action process for people to gain mastery over their lives and the lives of their communities" (Minkler, Wallerstein, & Wilson, 2008, p. 294). The neighborhood watch program provides a good example of empowerment. Obviously, police can make a neighborhood safer by regularly patrolling the area. However, because of limited resources, the police cannot be present in every neighborhood.

Empowering neighborhood residents, however, with the knowledge and skills (empowered) to provide an effective "watch" (be the eyes and ears of the police), can decrease crime and improve safety.

As you have probably gathered by now, there are many factors that impact the effectiveness of health education/promotion programming. Because of the health disparities that exist between and among the various subpopulations in the United States (Selig, Tropiano, & Greene-Moton, 2006) and because of the increasing diversification of the U.S. population (Pérez & Luquis, 2008), much more attention has been placed on understanding the impact of culture (i.e., values, beliefs, attitudes, traditions, and customs) on health and providing culturally appropriate programs (Davis & Rankin, 2006). Cultural factors arise from guidelines (both explicit and implicit) that individuals "inherit" from being a part of a particular society, racial or ethnic group, religious community, or other group. In order for health education specialists to be effective in a variety of communities, they need to strive to be culturally competent (Davis & Rankin, 2006; Luquis, Pérez, & Young, 2006; Selig et al., 2006). Being **culturally competent** means having the ability "to understand and respect values, attitudes, beliefs, and mores that differ across cultures, and to consider and respond appropriately to these differences in planning, implementing, and evaluating health education and health promotion programs and interventions" (Joint Committee, 2001, p. 99). Even services that are provided to all in an equal and nondiscriminatory manner may not take into account the needs of those in the priority population and therefore be culturally inappropriate (Davis & Voegtle, 1994).

## SUMMARY

In this introductory chapter, many of the basic principles of the profession of health education/promotion were presented including definitions of many of the key words and terms used in the profession, including *health, health education, health promotion, disease prevention, community health, global health, population health, coordinated school health program,* and *wellness;* a brief discussion of why health education/promotion is referred to as an emerging profession; a look at the current status of health education/promotion; an explanation of how health or health status has been measured, including mortality rates, life expectancy, YPLL, DALYs, HALE, HRQOL, and health surveys; an outline of the goal and purpose of the profession; the practice of health education/promotion, including planning, implementing, and evaluating programs; some of the basic underlying concepts and principles of the profession, including the health field concept, determinants of health, levels of prevention, risk factors, health risk reduction via understanding disease; and the principles of participation, empowerment, ecological approach, advocacy, and culturally competent.

## REVIEW QUESTIONS

1. Define—*health, health education, health promotion, disease prevention, public health, community health, global health, population health, coordinated school health program,* and *wellness.*

2. Why have the authors chosen to describe health education/promotion as an emerging profession?

3. What is the current status of health education/promotion?

4. Explain each of the following means of measuring health or health status.

   • Mortality rates. What is the difference among crude, adjusted, and specific rates?
   • Life expectancy
   • Years of potential life lost (YPLL)
   • Disability-adjusted life years (DALYs)
   • Health-adjusted life expectancy (HALE)
   • Health-related quality of life (HRQOL)
   • Health surveys

5. Of all the different measures of health presented in this chapter, which one do you think is the best indicator of health? Why?

6. Why are health-related data and epidemiology such an important discipline for health education/promotion?

7. In a given community with a midyear population estimate of 50,000, there were 21 deaths due to strokes in the year. What is the rate of stroke deaths per 100,000 population?

8. What is the goal of health education/promotion? What is its purpose?

9. What constitutes the basic practice of health education/promotion?

10. Briefly explain the following concepts and principles of health education/promotion.

    • Health Field Concept; Determinants of health
    • Levels of prevention
    • Risk factors
    • Health risk reduction
    • Chain of infection
    • Communicable disease model
    • Multicausation disease model
    • Selected principles of health education/promotion—participation, socio-ecological approach, advocacy, empowerment, and culturally competent.

## CASE STUDY

As a health education specialist with the Delaware County Health Department, Matt has been asked by a local religious leader to give a presentation on HIV/AIDS to the ecumenical youth group (ninth to twelfth graders) of the community. The request has taken Matt by surprise because for the past couple of years he has attempted to make similar presentations in the local schools but has been turned away because the superintendent said "the community was too conservative for such matters." Knowing that at least some of the people in the community think HIV/AIDS is too controversial to talk about, but also knowing the information is important for youth to have, Matt wants to make sure he prepares and delivers a program that is well received. This is finally the chance he has been waiting for to make his entry into the youth population of the community. Matt has decided to create a presentation on HIV/AIDS that incorporates information on both risk factors and the chain of infection. To make sure that his presentation is on target he has asked several other employees of the health department to sit down with him and brainstorm some ideas for his presentation. He begins his session with his colleagues by asking them all to write down information they think he should include in his presentation. Assume that you are one of these other employees of the health department in this meeting. What would you include on your list for Matt? What would you advise Matt not to include? Why? He then asks his colleagues for ideas on how to present the information (e.g., lecture, video, role playing). What do you think would be the best method to use? Why did you select this method? How long do you think Matt's presentation should be? Why?

## CRITICAL THINKING QUESTIONS

1. In this chapter, the term *public health* was defined. To what extent do you think that the government, at any level, has the right to legislate good health? For example, do you think a governmental body has the responsibility (or right) to require all motorcycle drivers to wear helmets because statistics show that wearing helmets can save lives? Defend your answer.

2. If you were asked by the Centers for Disease Control and Prevention to come up with a new measure to describe the health status of an individual, what would you include in such a measure and why?

3. If you had the opportunity to develop three new health education/promotion programs, one at each level of the three levels of prevention (primary, secondary, and tertiary) for the community in which you live, what would they be? Who would be the priority population? Why did you pick the three that you did?

## ACTIVITIES

1. If you have not already done so, locate and read a copy of the government document *Healthy People: The Surgeon General's Report on Health Promotion and Disease Prevention*. It provides a good background on the health promotion era in the United States.

2. Do you agree with the authors that health education/promotion is an emerging profession? Defend your response in a one- to two-page paper.

3. Write your own definitions for *health*, *health education*, and *health promotion* using the concepts presented in the chapter.

4. Write one paragraph for each of the following:
   - Why do you think the Health Field Concept was so important in getting people to think about health promotion?
   - At what level of prevention do you think it would be most difficult to change health behavior? Why?

5. In a one-page paper, use the chain of infection to outline three different means for preventing the spread of HIV.

6. In a one-page paper, use the multicausation disease model to explain how a person develops heart disease.

## WEBLINKS

1. http://www.cdc.gov/nchs/

   National Center for Health Statistics (NCHS)

   This site is a rich source of data about health in the United States and the instruments used to collect the data.

2. http://www.cdc.gov/brfss/

   Behavioral Risk Factor Surveillance System (BRFSS)

   The BRFSS, the world's largest telephone survey, tracks health risks in the United States. Information from the survey is used to improve the health of U.S. citizens. At this site, you will find general information about the BRFSS, data generated by the BRFSS, copies of the data collection instruments, and more.

3. http://www.cdc.gov/healthyyouth/yrbs/index.htm

   Youth Risk Behavioral Surveillance System (YRBSS)

   At this site, you will find general information about the YRBSS, data generated by the YRBSS, copies of the data collection instruments, and more.

4. http://www.iom.edu/

   Institute of Medicine (IOM)

   The IOM is a nonprofit organization specifically created to provide science-based advice on matters of biomedical science and medicine and health, as well as an honorific membership organization that was chartered in 1970 as a component of the National Academy of Sciences. The IOM's mission is to serve as adviser to the nation to improve health. The Institute provides unbiased, evidence-based, and authoritative information and advice concerning health and science for all. At this site you can find many of their reports cited in this chapter.

5. http://www.healtheducationadvocate.org

   Health Education Advocate

   The Health Education Advocate site is sponsored by the Coalition of National Health Education Organizations (CNHEO). It was designed to provide a timely source of advocacy information related to the field of health education/promotion. It also includes a number of items to health planners with advocacy activities. The site includes, but is not limited to, information about how to identify and contact senators and congressional representatives, the status of specific bills, health resolutions and policy statements of sponsoring agencies, and advocacy resources.

6. https://www.thinkculturalhealth.hhs.gov/

   Think Cultural Health

   This is a page at the United States Department of Health and Human Services, Office of Minority Health Web site that presents information on cultural competence for health professionals. The site has a tag line of "bridging the health care gap through cultural competency continuing education programs." Included at the site are educational programs, resources, and other materials.

7. http://www.bls.gov/oco/ocos063.htm#training

   Occupational Outlook Handbook, 2010-11: Health Educators

   This is a page at the United States Department of Labor, Bureau of Labor Statistics Web site that provides the occupational outlook for health education specialists. The site includes short explanations of: nature of the work; training, other qualifications, and advancement; employment; job outlook and projections; earnings; wages; and sources of additional information about health education specialists.

8. http://www.countyhealthrankings.org/

   County Health Rankings

   This Web site presents the *County Health Rankings*, which are a key component of the Mobilizing Action Toward Community Health (MATCH) project. MATCH is a collaboration between the Robert Wood Johnson Foundation and the University of Wisconsin Population Health Institute.

9. http://www.teachepidemiology.org

   Teach Epidemiology

   This is a Web site sponsored by the Robert Wood Johnson Foundation that provides middle and high school teachers with ideas about how to incorporate the teaching of epidemiology into their curriculum.

## REFERENCES

American College Health Association (ACHA). (2009). *About ACHA-NCHA*. Retrieved August 18, 2010 from http://www.acha-ncha.org/overview.html

Association of Schools of Public Health. (n. d.). What is public health? Retrieved on August 24, 2010 from http://www.whatispublichealth.org/

Auld, M. E., & Dixon-Terry, E. (2010). The role of health education associations in advocacy. In J. M. Black, S. Furney, H. M. Graf, & A. E. Nolte (Eds.), *Philosophical foundations of health education* (pp. 311–318). San Francisco, CA: Jossey-Bass.

Barber, B. (1988). Professions and emerging professions. In J. C. Callahan (Ed.), *Ethical issues in professional life* (pp. 35–39). New York: Oxford University Press.

Breslow, L. (1999). From disease prevention to health promotion. *Journal of the American Medical Association, 281* (11), 1030–1033.

Centers for Disease Control and Prevention. (2009). *Smoking & tobacco use*. Retrieved August 19, 2010 from http://www.cdc.gov/tobacco/data_statistics/fact_sheets/health_effects/tobacco_related_mortality/

Centers for Disease Control and Prevention (CDC). (2000). *Measuring healthy days*. Atlanta, GA: Author.

Centers for Disease Control and Prevention (CDC). (1994). *Chronic disease in minority populations*. Atlanta, GA: Author.

Centers for Disease Control and Prevention (CDC). (2010a). *Behavioral Risk Factor Surveillance System*. Retrieved August 18, 2010 from http://www.cdc.gov/brfss/

Centers for Disease Control and Prevention. (2010b). *Chronic diseases and health promotion*. Retrieved August 17, 2010 from http://www.cdc.gov/chronicdisease/overview/index.htm#1

Centers for Disease Control and Prevention. (2010c). *Health-related quality of life*. Retrieved August 18, 2010 from http://www.cdc.gov/hrqol/index.htm

Centers for Disease Control and Prevention (CDC). (2010d). *Youth Risk Behavior Surveillance System*. Retrieved August 18, 2010 from http://www.cdc.gov/healthyyouth/yrbs/index.htm

Cleary, M. J., & Neiger, B. L. (1998). *The certified health education specialist: A self-study guide for professional competency* (3rd ed.). Allentown, PA: The National Commission for Health Education Credentialing.

Coalition for National Health Education Organizations (CNHEO). (2007). *Employer's guide*. Retrieved August 18, 2010 from http://www.cnheo.org/index.html

Cottrell, R. R., & McKenzie, J. F. (2011). *Health promotion & education research methods: Using the five chapter thesis/dissertation model* (2nd ed.). Sudbury, MA: Jones and Bartlett Publishers.

Davis, B. J., & Voegtle, K. H. (1994). *Culturally competent health care for adolescents*. Chicago: American Medical Association.

Davis, P. C., & Rankin, L. L. (2006). Guidelines for making existing health education programs more culturally appropriate. *American Journal of Health Education, 37* (4), 250–252.

Feeney, S., & Freeman, N. K. (1999). *Ethics and the early childhood educators: Using the NAEYC code*. Washington, DC: National Association for the Education of Young Children.

Galli, N. (1976). Foundations of health education. *Journal of School Health, 46* (3), 158–165.

Glanz, K., & Rimer, B. K. (2008). Perspectives on using theory: Past, present, and future. In K. Glanz, B. K. Rimer, & K. Viswanath (Eds.), *Health behavior and health education: Theory, research, and practice* (pp. 509–517). San Francisco, CA: Jossey-Bass.

Green, L. W., & McKenzie, J. F. (2002). Community and Population Health. In L. Breslow, L. Green, W. Keck, J. Last, & J. M. McGinnis (Eds.), *Encyclopedia of public health* (pp. 247–255). New York: Macmillan Reference.

Green, L. W., & Ottoson, J. M. (1999). *Community and population health* (8th ed.). Boston: WCB/McGraw-Hill.

Hancock, T., & Minkler, M. (2005). Community health assessment or healthy community assessment: Whose community? Whose health? Whose assessment? In M. Minkler (Ed.), *Community organizing and community building for health* (pp. 138–157) (2nd ed.). New Brunswick, NJ: Rutgers University Press.

Hanlon, J. J. (1974). *Public Health*. St. Louis, MO: Mosby.

Hezel Associates. (2007). *Marketing the health education profession: Knowledge, attitudes, and hiring practices of employers*. Retrieved August 24, 2010 from http://www.cnheo.org/

Institute of Medicine (IOM). (1988). *The future of public health*. Washington, DC: National Academy Press.

Institute of Medicine. (1997). *America's vital Interest in global health: Protecting our people, enhancing our economy, and advancing our international interests*. Washington, DC: National Academy Press. Retrieved August 17, 2010, from http://books.nap.edu/openbook.php?record_id=5717&page=3

Institute of Medicine (IOM). (2000). *Brief Report. Promoting health: Intervention strategies from social and behavioral research*. Retrieved March 25, 2004 from http://www.iom.edu/includes/dbfile.asp?id=4121

Institute of Medicine (IOM). (2001). *Health and behavior: The interplay of biological, behavioral, and societal influences*. Washington, DC: Academy Press.

Institute of Medicine (IOM). (2002). *Brief Report. The future of the public's health in the 21st century*. Retrieved March 25, 2004 from http://www.iom.edu/file.asp?id=4165

Johns, E. B. (1973). Joint Committee on Health Education Terminology: Report of the Joint Committee on Health Education Terminology. *Health Education, 4* (6), 25.

Joint Committee on Health Education Terminology. (1991a). Report of the 1990 Joint Committee on Health Education Terminology. *Journal of Health Education, 22* (2), 105–106.

Joint Committee on Health Education Terminology. (1991b). Report of the 1990 Joint Committee on Health Education Terminology. *Journal of School Health, 61* (6), 251–254.

Joint Committee on Health Education and Health Promotion Terminology. (2001). Report of the 2000 Joint Committee on Health Education and Health Promotion Terminology. *American Journal of Health Education, 32* (2), 89–103.

King, N. (2009). Health inequalities and health inequities. In E. E. Morrison (Ed.), *Health care ethics: Critical issues for the 21st century* (pp. 339–354). Sudbury, MA: Jones & Bartlett.

Laframboise, H. L. (1973). Health policy: Breaking it down into more manageable segments. *Journal of the Canadian Medical Association, 108* (Feb. 3), 388–393.

Lalonde, M. (1974). *A new perspective on the health of Canadians: A working document*. Ottawa, Canada: Ministry of National Health and Welfare.

Last, J. M. (Ed.). (2007). *A dictionary of public health*. New York, NY: Oxford University Press.

Livingood, W. C. (1996). Becoming a health education profession: Key to societal influence—1995 SOPHE presidential address. *Health Education Quarterly, 23* (4), 421–430.

Luquis, R., Perez, M., & Young, K. (2006). Cultural competence development in health education professional preparation programs. *American Journal of Health Education, 37* (4), 233–241.

Mason, J. O., & McGinnis, J. M. (1990). Healthy people 2000: An overview of the national health promotion disease prevention objectives. *Public Health Reports, 105* (5), 441–446.

Mathers, C. D., Sdana, R., Salomon, J. A., Murray, C. J. L., & Lopez, A. D. (2001). Healthy life expectancies in 191 countries, 1999. *Lancet, 357*, 1685–1691.

McGinnis, J. M. (1985). The limits of prevention. *Public Health Reports, 100* (3), 255–260.

McGinnis, J. M. (2001). United States. In C. E. Koop (Ed.), *Critical issues in global health* (pp. 80–90). San Francisco: Jossey-Bass.

McGinnis, J. M., & Foege, W. H. (1993). Actual causes of death in the United States. *Journal of the American Medical Association, 270* (18), 2207–2212.

McGinnis, J. M., Williams-Russo, P., & Knickman, J. R. (2002). The case for more active policy attention to health promotion. *Health Affairs, 21* (2), 78–93.

McKenzie, J. F., Neiger, B. L., & Thackeray, R (2009). *Planning, implementing, and evaluating, health promotion programs: A primer* (5th ed.). San Francisco, Benjamin Cummings.

McKenzie, J. F., Pinger, R. R., & Kotecki, J. E. (2012). *An introduction to community health* (7th ed.). Boston: Jones and Bartlett Publishers.

McLeroy, K. R., Bibeau, D., Steckler, A., &. Glanz, K. (1988). An ecological perspective for health promotion programs. *Health Education Quarterly, 15* (4): 351–378.

Merriam-Webster, Inc. (2010a). Discipline. In *Merriam-Webster online dictionary*. Retrieved August 17, 2010, from http://www.merriam-webster.com/dictionary/discipline

Merriam-Webster, Inc. (2010b). Professional. In *Merriam-Webster online dictionary*. Retrieved August 17, 2010, from http://www.merriam-webster.com/dictionary/profession

Merriam-Webster, Inc. (2010c). Profession. In *Merriam-Webster online dictionary*. Retrieved August 17, 2010, from http://www.merriam-webster.com/dictionary/professional

Minkler, M., Wallerstein, N., & Wilson, N. (2008). Improving health through community organizing and community building. In K. Glanz, B. K. Rimer, & K. Viswanath (Eds.), *Health behavior and health education practice: Theory, research, and practice* (4th ed.) (pp. 287–312). San Francisco, CA: Jossey-Bass.

Mokdad, A. H., Marks, J. S., Stroup, D. F., & Gerberding, J. L. (2004). Actual causes of death, in the United States, 2000. *Journal of the American Medical Association, 291* (10), 1238–1245.

Montagu, A. (1968). *Man observed*. New York: G. P. Putnam.

Moss, B. (1950). Joint Committee on Health Education Terminology. *Journal of Physical Education, 21*, 41.

Murray, C. J. L., & Lopez, A. D. (Eds.). (1996). *Summary of the global burden of disease: A comprehensive assessment of mortality and disability from diseases, injuries, and risk factors in 1990 and projected to 2020*. Geneva, Switzerland: World Health Organization.

National Center for Health Statistics (NCHS). (2006). *Health, United States, 2006 with chartbook on trends in the health of Americans*. Hyattsville, MD: Author.

National Center for Health Statistics (NCHS). (2009). *National health care surveys*. Retrieved August 18, 2010 from http://www.cdc.gov/nchs/nhcs.htm/nhcs_surveys.htm

National Center for Health Statistics. (2010). *Health, United States, 2009: With special feature on medical technology*. Hyattsville, MD: Author.

National Commission for Health Education Credentialing, Inc. (NCHEC). (1996). *A competency-based framework for professional development of certified health education specialists*. Allentown, PA: Author.

Pellmar, T. C., Brandt, Jr., E. N., & Baird, M. (2002). Health and behavior: The interplay of biological, behavioral, and social influences: Summary of an Institute of Medicine Report. *American Journal of Health Promotion, 16* (4), 206–219.

Perez, M. A., & Luquis, R. R. (2008). Changing U.S. demographics: Challenges and opportunities for health educators. In M. A. Perez & R. R. Luquis (Eds.) *Cultural competence in health education and health promotion*. San Francisco, CA: Jossey-Bass, 1–21.

Pinzon-Perez, H., & Perez, M. A. (1999). Advocacy groups for Hispanic/Latino health issues. *The Health Educator Monograph Series, 17* (2), 29–31.

Raphael, D., Brown, I., Renwick, R., & Rootman, I. (1997). Quality of life: What are the implications for health promotion? *American Journal of Health Behavior, 21* (2), 118–128.

Rimer, B. K., & Glanz, K. (2005). *Theory at a glance: A guide for health promotion practice* (2nd ed). [NIH Pub. No. 05-3896]. Washington, DC: National Cancer Institute.

Rugen, M. (1972). *A fifty year history of the public health section of American Public Health Association; 1922–1972*. Washington, DC: American Public Health Association, Inc.

Sallis, J. F., Owen, N., & Fisher, E. B. (2008). Ecological models of health behavior. In K. Glanz, B. K. Rimer, & K. Viswanath (Eds.), *Health behavior and health education practice: Theory, research, and practice* (4th ed.) (pp. 465–485). San Francisco, CA: Jossey-Bass.

Selig, S., Tropiano, E., & Greene-Moton, E. (2006). Teaching cultural competence to reduce health disparities. *Health Promotion Practice, 7* (3), 247S–255S.

Slee, D. A., Slee, V. N., & Schmidt, H. J. (2008). *Slee's health care terms* (5th ed.). Sudbury, MA: Jones & Bartlett

Smith, B., & Bauman, A. (2005). Physical environments. In J. Kerr, R. Weitkunat, & M. Moretti (Eds.), *ABC of behavior change: A guide to successful disease prevention and health promotion* (pp. 139–152). Edinburgh: Elsevier.

Stokols, D. (1992). Establishing and maintaining healthy environments: Toward a social ecology of health promotion. *American Psychologist, 47* (1), 6–22.

Turnock, B. J. (2006). *Public health: Career choices that make a difference.* Sudbury, MA: Jones & Bartlett.

Ubbes, V. A., & Watts, P. R. (1995). Terminology, tolerance, and flexibility: Communication challenges for health education. *Journal of Health Education, 26* (4), 251–253.

U.S. Department of Health, Education, and Welfare (USDHEW). (1980). *Promoting health/ preventing disease: Objectives for the nation.* Washington, DC: U.S. Government Printing Office.

U.S. Department of Health and Human Services (USDHHS). (1991). *Health status of minorities and low-income groups* (3rd ed.). Washington, DC: U.S. Government Printing Office.

U.S. Department of Health and Human Services (USDHHS) (2000). *Healthy People 2010.* (Conference Edition, in Two Volumes). Washington, DC: U.S. Government Printing Office.

Williams, J. F. (1934). Report of the Health Education Section of the American Physical Education Association: Definitions of terms in health education. *Journal of Physical Education, 5* (16–17), 50–51.

World Health Organization. (1947). *Constitution of the World Health Organization.* Retrieved August 17, 2010, from http://www.who.int/governance/eb/constitution/en/

World Health Organization. (1986). *Health promotion sante: Ottawa charter.* Retrieved August 17, 2010, from http://www.euro.who.int/en/who-we-are/policy-documents/ottawa-charter-for-health-promotion,-1986

World Health Organization. (2008). *The global burden of disease: 2004 update.* Retrieved August 18, 2010 from http://www.who.int/healthinfo/global_burden_disease/GBD_report_2004update_full.pdf

Yoho, R. (1962). Joint Committee on Health Education Terminology: Health education terminology. *Journal of Physical Education and Recreation, 33* (Nov.), 27–28.

Young, K. J., & Perko, M. (2009). Developing professionalism as a health educator. In R. J. Bensley & J. Brookins-Fisher (Eds.). *Community health methods: A practical guide* (pp. 51–71). Sudbury, MA: Jones & Bartlett.

## CHAPTER 2

# The History of Health and Health Education/Promotion

After reading this chapter and answering the questions at the end, you should be able to:

- Discuss how health beliefs and practices have changed from the earliest humans to the present day.
- Identify the dual roots of modern health education/promotion.
- Explain why a need for professional health education specialists emerged.
- Trace the history of public health in the United States.
- Relate the history of school health from the mid-1800s to the present.
- Identify important governmental publications from 1975 to the present, and describe how these publications have impacted health promotion and education.

While the history of health education/promotion as an emerging profession is just over 100-years old, the concept of educating about health has been around since the dawn of humans. This chapter tells the historical story of health, health care, and health education/promotion, from the earliest human records to the present. The main focus is on Northern Africa and Europe. These areas had the greatest influence on the development of health knowledge and health care in the United States. Although other parts of the world—for example, the Far East, Africa, Central America, and South America—contributed to the history of health and health care, their accounts are not as directly relevant to the United States' health history.

It is important that students recognize the difference between "educating about health," which can be done by anyone who believes he/she has knowledge about health to share with someone else, and "health education/promotion," which is done by a professionally trained health education specialist. The need for professional health education specialists emerged as human knowledge of health and health care increased. This chapter emphasizes the health education/promotion profession during the past 150 years, as it evolved from the dual roots of school health and public health. You cannot fully appreciate the health education/promotion profession without understanding its origin. History reveals how progress was made over time. It also depicts the obstacles faced by those who promoted health improvements throughout the years. "At the same time, historical study shows us that despite the difficulties, change is possible, given dedication, organization and persistence. . . . Historical case studies may be able to teach us useful lessons about successful strategies used by public health reformers in the past" (Fee & Brown, 1997, p. 1763).

## Early Humans

We assume that the earliest humans learned by trial and error to distinguish between things that were healthful and those that were harmful. "By observing animals he learned that bathing not only cooled and refreshed his body, but helped remove external parasites; he learned that application of mud assuaged insect bites; and by determining the actions of certain herbs, he learned their various medicinal or poisonous characteristics" (Goerke & Stebbins, 1968, p. 5).

It does not stretch the imagination too far to see how education about health first took place. Someone may have eaten a particular plant or herb and become ill. That person would then warn (educate) others against eating the same substance. Conversely, someone may have ingested a plant or an herb that produced a desired effect. That person would then encourage (educate) others to use this substance. Through observation, trial, and error, other types of health-related knowledge were discovered. Eventually, this knowledge was transformed into rules or taboos for a given society. Rules about preserving food and how to bury the dead may have been implemented. Perhaps taboos against defecation within the tribe's communal area or near sources of drinking water were established (McKenzie, Pinger, & Kotecki, 2008). The trial and error method, which undoubtedly produced serious illness and even death among some early humans, gradually became less needed. Knowledge was passed verbally from one generation to the next, preventing at least some of the potential ill effects of everyday life. As society progressed even further, this knowledge was written down and saved (see **Figure 2.1**).

There was still much more unknown than known about protecting health. Disease and death were probably much more common than health and longevity. To early humans, it was puzzling when disease and death occurred for no apparent reason. In an attempt to make these events seem more rational, "disease and infirmity were believed to be caused by the influence of magic or malevolent spirits that inhabited streams, trees, animals, the earth, and the air. Purposively or accidentally provoking any of the spirits, it was thought, would result in dire consequences for the individual or his/her community" (Goerke & Stebbins, 1968, p. 5). To prevent disease, sacrifices were made to the gods, taboos were obeyed, amulets were worn, and "haunted" places were avoided. Charms, spells, and chants were also used to protect from disease (Duncan, 1988). Again, it is likely that some form of rudimentary education about health was taking place to inform people how to keep from provoking the spirits and, thus, prevent disease.

## Early Efforts at Public Health

Evidence of broad-scale public health activity has been found in the very earliest of civilizations. In India, sites excavated at Mohenjo-Daro and Harappa dating back 4,000 years indicate that bathrooms and drains were common. The streets were broad, paved,

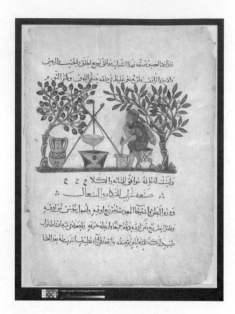

**Figure 2.1** Preparation of medicine from honey (the leaf from an Arabic translation of the Materia Medica of Dioscorides, dated 1224 Iraq, Baghdad School)

(© The Metropolitan Museum of Art/Art Resources, NY)

and drained by covered sewers (Rosen, 1958). Archeological evidence also shows that the Minoans (3000–1430 B.C.) and Myceneans (1430–1150 B.C.) built drainage systems, toilets, and water flushing systems (Pickett & Hanlon, 1990). The oldest written documents related to health care are the **Smith Papyri**, dating from 1600 B.C., which describe various surgical techniques. The earliest written record concerning public health is the **Code of Hammurabi** (see **Box 2.1**), named after the king of Babylon. It contained laws pertaining to health practices and physicians, including the first known fee schedule (Rubinson & Alles, 1984).

## Early Cultures

The medical lore of the distant past was handed down from generation to generation. In virtually every culture for which there are documented historical accounts, people turned to some type of a physician or medicine man for health information (education about health), treatments, and cures (Green & Simons-Morton, 1990). In Egypt, as in many other cultures, this role was held by the priests. Eventually, the various incantations, spells, exorcisms, prescriptions, and clinical observations were compiled into written format, some of which survive in our museums and libraries (Libby, 1922).

The Egyptians made substantial progress in the area of public health. They possessed a strong sense of personal cleanliness and were considered to be the healthiest people of their time (see **Figure 2.2**). They used numerous pharmaceutic preparations and constructed earth privies for sewage, as well as public drainage pipes (Pickett & Hanlon, 1990). Nevertheless, they relied primarily on priests for their health information and used remedies such as "dung of the gazelle and the crocodile, the fat of a serpent, mammalian entrails and other excreta, tissues and organs" (Libby, 1922, p. 6).

In approximately 1500 B.C. the Hebrews extended Egyptian hygienic thought and formulated (in the biblical book of Leviticus) what is probably the world's first written

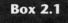 **Box 2.1**  THE RIGHTS AND DUTIES OF THE SURGEON OF 2080 B.C.: FROM THE CODE OF HAMMURABI

"If a physician operate on a man for a severe wound (or make a severe wound upon a man), with a bronze lancet, and save the man's life; or if he open an abscess (in the eye) of a man, with a bronze lancet, and save the man's eye, he shall receive ten shekels of silver (as his fee)."

"If he be a freeman,* he shall receive five shekels."

"If it be a man's slave, the owner of the slave shall give two shekels of silver to the physician."

"If a physician operate on a man for a severe wound, with a bronze lancet, and cause the man's death; or open an abscess (in the eye) of a man with a bronze lancet, and destroy the man's eye, they shall cut off his hands."

"If a physician operate on a slave of a freeman for a severe wound, with a bronze lancet, and cause his death, he shall restore a slave of equal value."

"If he open an abscess (in his eye), with a bronze lancet, and destroy his eye, he shall pay silver to the extent of one half of his price."

"If a physician set a broken bone for a man or cure his diseased bowels, the patient shall give five shekels of silver to the physician."

"If he be a freeman, he shall give three shekels."

"If it be a man's slave, the owner of the slave shall give two shekels of silver to the physician."

"If a veterinary physician operate on an ox or ass for a severe wound and save its life, the owner of the ox or ass shall give the physician, as his fee, one sixth of a shekel of silver."

"If he operate on an ox or an ass for a severe wound, and cause its death, he shall give to the owner of the ox or ass one fourth its value."

*Freeman indicates a rank intermediate between that of "man" (or gentleman) and that of "slave."
Source: From R. F. Harper, The Code of Hammurabi, 1904, Chicago.

hygienic code. It dealt with a variety of personal and community responsibilities, including cleanliness of the body, protection against the spread of contagious diseases, isolation of lepers, disinfection of dwellings after illness, sanitation of campsites, disposal of excreta and refuse, protection of water and food supplies, and specific hygiene rules for menstruating women and women who had recently delivered a child.

The history of health and health care in the Greek culture (1000–400 B.C.) is intriguing as well as relevant to modern health care philosophy. The Greeks were perhaps the first people to put as much emphasis on disease prevention as they did on the treatment of disease conditions. Balance among the physical, mental, and spiritual aspects of the person was emphasized. Among the early Greeks, religion played an important role in health care. However, the role of physician began to take on a more defined shape, and a more scientific view of medicine emerged.

In the early stages of Greek culture, as represented in the *Iliad* and the *Odyssey*, the priesthood played a role in the healing arts. In the *Iliad*, **Asclepius** was a Thessalian chief

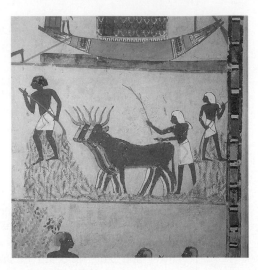

**Figure 2.2** The Egyptians were known for their cleanliness and were considered the healthiest people of the time.
("Tomb Menna"/The Ancient Art & Architecture Collection)

who had received instruction in the use of drugs. By the beginning of the eighth century B.C., tradition had enshrined him as the god of medicine (see **Box 2.2**). He had two daughters who also had health-related powers. **Hygeia** was given the power to prevent disease, while **Panacea** was given the ability to treat disease. Hygeia was the more prominent figure and was often pictured with her father in sculptures and illustrations of the time (Schouten, 1967) (see **Figure 2.3**). The words *hygiene* and *panacea* can be traced back to these daughters of Asclepius (Libby, 1922).

Eventually, hundreds of elaborate temples were built throughout Greece to worship Asclepius. These temples were typically on beautiful sites overlooking the sea or beside healing fountains. The temple priests practiced their healing arts, which often involved fraud. The temple priests should not be confused with the **Asclepiads**. The Asclepiads were a brotherhood of men present at the temples who initially claimed descent from Asclepius. While some of the Asclepiads probably helped the priests with their trickery, others broke away from the priests and began to practice medicine based on more rational

---

**Box 2.2**  THE STORY OF ASCLEPIUS

"According to Greek mythology, Asclepius, the son of Apollo, was a god of healing whose powers were so great that he could bring the dead back to life. When Hades, the god of the dead, jealously complained to Zeus that Asclepius was cheating the kingdom of the dead, Zeus agreed with Hades that Asclepius had violated a basic law of nature by saving mortals from death. Consequently, Asclepius was killed with a thunderbolt. Before he died, however, he gave his healing powers to two of his daughters: Panacea, goddess of healing, who administered medication to the sick, and Hygeia, goddess of health, who taught mortals to live wisely and preserve their bodies."

*Source:* Bates, I.J., and Winder, A.E., *Introduction to Health Education.* San Francisco: Mayfield Publishing, 1984.

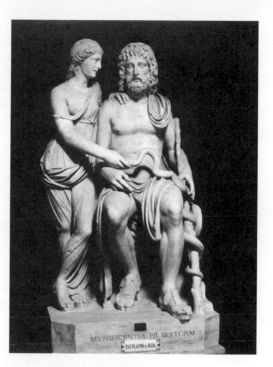

**Figure 2.3** Asclepius and Hygeia
(Museo Vaticano/Art Resource)

principles. These ancient temples of Asclepius left their symbol as a permanent reminder of the past—the staff and serpent of the physician, known as the **caduceus** (Rubinson & Alles, 1984) (see **Figure 2.4**).

The famous Greek physician **Hippocrates** came from the Asclepian tradition. He lived from about 460 B.C. until 377 B.C. Hippocrates developed a theory of disease causation consistent with the philosophy of nature held by leading philosophers of his day. Hippocrates taught that health was the result of balance, and disease was the result of

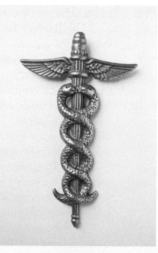

**Figure 2.4** Illustration of a caduceus, a symbol that shows two snakes braided around a staff. It is representative of the medical profession and has its earliest association with Asclepius, the Greek healer.

(Garry Gay/Alamy)

an imbalance. To the Greeks, the ideal person was perfectly balanced in mind, body, and spirit. Thus, study and practice related to philosophy, athletics, and theology were all important to maintain balance. To do this, however, took a tremendous commitment of time and energy. Each day required physical activity, study, and philosophical discussion while maintaining proper nutrition and rest. Few people could afford to lead such a life. Those who did were the aristocratic upper class leading a life of leisure supported by a slave economy (Rosen, 1958). The ideal Greek human being that is so often mentioned was, in fact, a small percentage of the Greek population.

Hippocrates holds an important place in the history of medicine. His theory of health and disease was still being taught in medical schools as a valid theory of disease causation as recently as the first quarter of the twentieth century. Hippocrates, however, did more than just theorize about disease. He carefully observed and recorded associations between certain diseases and such factors as geography, climate, diet, and living conditions. Duncan (1988) noted, "One of his [Hippocrates's] most noteworthy contributions is the distinction between 'endemic' diseases, which vary in prevalence from place to place, and 'epidemic' diseases, which vary in prevalence over time" (p. 12). The traditional Hippocratic Oath is still used today and is the basis for medical ethics. Hippocrates and the Asclepiads moved health care away from religion and priests and attempted to establish a more rational basis to explain health and disease. Hippocrates's concept of balance in life is still promoted today as the best means for maintaining health and well-being.

Hippocrates has been credited as being the first epidemiologist and the father of modern medicine (Duncan, 1988). It is not hard to imagine that he was also a health educator. One can easily see Hippocrates educating his friends and patients about diet, exercise, rest, and the importance of balance in preventing disease and promoting health.

The Romans conquered the Mediterranean world, including the Greeks. In doing so, however, the Romans did not destroy the cultures they conquered but learned from them. The Romans accepted many Greek ideas, including those related to health and medicine. "As clinicians, the Romans were hardly more than imitators of the Greeks, but as engineers and administrators, as builders of sewerage systems and baths, and as providers of water supplies and other health facilities, they set the world a great example and left their mark in history" (Rosen, 1958, p. 38). (See **Figure 2.5**.)

The Roman Empire (500 B.C.–A.D. 500) built an extensive and efficient aqueduct system. "Evidence of some 200 Roman aqueducts remains today, from Spain to Syria and from Northern Europe to North Africa" (McKenzie et al., 2008, p. 12). The total capacity of the thirteen aqueducts delivering water to the city of Rome has been estimated at 222 million gallons per twenty-four hours. At the height of the empire, this would have been enough to provide each citizen of Rome with at least forty gallons of fresh water per day. Additionally, attention was paid to water purity. At specific points along the aqueduct, generally near the middle and end, settling basins were located, in which sediment might be deposited (Rosen, 1958).

The Romans also developed an extensive system of underground sewers. These served to carry off both surface water and sewage. The main sewer in Rome that emptied into the Tiber River was 10 feet wide and 12 feet high; it was still part of the Roman sewer system during the twentieth century.

The Romans made other health advancements. They observed the effect of occupational hazards on health, and they were the first to build hospitals. By the second century

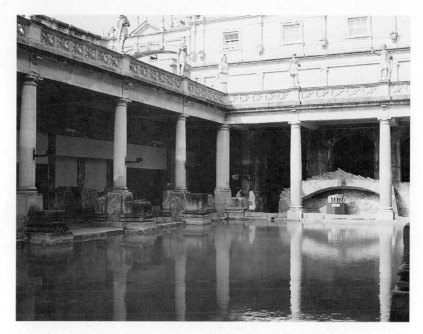

**Figure 2.5** The Romans enjoyed a system of public baths that were supplied with fresh water. This picture shows the Roman baths in Bath, England.
(Pierre Berger/Photo Researchers)

A.D., a public medical service was set up whereby physicians were appointed to various towns and institutions. A system of private medical practice also developed during the Roman era (Rosen, 1958).

The Romans furthered the work of the Greeks in the study of human anatomy and the practice of surgery. Some Roman anatomists even dissected living human beings to further their knowledge of anatomy (Libby, 1922). In quoting the Latin writer Cornelius, Libby found that these anatomists "procured criminals out of prison, by royal permission, and dissecting them alive, contemplated, while they were still breathing, the parts which nature had before concealed, considering their position, color, figure, size, order, hardness, softness, smoothness, and asperity" (Libby, 1922, p. 54). While some opposed this hideous practice, others supported it, holding "it is by no means cruel as most people represent it, by the tortures of a few guilty, to search after remedies for the whole innocent race of mankind in all ages" (Libby, 1922, p. 54).

## Middle Ages

The era from the collapse of the Roman Empire to about A.D. 1500 is known as the Middle Ages or Dark Ages. This was a time of political and social unrest, when many health advancements of earlier cultures were lost. Rosen (1958) notes that "the problem that confronted the medieval world was to weld together the culture of the barbarian invaders with the classical heritage of the defunct [Roman] Empire and with the beliefs and teachings of the Christian religion" (p. 52). This proved to be no easy task.

With the Roman Empire no longer able to protect settlements, each city had to defend itself against its enemies. For safety, people lived within city walls along with their domesticated animals. As the population grew, expansion was difficult and overcrowding common (Rosen, 1958). Lack of fresh water and sewage removal were major problems for many medieval cities; Roman public health advancements were lost.

To make matters worse, there was little emphasis on cleanliness or hygiene. The new religion, Christianity,

> found its disciples among the lower classes, where personal hygiene was not practiced, and as a consequence, an entirely different attitude toward the human body developed. Excessive care of the body, that is, man's earthly and mutable part, was unimportant in the Christian dualistic concept, which separated body from soul. For some Eastern churchmen and holy men, living in filth was regarded as evidence of sanctity: cleanliness was thought to betoken pride, and filthiness humility. (Goerke & Stebbins, 1968, p. 9)

Fortunately, as Christianity matured so did its concept of the human body. Eventually, Christians came to believe that the body is the soul's earthly dwelling, permitting better care of it.

Early Christians also reinforced the notion that disease was caused by sin or disobeying God. This propelled priests and religious leaders back into the position of preventing and treating disease. The health-related advancements of the Greco-Roman era were abandoned and shunned. Entire libraries were burned, and knowledge about the human body was seen as sinful.

The Middle Ages were characterized by great epidemics. Perhaps the cruelest of these was leprosy, a disease characterized by severe facial disfigurement. A highly contagious and virulent disease, all Western countries issued edicts against anyone suspected of having leprosy and regulated every aspect of the sufferer's life. In some communities, lepers were given the last rites of the church, forced to leave the city, made to wear identifying clothing, and required to carry a rod identifying them as lepers. Other lepers were forced to wear a bell around their necks and to ring it as a warning when other people came near. Such isolation usually brought about a relatively quick death due to hunger and exposure (Goerke & Stebbins, 1968). Eventually, leprosy hospitals were founded to treat the inflicted. It has been estimated that by A.D. 1200, there were 1,900 leper houses and leprosaria in Europe (Rosen, 1958).

The bubonic plague, known as the Black Death, may have been the most severe epidemic the world has ever known. The death toll was higher and the disruption of society greater than from any war, famine, or natural disaster in history. "At Constantinople, the plague raged with such violence that 5,000, and even 10,000 persons are said to have died in a single day" (Donan, 1898, p. 94). Estimates of casualties vary from 20 to 35 million, with Europe losing one quarter to one third of its entire population. In Avignon, France, 60,000 people died. As a result, the pope was forced to consecrate the Rhone River so that bodies might be thrown into it, because the churchyards were filled (Goerke & Stebbins, 1968).

Imagine what it must have been like to live through the plague. Literally one out of every three or four people you knew contracted the disease and died. The cause of the disease was unknown, causing widespread fear and superstition. Often, religious leaders and doctors were some of the first victims. They were exposed to the disease early in the epidemic through their contact with infected sufferers. This left many communities with no religious or medical leadership.

Goerke and Stebbins (1968) note, "Many people reacted to the plague either by becoming licentious and hedonistic or by becoming severely ascetic . . .," (p. 11). The Brotherhood of the Flagellants was a group of religious zealots who believed the plague could be avoided by admitting to their sins and then ritualistically beating themselves in atonement. Today, such a group would most likely be labeled a religious cult. Members of this group marched in long, two-column lines from city to city. In each city, they would chant a litany and conduct their ritualistic ceremony. At a signal from the group's master, the Flagellants would strip to the waist and march in a circle until they received another signal from the master. Upon receiving the second signal, they would throw themselves to the ground with their body position indicating the specific sin they had committed. The master would move among the bodies, thrashing those who had committed certain sins or had offended the discipline of the Flagellants in some way. This would be followed by a collective flagellation in which the group members would rhythmically beat their own backs and breasts with a heavy scourge made of three or four leather thongs tipped with metal studs. According to eyewitness accounts, the Flagellants lashed themselves until their bodies became swollen and blue, and blood dripped to the ground. Further complicating the health consequences of such punishment was a rule prohibiting bathing, washing, or changing clothes. When joining the Brotherhood, group members had to pledge to scourge themselves three times daily for thirty-three days and eight hours, which represented one day for each year of Christ's earthly life (Ziegler, 1969).

Debate existed during the Middle Ages concerning the cause of the plague. In 1348, Jehan Jacme wrote that the disease was caused by five factors: (1) the wrath of God, (2) the corruption of dead bodies, (3) waters and vapors formed in the interior of the earth, (4) unnatural hot and humid winds, and (5) the conjunction of stars and planets (Winslow, 1944).

Another story concerning the origins of the disease had Italian merchants trapped in a city on the Black Sea that was under siege by a local Mongol prince. The prince was forced to call off the siege because large numbers of his army were dying of a strange disease. Before leaving, the prince ordered his army to catapult the dead, diseased bodies into the city. Within days, the people inside the city began to die. Afraid, the Italian merchants set sail for Italy, but not before infected rats had boarded the ship. Soon many of the sailors became sick. The ship tried to dock in several cities but was denied permission because of the illness. Finally permission was granted to dock in Sicily where the rats came on shore and the plague began (De'ath, 1995).

Despite the disagreement that existed on the cause of the disease, contemporaries believed that the disease was contagious. In other words, it was passed from person to person in some unknown way. While this concept of contagion had been around for many years and was discussed in the Bible, it was not until the Middle Ages and the epidemics of leprosy and bubonic plague that it started to become more universally accepted. The contagion concept opened the door to new interest in science and severely weakened the argument of those promoting the sin-disease theory.

The Middle Ages also saw epidemics of other communicable diseases, including smallpox, diphtheria, measles, influenza, tuberculosis, anthrax, and trachoma. The last major epidemic disease of this period was syphilis, which appeared in 1492. As with other epidemics, syphilis killed thousands of people (McKenzie et al., 2008).

Although there were no professional health education specialists during the Middle Ages, education about health continued to exist. Priests, medical doctors, and community leaders attempted to "educate" anyone who would listen to their ideas about health and disease prevention. Given the rudimentary level of health knowledge and the lack of consensus on prevention and causation of disease, a professional health education specialist would probably have contributed little to the general population's health in the Middle Ages.

## Renaissance

The Renaissance, which means "rebirth," lasted roughly from A.D. 1500 to 1700. This time period was characterized by a gradual change in thinking. People began to view the world and humankind in a more naturalistic and holistic fashion. Although progress was slow, science again emerged as a legitimate field of inquiry, and numerous scientific advancements were made. The world did not change overnight from the superstitious and backward beliefs of the Dark Ages to a completely enlightened society in the Renaissance. Disease and plague still ravaged Europe and overall medical care was still rudimentary. Bloodletting was a major form of treatment for everything from the common cold to tuberculosis. Popular remedies included crabs' eyes, foxes' lungs, oil of anise, oil of spiders, and oil of earthworms. A major means of diagnosing a patient's condition consisted of examining the urine for changes in color. The inspection of a patient's urine by a true physician was known as "water casting." For many years, this was the principal occupation of the medical profession.

Much surgery and dentistry was performed by barbers because they had the best chairs and sharpest instruments available. Some barbers dispensed health information, as can be seen in the following example from a Danish barber-surgeon: "It is very good for persons to drink themselves intoxicated once a month for the excellent reasons that it frees their strength, furthers sound sleep, eases the passing of water, increases perspiration, and stimulates general well-being" (Durant, 1961, pp. 495–496). Unfortunately, few were probably moderate enough to restrict their binges to once a month.

Rosen (1958) notes that, while the Renaissance "is characterized by the rapid growth and spread of science in various fields, public health as a practiced activity received very little, if any, direct benefit from these advances" (p. 84). Evidence of the poor public health conditions can be seen in this note describing the average English household floor of the sixteenth century:

> As to floors, they are usually made with clay, covered with rushes that grow in the fens and which are so seldom removed that the lower part remains sometimes for twenty years and has in it a collection of spittle, vomit, urine of dogs and humans, beer, scraps of fish and other filthiness not to be named. (Pickett & Hanlon, 1990, p. 25)

Although living conditions among the English royalty were certainly better than for those of the laboring class, health-related problems still were prevalent. Disposal of human waste was a major problem. Those who lived in old castles located their latrines in large projections on the face of walls. The excrement was discharged from these projections into deep-walled pits, moats, or streams near the walls of the castle. Those less fortunate used chamber pots and simply tossed their contents out the nearest window. Even among royalty, basic hygiene left much to be desired. Few monarchs bathed more frequently than once a week. Much of the material used in royal apparel, such as silk, velvet, and ermine, could not be washed; thus, it simply accumulated dirt and perspiration.

Cloaking scents were used to try to renew the clothing, but they were not effective (Hansen, 1980).

On the positive side, the Renaissance was a period of exploration and expanded trade. The search for knowledge, characteristic of the Greek and Roman eras, was revitalized. Superstitions of the Middle Ages were slowly replaced with a more systematic inquiry into cause and effect. In the middle of the fifteenth century, learning gained momentum due to Johannes Gutenberg's invention of the printing press with moveable type. This allowed the great classical works of Hippocrates and Galen to be reproduced and distributed to larger audiences (Gordon, 1959).

There were also scientific advancements during the Renaissance. The human body was again considered appropriate for study, and realistic anatomical drawings were produced. John Hunter, the father of modern surgery, undertook a more orderly exploration of the workings of the human body. Antonie van Leeuwenhoek discovered the microscope and proved there were life forms too small for the human eye to see. These life forms, however, were not yet associated with disease. John Graunt forwarded the fields of statistics and epidemiology. Through studying the *Bills of Mortality,* published weekly in London, "he determined the excess of male over female births, the high rate of mortality during the earlier years of life, the approximate numerical equality of the sexes, and the excess of urban over the rural death rate" (Goerke & Stebbins, 1968, p. 16).

In Italy, many cities had instituted health boards to fight the plague. It did not take long, however, for their responsibilities to be expanded. By the middle of the sixteenth century, numerous matters had fallen under the control and jurisdiction of these health boards. These included "the marketing of meat, fish, shellfish, game, fruit, grain, sausages, oil, wine and water; the sewage system; the activity of the hospitals; beggars and prostitutes; burials, cemeteries, and pesthouses; the professional activity of physicians, surgeons and apothecaries; the preparation and sale of drugs; the activity of hostelries and the Jewish community" (Cipolla, 1976, p. 32).

## Age of Enlightenment

The 1700s were a period of revolution, industrialization, and growth of cities. Both the French and American Revolutions took place during this century. Plague and other epidemics continued to be a problem. Science had not yet discovered that these diseases were produced by microscopic organisms. The general belief was that disease was formed in filth and that epidemics were caused by some type of poison that developed in the putrefaction process. The vapors, or "miasmas," rising from this rotting refuse could travel through the air for great distances and were believed to result in disease when inhaled. This concept, known as the **miasmas theory**, remained popular throughout much of the nineteenth century. As preventive measures, herbs and incense were often used to perfume the air, supposedly filling the nose and crowding out any miasmas (Duncan, 1988). It was still not known that contaminated water could cause disease infection.

Scientific advancements continued throughout the period. Dr. James Lind, a Royal Navy surgeon, discovered that scurvy could be controlled on long sea voyages by having sailors consume lime juice. To this day, British sailors are known as "limeys." Edward Jenner discovered a vaccine procedure against smallpox. Bernardino Ramazzini wrote on trade and industrial diseases. Theorists of the time conceived of the mind and body not as separate entities, but as dependent on each other. Eighteenth-century philosophers such as Diderot, Locke, Rousseau, and Voltaire all "promoted the worth of each human life and the importance of individual health for the well being of society" (Rubinson & Alles, 1984, p. 5).

Although progress was made during this time, health education/promotion in itself still did not emerge as a profession. With the rudimentary state of medical knowledge in the sixteenth, seventeenth, and even eighteenth centuries, there would have been little for a health education specialist to do other than promote the misconceptions and half-truths that predominated during the time period. However, health boards, the forerunner of today's health departments, did develop as scientific and medical knowledge increased. The roots of modern health education/promotion were planted, and the first sprouts would soon emerge.

## The 1800s

In the first half of the 1800s, little happened to improve the public's health. In England, the streets of London were filthy with animal and human waste. Overcrowding and industrialization added to the problem. These conditions, under which so many people lived and worked, had dire results. Smallpox, cholera, typhoid, tuberculosis, and many other diseases reached high endemic levels (Pickett & Hanlon, 1990).

In 1842, a momentous event occurred in the history of public health when Edwin Chadwick published his *Report on an Inquiry into the Sanitary Conditions of the Labouring Population of Great Britain.* In the report, he documented the deplorable living conditions of Britain's laboring class, made a strong case that these conditions were the cause of much disease and suffering, and called for government intervention. This report eventually led to the formation of a General Board of Health for England in 1848 (Goerke & Stebbins, 1968).

Extraordinary advancements in biology and bacteriology took place by the middle of the nineteenth century in England and throughout Europe. In 1849, Dr. John Snow, who laboriously studied epidemiological data related to a cholera epidemic in London, hypothesized that the disease was caused by microorganisms in the drinking water from one particular water pump located on Broad Street (see **Figure 2.6**). He removed the pump's handle to keep people from using the water source, and the epidemic abated. Snow's action was remarkable, as it predated the discovery that microorganisms cause disease and was in opposition to the prevailing miasmas theory of the time.

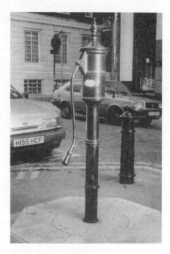

**Figure 2.6** By removing the handle of this pump, which is still in place on Broad Street in London, John Snow interrupted a cholera epidemic.

(Robert Hardy Picture Library Ltd., London)

In 1862, Louis Pasteur of France proposed his germ theory of disease. After this, advancements in bacteriology greatly accelerated. Over the next twenty years, Pasteur discovered how microorganisms reproduce, introduced the first scientific approach to immunization, and developed a technique to pasteurize milk. Robert Koch, a German scientist, developed the criteria and procedures necessary to establish that a particular microbe, and no other, caused a particular disease. Joseph Lister, an English surgeon, developed the antiseptic method of treating wounds by using carbolic acid, and he introduced the principle of asepsis to surgery. These are just a few of the tremendous advancements in bacteriology made during the second half of the nineteenth century. As a result, the years from 1875 to 1900 became known as the **bacteriological period of public health** (McKenzie et al., 2008).

## Public Health in the United States

### 1700s

During the 1700s, health conditions in the United States were similar to those in Europe—deplorable. Diseases such as smallpox, cholera, and diphtheria were prevalent. Because of the slave trade, diseases such as yaws, yellow fever, and malaria were common in southern states (Marr, 1982). Large numbers of immigrants were entering the ports, cities were growing, overcrowding was common, and the Industrial Revolution was about to begin.

The primary means of controlling disease were quarantine and regulations on environmental cleanliness. For example, as early as 1647, the Massachusetts Bay Colony enacted regulations to prevent pollution of Boston Harbor. In 1701, Massachusetts passed laws allowing for the isolation of smallpox patients and for ship quarantine, as needed. However, there was no overseeing body or agency to enforce compliance.

In an attempt to address health problems, some cities formed local health boards (Pickett & Hanlon, 1990). Prominent citizens who advised elected officials on health-related matters made up these boards. They had no paid staff, no budget, and no authority to enforce regulations. According to tradition, the first health board was formed in Boston in 1799, with Paul Revere as chairman. This is contested, however, by other cities claiming earlier health boards, including Petersburg, Virginia (1780), Baltimore (1793), Philadelphia (1794), and New York (1796).

Life expectancy is one measure of health status for a given population. It is defined as "the average number of years a person from a specific cohort is projected to live from a given point in time" (McKenzie et al., 2008, p. 76). The first life expectancy tables were developed for the United States in 1789 by Dr. Edward Wigglesworth (Ravenel, 1970). **Table 2.1** shows Wigglesworth's table. It provides strong evidence of the prevailing health conditions. In 1789, life expectancy at birth was only 28.15 years. In 2006, life expectancy at birth was 77.7—the highest ever in the United States. By 2020, the projected life expectancy at birth in the United States will be 79.5 years (U.S. National Center for Health Statistics, 2009).

### 1800s

From 1800 to 1850, health status improved little. Conditions of overcrowding, poverty, and filth worsened as the Industrial Revolution encouraged more and more people to move to the cities. Epidemics of smallpox, yellow fever, cholera, typhoid, and typhus were common. Tuberculosis and malaria also reached exceptionally high levels. For example, in 1850, the Massachusetts tuberculosis death rate was 300 per 100,000 population, and

**Table 2.1**  Expectation of life according to Wigglesworth life table—1789

| Expectation | Years | Expectation | Years |
|---|---|---|---|
| At birth | 28.15 | At age 50 | 21.16 |
| At age 5 | 40.87 | At age 55 | 18.35 |
| At age 10 | 39.23 | At age 60 | 15.43 |
| At age 15 | 36.16 | At age 65 | 12.43 |
| At age 20 | 34.21 | At age 70 | 10.06 |
| At age 25 | 32.32 | At age 75 | 7.83 |
| At age 30 | 30.24 | At age 80 | 5.85 |
| At age 35 | 28.22 | At age 85 | 4.57 |
| At age 40 | 26.04 | At age 90 | 3.73 |
| At age 45 | 23.92 | At age 95 | 1.62 |

*Source:* Ravenel, M. P. (Ed.). (1970). *A Half Century of Public Health.* New York: Arno Press and *The New York Times.* Originally published in 1921 by American Public Health Association.

the infant mortality was about 200 per 1,000 live births. Conditions were so bad that life expectancy actually decreased in some cities during this period of time. In Boston, the average age at death dropped from 27.85 years in 1820–1825 to 21.43 in 1840–1845. In New York during the same period, the average age of death decreased from 26.15 to 19.69 (Shattuck, 1850).

Public health reform in the United States was slow to begin. Interestingly, a major report helped jump-start the public health reform movement in the United States, just as Chadwick's landmark 1842 report stimulated public health reform in Britain. Lemuel Shattuck's 1850 *Report of the Sanitary Commission of Massachusetts* contained remarkable insights about the public health issues of Massachusetts, including how to approach and solve these problems. In describing the content of this famous report, Pickett and Hanlon (1990) noted:

> Among the many recommendations made by Shattuck were those for the establishment of state and local boards of health; a system of sanitary police or inspectors; the collection and analysis of vital statistics; a routine system for exchanging data and information; sanitation programs for towns and buildings; studies of the health of school children; studies of tuberculosis; the control of alcoholism; the supervision of mental disease; the sanitary supervision and study of problems of immigrants; the erection of model tenements, public bathhouses, and washhouses; the control of smoke nuisances; the control of food adulteration; the exposure of nostrums; the preaching of health from pulpits; the establishment of nurses' training schools; the teaching of sanitary science in medical schools; and the inclusion of preventive medicine in clinical practice, with routine physical examinations and family records of illness. (p. 31)

This report is remarkable because no national or state public health programs existed at the time, and local health agencies that did exist were functioning at a minimal level. Shattuck visualized how to improve the public's health. "Of the 50 recommendations which Shattuck listed, 36 have become accepted principles of public health practice" (Goerke & Stebbins, 1968, p. 28).

The publication of Shattuck's report did not mean an end to the public health problems in the United States. In fact, the report went unnoticed for nineteen years until

1869, when the Commonwealth of Massachusetts established a state board of health made up of physicians and laymen exactly as Shattuck had envisioned. One year later, Virginia and California formed their own state boards of health (Ravenel, 1970). By 1900, thirty-eight states had established state boards of health. Today, every U.S. state has a state board or department of health.

Despite the formation of state boards of health, state-level health departments could not meet health needs on a more local level. With limited resources, there was simply too much to accomplish. As a result, the first full-time county health departments were formed in Guilford County, North Carolina, and Yakima County, Washington, in 1911. Some sources have cited Jefferson County, Kentucky, as the first county health department, set up in 1908 (Pickett & Hanlon, 1990).

As states initiated boards of health, board members had to interact, communicate, and develop their skills. These needs led to the founding of the American Public Health Association. (See Chapter 8 for more information on the APHA.) Following a series of national conventions on quarantine held from 1857 through 1860, "Stephen Smith invited a group of 'refined gentlemen' to discuss informally the possibility of a national sanitary association" (Bernstein, 1972, p. 2). Smith's suggestion of an association for health officials and interested citizens was well received. A decision was made to establish a committee to work on a permanent organization. One year later, in 1873, the first annual meeting was held in Cincinnati, Ohio, and seventy new members were elected. Smith remained active in the association throughout his life. At the age of ninety-nine, he walked to the podium unassisted to speak at the fiftieth anniversary celebration of the APHA.

The federal government started a public health service that dates back to 1798, when Congress passed the Marine Hospital Service Act. Previously, sailors in the merchant marine had nowhere to turn for health care. Since they paid no local or state taxes, ill or injured sailors generally were not welcomed in port cities. The Marine Hospital Service Act required the owners of every ship to pay the tax collector twenty cents per month for every seaman they employed. This money was used to build hospitals and provide medical services in all major seaport cities (see **Figure 2.7**). This Act "represented the first prepaid medical and hospital insurance plan in the world, under the administrative supervision of what eventually became a public health agency" (Pickett & Hanlon, 1990, p. 34).

Successive legislation throughout the nineteenth century gradually expanded the scope of the Marine Hospital Service. In 1902, Congress retitled it the Public Health and Marine Hospital Service and gave it a definite organizational structure under the direction of the surgeon general. In 1912, "Marine Hospital" was dropped from the name, and the service became known as it is today, the U.S. Public Health Service. "The mission of the U.S. Public Health Service Commissioned Corps is to protect, promote, and advance the health and safety of our Nation" (U.S. Public Health Service, 2010).

In 1879, Congress created the National Board of Health. The board was comprised of seven members appointed by the president, including representatives of the army, navy, Marine Hospital Service, and Justice Department. Its functions were to obtain information on all matters related to public health, and provide grants-in-aid to state boards of health. The National Board also provided money to university scientists for health-related research. Unfortunately, the board was short-lived. In administering quarantine functions, the board incurred opposition from state agencies and private shipping concerns. Others in positions of power were not in favor of the research grant program

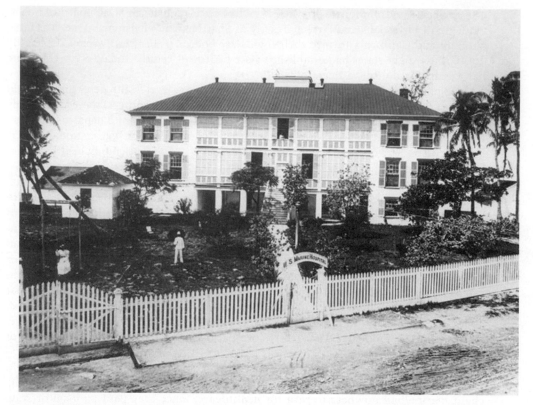

**Figure 2.7** Key West U.S. Marine Hospital in Key West, FL, early 1900s
(Courtesy of Special Collections Department, University of South Florida. Digitization provided by USF Libraries Digitization Center.)

and felt such expenditures were extravagant. Thus, in 1882, the board's appropriations were transferred to the Marine Hospital Service, which carried on with the quarantine functions but discontinued the grant program (USDHEW, 1976).

## 1900 to Present

The period from 1900 to 1920 is known as the reform phase of public health (McKenzie et al., 2008). During this time, urban areas expanded, and many people lived and worked in deplorable conditions. To address these concerns, federal regulations were passed concerning the food industry, states passed workers' compensation laws, the U.S. Bureau of Mines and the U.S. Department of Labor were created, and the first clinic for occupational diseases was established. By the end of the 1920s, the movement for healthier workplace conditions was well established, and the average life expectancy had risen to 59.7 years.

Also during this period, the first national voluntary agencies were formed. They were run primarily by volunteers and a few paid staff. Each of these agencies was designed to address a specific health problem. For example, the National Association for the Study and Prevention of Tuberculosis was established in 1902, and the American Cancer Society was founded in 1913. Today, volunteer agencies continue to be important players in the prevention of disease and the promotion of health (McKenzie et al., 2008).

The 1920s were a relatively quiet period in public health. Progress continued, but at a slower pace. However, the Public Health Education Section of the American Public Health Association was founded in 1922 (Bernstein, 1972). This is the APHA section to which most health education specialists belong. It "promotes the advancement of the health promotion and education profession and provides a forum for public health educators and those involved in health promotion activities to discuss ideas, research, and training; promotes activities related to training public health professionals" (APHA 2010).

The need for health education/promotion existed in the early twentieth century. Moore's book about public health in the United States (1923) included two chapters on questionable and unreliable health activities. One of the most interesting examples involved a cure-all product known as Tanlac. The May 11, 1917, edition of the *Holyoke Daily Transcript* contained Fred Wicks' testimonial in a Tanlac advertisement, as well as his obituary (Moore, 1923, pp. 173–174).

Other examples of questionable health practices also abound. William Harvey Kellogg and his younger brother W.K., founders of the Kellogg cereal company, were best known in the early 1900s for the sanitarium they established and operated in Battle Creek, Michigan. The rich and famous came from all over the world to be treated at the sanitarium. Many of the treatment modalities, however, would be considered questionable and even quackery by today's standards. For example, they utilized some 200 different types of hydrotherapy along with therapeutic enemas, electric horses, vibrators, and cold air (Butler, Thornton, & Stoltz, 1994). However, the sanitarium did promote exercise and good nutrition as ways to prevent and treat disease. The concept of prevention was beginning to take hold.

Tension between preventive medicine and curative medicine began to appear in the United States during the early twentieth century. Moore (1923) related a story about a town in which public health work had banished malaria. A physician was asked how his profession had been affected by this public health advancement. He replied off-handedly, "If it hadn't been for the influenza, I'd have gone broke. That saved us" (p. 373).

In a more rational manner, Newsholme (1936) noted three reasons that treatment formed a larger part of public health efforts and why it would continue to do so in the future. First, the knowledge to prevent "a large proportion of the total sickness and mortality in the community is only partial" (p. 169). Second, "even when knowledge exists which if applied would reduce avoidable illness, it has not become vitally realized by most of us, and many among us are completely ignorant concerning it. Many more are unwilling to live in accord with this knowledge or are so circumstanced that their knowledge cannot be applied in their lives" (p. 169). Third, "physicians, hygienists, and Public Health Authorities find themselves confronted by an embarrassing multitude of sick people needing immediate aid; and their primary duty obviously is to give adequate and complete treatment of already existent sickness. Ambulance work must precede work to prevent future accidents, though no ambulance work is fully satisfactory which does not include thorough investigation of the origin of the accident and the full application of the conclusions from inquiry to the prevention of recurrent accidents" (pp. 169–170). Many of the same arguments are used today to account for the emphasis on traditional medical interventions instead of prevention.

From 1930 through World War II, the role of federal government in social programs expanded. Prior to the Great Depression, medical services were provided by relatives and friends, as well as by religious organizations and some voluntary agencies.

During the Depression, however, private resources could not meet the demands of those requiring assistance. In 1933, President Franklin D. Roosevelt created numerous agencies and programs as part of his New Deal, which improved the plight of the disadvantaged. Much of the money was used for public health efforts, including the control of malaria, the building of hospitals, and the construction of municipal water and sewage systems.

The Social Security Act of 1935 was a real milestone and the beginning of the federal government's involvement in social issues, including health. The act provided support for state health departments and their programs. Funding was made available to develop sanitary facilities and to improve maternal and child health.

Two major public health agencies were formed at this time. On May 26, 1930, the Ransdell Act converted the Hygienic Laboratory to the National Institute of Health, with a broad mandate to learn the cause, prevention, and cure of disease (USDHEW, 1976). The National Institutes of Health, as it is called today, is now one of the premiere—if not *the* premiere—medical research facilities in the world. In 1946, the Communicable Disease Center was established in Atlanta, Georgia. Now called the Centers for Disease Control and Prevention (CDC), it is one of the world's leading epidemiological centers. The CDC is also a major training facility for health communications and educational methods (Pickett & Hanlon, 1990). The CDC's vision for the twenty-first century is "Health Protection . . . Health Equity" (CDC, 2010). Its mission is "Collaborating to create the expertise, information, and tools that people and communities need to protect their health—through health promotion, prevention of disease, injury and disability, and preparedness for new health threats" (CDC, 2010).

Following World War II, concern rose over the number of health care facilities and the adequacy of the care they provided. In 1946, Congress passed the National Hospital Survey and Construction Act, also known as the Hill-Burton Act, to improve the distribution and enhance the quality of hospitals. From the passage of the Hill-Burton Act through the 1960s, new hospital construction occurred rapidly. Little thought, however, was given to planning. As a result, hospitals were built too close together and provided overlapping and unnecessary services (McKenzie et al., 2008).

In 1954, Dr. Mayhew Derryberry, the first chief of health education in the federal government, noted, "The health problems of greatest significance today are the chronic diseases. . . . The extent of chronic diseases, various disabling conditions, and the economic burden that they impose have been thoroughly documented" (*Voices From the Past*, 2004, p. 368). Prior to the 1950s, the major emphasis of public health had been on communicable or contagious diseases. However, through improved public health services, medical care, and immunization programs, many contagious diseases no longer threatened as they once had, and the focus shifted ever so slowly to the prevention of chronic diseases. Derryberry predicted how this change of focus would impact health education: "Health education and health educators will be expected to contribute to the reduction of the negative impact of such major health problems as heart disease, cancer, dental disease, mental illness and other neurological disturbances, obesity, accidents and the adjustments necessary to a productive old age" (*Voices From the Past*, 2004, p. 368). While the seed may have been planted for health education specialists to play a greater role in the prevention of chronic diseases, it was not until the 1970s that the seed finally sprouted.

In 1965, the federal government again passed major legislation designed to improve the health of the U.S. population. While major improvements were made in health facilities and the quality of health care, there were still many underserved people. Most of these people were either poor or elderly. In response, Congress passed the Medicare and Medicaid bills as amendments to the Social Security Act of 1935. **Medicare** was created to assist in the payment of medical bills for the elderly, while **Medicaid** did the same for the poor. These bills provided medical care for millions of people who could not otherwise have obtained such services. Unfortunately, these bills also created an influx of federal dollars to the health care system, ultimately increasing the cost of health care for everyone.

It was evident by the 1970s that disease prevention held the greatest potential for improving Americans' health and reducing health care costs. The first national effort to promote the health of citizens through a more preventive approach took place in Canada. In 1974, the Canadian Ministry of Health and Welfare released a publication entitled *A New Perspective on the Health of Canadians* (Lalonde, 1974). This document, often called the Lalonde Report, presented epidemiological evidence that supported the importance of lifestyle and environmental factors. It called for numerous national health promotion strategies that encouraged Canadians to be more responsible for their own health. (See Chapter 1 for information on the Health Field Concept associated with this publication.) The Lalonde Report influenced many U.S. health professionals to rethink current assumptions that focused on high-technology, treatment-based medicine. So important was this report that Bates and Winder (1984) likened it to a reemergence of Hygeia and the beginning of the second public health revolution (p. 24).

**Healthy People Initiatives and Public Health Standards**    In the United States, the government publication *Healthy People* was the first major recognition of the importance of lifestyle in promoting health and well-being (U.S. Public Health Service, 1979). This publication supported a shift from the traditional medical model toward lifestyle and environmental strategies that emphasized prevention.

In 1980, *Promoting Health/Preventing Disease: Objectives for the Nation* was released. This federal document contained 226 U.S. health objectives for the United States, divided into three areas: preventive services, health protection, and health promotion. These objectives provided the framework for public health efforts during the 1980s. They allowed public health professionals to focus on key areas while providing baseline data for measuring progress (USDHHS, 1980). Although not all of these objectives were met, the planning and evaluation process used to develop them became a valuable way to measure progress in U.S. health and health care services. This led to the practice of developing U.S. health objectives each decade. In 1990, *Healthy People 2000: National Health Promotion and Disease Prevention Objectives* was released, and in 2000, *Healthy People 2010: Understanding and Improving Health* was released.

The Healthy People initiative has evolved into an important strategic planning tool for public health professionals at the federal, state, and local levels. Formal reviews measure the progress of these objectives at mid-course (halfway through the ten-year period) and again at the end of ten years. The mid-course review provides an opportunity to update the document based on events that may impact the objectives. For example, in Healthy People 2010, a number of objectives were changed, updated, or deleted because of the 9/11 event (2001) and Hurricanes Katrina and Rita (2005). The results of both the mid-course and end reviews along with other available data are used to help create the next set of goals and objectives.

**Table 2.2**    *Healthy People 2020* Vision, Mission, and Goals

---

*Vision*

A society in which all people live long, healthy lives.

*Mission*

*Healthy People 2020 strives to:*

- Identify nationwide health improvement priorities;
- Increase public awareness and understanding of the determinants of health, disease, and disability and the opportunities for progress;
- Provide measurable objectives and goals that are applicable at the national, state, and local levels;
- Engage multiple sectors to take actions to strengthen policies and improve practices that are driven by the best available evidence and knowledge;
- Identify critical research, evaluation and data collection needs.

*Overarching Goals*

- Attain high quality, longer lives free of preventable disease, disability, injury, and premature death.
- Achieve health equity, eliminate disparities, and improve the health of all groups.
- Create social and physical environments that promote good health for all.
- Promote quality of life, healthy development and healthy behaviors across all life stages.

---

*Source:* U.S. Department of Health and Human Services. (2010). *Developing Healthy People 2020.*

*Healthy People 2020,* with a release date in December 2010, will guide U.S. public health practice and health education specialists for the next ten years. A preliminary advisory on *Healthy People 2020* includes a vision statement, a mission statement, four overarching goals (see **Table 2.2**), and numerous objectives spread over 38 different topic areas (see **Table 2.3**) (CDC, 2010e).

The *Healthy People 2020* developers feel that the best way to achieve the goals is through a feedback loop of intervention, assessment, and results distribution. The Action Model to Achieve Healthy People Goals (see **Figure 2.8**) "represents the impact of interventions (i.e., policies, programs, and information) on determinants of health at multiple levels (e.g., individual; social, family and community; living and working conditions; and broad social, economic, cultural, health, and environmental conditions) to improve outcomes. The results of such interventions can be demonstrated through assessment, monitoring, and evaluation. Through dissemination of evidence-based practices and best practices, these findings would feed back to intervention planning to enable the identification of effective prevention strategies in the future" (CDC, 2010e).

Another important initiative designed, in part, to improve the effectiveness of public health departments working on Healthy People objectives is the National Public Health Performance Standards Program (NPHPSP) (CDC, 2010d). This is a partnership initiative to develop performance standards; collect, monitor, and analyze data; and ultimately improve public health performance. It is the first time that a common, systematic strategy for measuring public health performance has been available. The goals of the program are to

- provide performance standards for public health systems and encouraging their widespread use;
- encourage and leverage national, state, and local partnerships to build a stronger foundation for public health preparedness;

**Table 2.3**    *Healthy People 2020* Topic Areas

| | |
|---|---|
| 1. | Access to Health Services |
| 2. | Adolescent Health |
| 3. | Arthritis, Osteoporosis, and Chronic Back Conditions |
| 4. | Blood Disorders and Blood Safety |
| 5. | Cancer |
| 6. | Chronic Kidney Diseases |
| 7. | Diabetes |
| 8. | Disability and Secondary Conditions |
| 9. | Early and Middle Childhood |
| 10. | Educational and Community-Based Programs |
| 11. | Environmental Health |
| 12. | Family Planning |
| 13. | Food Safety |
| 14. | Genomics |
| 15. | Global Health |
| 16. | Health Communication and Health IT |
| 17. | Healthcare-Associated Infections |
| 18. | Hearing and Other Sensory or Communication Disorders (Ear, Nose Throat—Voice, Speech, and Language) |
| 19. | Heart Disease and Stroke |
| 20. | HIV |
| 21. | Immunization and Infectious Diseases |
| 22. | Injury and Violence Prevention |
| 23. | Maternal, Infant, and Child Health |
| 24. | Medical Product Safety |
| 25. | Mental Health and Mental Disorders |
| 26. | Nutrition and Weight Status |
| 27. | Occupational Safety and Health |
| 28. | Older Adults |
| 29. | Oral Health |
| 30. | Physical Activity and Fitness |
| 31. | Public Health Infrastructure |
| 32. | Quality of Life and Well-Being |
| 33. | Respiratory Diseases |
| 34. | Sexually Transmitted Diseases |
| 35. | Social Determinants of Health |
| 36. | Substance Abuse |
| 37. | Tobacco Use |
| 38. | Vision |

*Source:* U.S. Department of Health and Human Services. (2010). *Developing Healthy People 2020.*

**Action Model to Achieve Healthy People 2020 Overarching Goals**
Determinants of Health

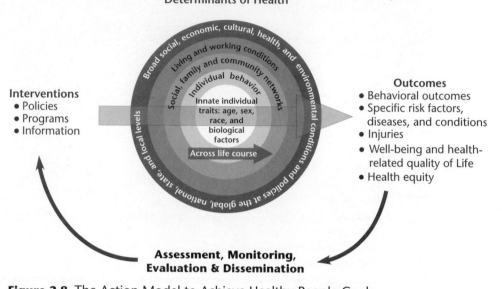

**Figure 2.8** The Action Model to Achieve Healthy People Goals
*Source:* U.S. Department of Health and Human Services. (2010). *Developing Healthy People 2020.*

- promote continuous quality improvement of public health systems;
- strengthen the science base for public health practice improvement (CDC, 2010d).

Local and state health departments are encouraged to utilize these performance standard assessments to conduct their own self-assessments. Through this process, weaknesses can be identified and improvements made to enhance the overall performance of public health departments (CDC, 2010d).

**Health Education/Promotion—A Recognized Profession**    One more important historical event for health education/promotion occurred on October 27, 1997, when the Standard Occupational Classification (SOC) Policy Review Committee approved the creation of a new, distinct classification for the occupation of health educator (Auld, 1997/1998). Health educators had pursued this goal for over twenty-five years. Health educators were previously included in the category "Instructional Coordinator," a broad, primarily education-related category that failed to consider the many varied and unique responsibilities of health educators. Approval of health education as a separate occupational classification means that the Department of Labor's Bureau of Labor Statistics, the Department of Commerce's Bureau of the Census, and all other federal agencies that collect occupational data now collect data on health education specialists. Many state and local governments also maintain data on health education/promotion. For the first time, it is possible to determine the number of health education specialists employed and the outlook for future health education/promotion positions. This approval is one more sign that health education/promotion is gaining the respect and recognition it deserves.

| **Box 2.3** | TEN GREAT PUBLIC HEALTH ACHIEVEMENTS—UNITED STATES, 1900–1999 |

- Vaccination
- Motor vehicle safety
- Safer workplaces
- Control of infectious diseases
- Decline in deaths from coronary (heart) disease and stroke
- Safer and healthier foods
- Healthier mothers and babies
- Family planning
- Fluoridation of drinking water
- Recognition of tobacco use as a health hazard

Source: U.S. Department of Health & Human Services; Centers for Disease Control and Prevention (1999). "Changes in the Public Health System," *Morbidity and Mortality Weekly Report,* 48, 50, 1141.

In summary, tremendous advancements in public health and health education/promotion took place during the twentieth century. It could reasonably be argued that the total number of advancements in public health during the twentieth century were equal to or greater than the total number of public health advancements in all prior time. In reflecting on these great successes of public health, the Department of Health and Human Services identified ten public health achievements they believed had the greatest impact on major causes of morbidity and mortality of the twentieth century. **Box 2.3** lists these ten achievements. Imagine what life would be like today if none of these achievements had been realized. Think of the role health education/promotion has played in these advancements.

## School Health in the United States

Life in early America was hard, and there was little time for education. The labor of building homes, clearing forests, tilling fields, hunting, and preparing food filled the days. Most people lived under primitive conditions. Settlements were few and far apart. Travel and transportation were costly, slow, and limited to foot, horseback, boat, or wagon.

In the mid-1600s, as communities became more established, the call for education was soon heard. Religion had always been an important part of life in America, and it was the religious leaders who led the drive for education. They believed that Satan benefited when people were illiterate, because they could not read the Scriptures. In 1647, Massachusetts passed the "Old Deluder" law to prevent Satan from deluding the people by keeping them from reading the Bible. The law specified that a town with fifty families should establish an elementary school, and a town with one hundred households should set up a Latin grammar secondary school (Means, 1962).

The curriculum in these early schools was largely derived from the educational practices in England. Essentially, reading, as the avenue to religious understanding, was

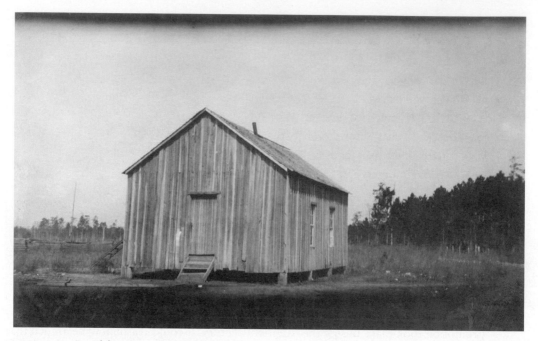

**Figure 2.9** An old one-room schoolhouse
(Courtesy of the Library of Congress, LC-DIG-nclc-02986)

the primary subject. Writing, spelling, grammar, and arithmetic supplemented reading. Later, geography and history were added, but the teaching of health was not part of the early education system in the United States.

Since only boys attended these early schools, and working for the family was still a major concern, daily sessions were by necessity of short duration. The length of the school term was usually only a few months. Teachers were lacking in preparation, with their basic qualifications being only to (1) read, (2) know more of the Bible than the students, (3) work cheap, and (4) keep the students under control. Teachers were totally dependent on the rod for classroom management (Means, 1962).

School buildings typically were inadequate (see **Figure 2.9**). They were poorly built, inaccessible, and sometimes temporary structures. Their interiors were inadequately lighted, were furnished with uncomfortable seating, had no sanitary facilities, and were heated with wood-burning stoves. These schools were not even close to meeting modern standards for school construction (Means, 1962).

The schools and their curricula remained much the same until the 1800s. By the mid-1800s, most schools had become tax supported, and attendance was compulsory. Those concerned about public health pointed out the numerous health and safety problems in the schools. These concerns helped bring attention to the conditions of the schools and ultimately paved the way for health instruction in the curriculum (Means, 1962).

Horace Mann, whose writings and speeches promoted the importance of education in general, was perhaps the first spokesperson for teaching health in schools. He was elected secretary of the Massachusetts State Board of Education in 1837. Beginning in 1837 with the publication of his *First Annual Report* and continuing through the publication of the *Sixth Annual Report* in 1843, Mann called for mandatory hygiene programs that would help students understand their bodies and the relationship between their behaviors and health (Rubinson & Alles, 1984).

Another momentous event in the development of school health occurred in 1850, when Lemuel Shattuck from Massachusetts wrote his *Report on the Sanitary Commission of Massachusetts* (1850). (This is the same report discussed earlier in reference to public health.) While the report has become a classic in the field of public health, it also provided strong support for school health (Means, 1975). In the report, Shattuck (1850) eloquently supports the teaching of physiology, as the term *health education* had yet to be coined:

> It has recently been recommended that the science of physiology be taught in the public schools; and the recommendation should be universally approved and carried into effect as soon as persons can be found capable of teaching it. . . . Every child should be taught early in life, that to preserve his own life and his own health and the lives and health of others, is one of the most important and constantly abiding duties. By obeying certain laws or performing certain acts, his life and health may be preserved; by disobedience, or performing certain other acts, they will both be destroyed. By knowing and avoiding the causes of disease, disease itself will be avoided, and he may enjoy health and live; by ignorance of these causes and exposure to them, he may contract disease, ruin his health, and die. Every thing connected with wealth, happiness and long life depend upon health; and even the great duties of morals and religion are performed more acceptably in a healthy than a sickly condition. (pp. 178–179)

Aside from local and state attempts to promote the teaching of health-related curricula in the schools, no concerted national effort existed until that of the Women's Christian Temperance Union. Originally founded in 1874, the union expounded on the evils of alcohol, narcotics, and tobacco through every conceivable means and was one of the most effective lobbying organizations ever (Means, 1962). Between 1880 and 1890, every state in the union passed a law requiring instruction concerning the effects of alcohol and narcotics due to stimulus from the Temperance Movement (Turner, Sellery, & Smith, 1957).

Other national movements soon followed. In 1915, the National Tuberculosis Association introduced the "Modern Health Crusade" as a device for promoting the health of school children. It was based on promotion to "knighthood" for those that followed certain health habits. The Child Health Organization of America encouraged the nation to adopt more functional health education/promotion programs. One of its active leaders, Sally Lucas Jean, was ultimately responsible for changing the name from hygiene education to health education (Means, 1962). With this name change, the focus of health education shifted from that of physiology and hygiene, which was factual and unrelated to everyday living, to an emphasis on healthy living and health behavior.

Despite these advancements, health education from 1900 to 1920 was generally characterized by inconsistency and awkward progress. World War I provided the impetus for widespread acceptance of school health education as a discipline in its own right (Turner, Sellery, & Smith, 1957). Out of 2,510,706 men examined as potential military draftees during World War I, 730,756 (29 percent) were rejected on physical grounds. A large portion of these physical deficiencies could have been prevented if the schools had been doing their part to train children concerning health and fitness (Andress & Bragg, 1922). In the immediate postwar years, sixteen states required hygiene instruction in their public schools. Twelve of these states made provisions for the preparation of health teachers in the teacher training schools supported by the state (Rogers, 1936).

Significant research and demonstration projects related to school health education were conducted in the 1920s and 1930s. Examples include the Malden, Massachusetts, project, done in cooperation with the Massachusetts Institute of Technology; the Mansfield, Ohio, project supported by the American Red Cross; the Fargo, North Dakota, project sponsored by the Commonwealth Fund; and the Cattaraugus County, New York, project financed by the Milband Memorial Fund. According to Turner, Sellery, and Smith (1957), "these programs showed that habits could be changed and health improved through health education" (p. 27).

In the 1930s, the drive for health education from the public slowed. Health education continued to address the major health issues of the time but without the enthusiasm brought on by World War I. Notable research studies supplemented authoritative opinion in helping to point out difficulties and offer solutions related to the teaching of health education. Several important conferences were held on health education and youth health at the national level (Means, 1962). The profession was moving forward.

Professional organizations emerged during the 1900s that still exist today. School health education, long associated with physical education, received official recognition in 1937, when the American Physical Education Association became the American Association for Health and Physical Education. One year later, recreation was added to the association, and the name changed to the American Association for Health, Physical Education and Recreation (AAHPER). In the 1970s, dance was added to the organization, making the acronym AAHPERD. AAHPERD still exists today, but in the 1990s AAHPERD changed from an association to an alliance of national and district associations, each representing one of the AAPHERD professions or all professions in a particular district of the United States. The national association that represents health education specialists is the American Association for Health Education (AAHE).

The American Association of School Physicians, founded in 1927, had expanded its functions, interests, and scope of activity. As a result, it broadened its membership to include school health personnel other than physicians. In 1938, its name was changed to the American School Health Association to reflect these changes.

The American Public Health Association had long been an organization interested in and supportive of school health. In fact, many of the earliest supporters of health education in the schools had been leaders in public health. Appropriately, the organization established a separate section within its administrative structure to focus on school health interests. In 1942, the School Health Section of the American Public Health Association was formed. (Chapter 8 discusses in greater detail these professional associations.)

With the bombing of Pearl Harbor on December 7, 1941, the United States found itself at war. Once again, national focus turned to physical fitness and health. With no major threats of war in the previous twenty years, the physical status of young American men had again degenerated. Of the approximately 2 million men examined for induction into the nation's armed forces, almost 50 percent were disqualified. Of those disqualified, 90 percent were found to be physically or mentally unfit (American Youth Commission, 1942). This unfortunate situation helped greatly to stimulate interest in the health of high school students and provided strong motivation for health education/promotion classes.

Following the war years, many demonstration projects and studies were again completed to examine the impact of school health education. The Massachusetts High School Study, the Astoria Study, the New York City Study, and the Denver Study were just a few of the efforts that provided valuable information on school health education (Means, 1975).

After World War II, school health education continued to grow as a profession. As Means (1975) observed, "This period from 1940 into the 1970s was one of appraisal, re-evaluation, and consolidation with respect to research accomplished in school health education. During this time leaders in the field attempted to look back, review, and take stock of what was known as a determinant of future action" (p. 107).

The **School Health Education Study** was a major study of significance to school health education. Directed by Dr. Elena M. Sliepcevich (1964), the study included 135 randomly selected school systems involving 1,460 schools and 840,832 students in thirty-eight states. Health behavior inventories were administered to students in grades 6, 9, and 12. The results were appalling. Health misconceptions among students at all levels prevailed. Questionnaires were distributed to school administrators throughout the country to obtain data on organizational procedures and instructional practices related to school health education. Again the results indicated major problems in the organization and administration of health programs. Cortese (1993) noted, ". . . some health topics were omitted while others were repeated grade after grade at the same level of sophistication. No logical rationale placed learning exercises at various grade levels, and a need existed for a challenging and meaningful curriculum" (p. 21).

The second phase of the school Health Education Study established a curriculum writing team to develop a school health education curriculum based on needs identified from the first phase of the study. The team consisted of prominent names in school health education, including Gus T. Dalis, Edward B. Johns, Richard K. Means, Ann E. Nolte, Marion B. Pollock, and Robert D. Russell (Means, 1975). Over the next eight years, the writing team developed a comprehensive curriculum package that still influences school health curricula today.

The **School Health Education Evaluation Study** of the Los Angeles Area was one more important study. Its purpose was to evaluate the effectiveness of school health work in selected schools and colleges of the area. More specifically, the project aimed at the appraisal of the entire school health program, including administrative organization, school health services, health instruction, and healthful school environment. Further, it examined the students' health knowledge, attitudes, and behavior. The study resulted in eleven conclusions and seventeen important recommendations for the field. Of equal importance, the study's planning, design, and operational process established a research pattern that has provided a model for the development of subsequent similar studies (Means, 1975).

School health programs have continued to evolve from the mid-1970s to the present. Several important events and trends have impacted school health education and overall school health programs. In 1978, the Office of Comprehensive School Health was established within the U.S. Department of Education. The primary purpose of the office was policy development for health issues that affected children and youth. Although the office held great promise for school health education efforts, unfortunately, it was never fully funded. A director was named, Peter Cortese, but the office was finally

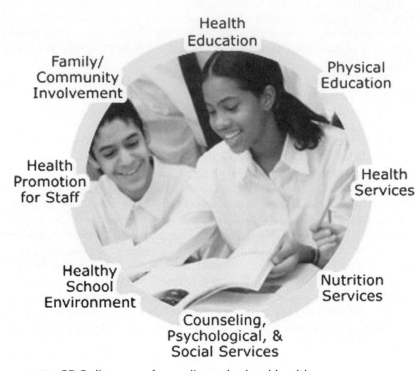

**Figure 2.10** CDC diagram of coordinated school health
*Source:* CDC

deactivated with the budget cuts during President Ronald Reagan's administration (Rubinson & Alles, 1984).

The 1980s saw the emergence of two important concepts: coordinated school health programs and comprehensive school health instruction. Based on the initial ideas of Turner, Sellery, and Smith (1957), and later refined by Allensworth and Kolbe (1987), a **coordinated school health program** consists of eight interactive components that work together to enhance the health and well-being of the students, faculty, staff, and community (see **Figure 2.10**). Leaders involved in each of these eight components work as an integrated team to coordinate the program (CDC, 2010b). Outside leadership is provided by a **school health advisory council** (SHAC). The SHAC is formed by community members (such as parents; medical, health, and safety professionals; and political, religious, and corporate or business leaders) to assist with the planning and promotion of school health initiatives.

**Comprehensive school health instruction** is actually the health education/promotion component of the coordinated school health program (see **Box 2.4**). It refers to the development and delivery of a planned, sequential grades K–12 health education/promotion curriculum. Topics include, but are not limited to personal health, family health, public health, consumer health, environmental health, sexuality education, mental and emotional health, injury prevention and safety, nutrition, prevention and control of disease, and substance use and abuse. The curriculum should be taught by a trained health

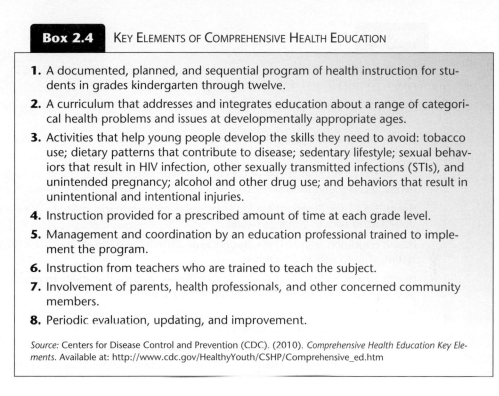

**Box 2.4**   KEY ELEMENTS OF COMPREHENSIVE HEALTH EDUCATION

1. A documented, planned, and sequential program of health instruction for students in grades kindergarten through twelve.

2. A curriculum that addresses and integrates education about a range of categorical health problems and issues at developmentally appropriate ages.

3. Activities that help young people develop the skills they need to avoid: tobacco use; dietary patterns that contribute to disease; sedentary lifestyle; sexual behaviors that result in HIV infection, other sexually transmitted infections (STIs), and unintended pregnancy; alcohol and other drug use; and behaviors that result in unintentional and intentional injuries.

4. Instruction provided for a prescribed amount of time at each grade level.

5. Management and coordination by an education professional trained to implement the program.

6. Instruction from teachers who are trained to teach the subject.

7. Involvement of parents, health professionals, and other concerned community members.

8. Periodic evaluation, updating, and improvement.

*Source:* Centers for Disease Control and Prevention (CDC). (2010). *Comprehensive Health Education Key Elements.* Available at: http://www.cdc.gov/HealthyYouth/CSHP/Comprehensive_ed.htm

education specialist and "designed to motivate and assist students to maintain and improve their health, prevent disease, and reduce health-related risk behaviors" (CDC, 2010b). The CDC (2010c) suggests placing emphasis on six specific adolescent risk behaviors "that research shows contribute to the leading causes of death and disability among adults and youth. These behaviors usually are established during childhood, persist into adulthood, are inter-related, and are preventable. In addition to causing serious health problems, these behaviors also contribute to the educational and social problems that confront the nation, including failure to complete high school, unemployment, and crime." These risk behaviors are as follows:

- Alcohol and drug use
- Injury and violence (including suicide)
- Tobacco use
- Nutrition
- Physical activity
- Sexual risk behaviors

In 2006, the American Cancer Society released the second edition of the National Health Education Standards (see **Box 2.5**). The goal of the National Health Education Standards is improved educational achievement for students and improved health in the United States. The standards promote **health literacy,** the capacity of individuals to access, interpret, and understand basic health information and services, and the skills to

**Box 2.5**    NATIONAL HEALTH EDUCATION STANDARDS

Health Education Standard 1—Students will comprehend concepts related to health promotion and disease prevention to enhance health.

Health Education Standard 2—Students will analyze the influence of family, peers, culture, media, technology, and other factors on health behaviors.

Health Education Standard 3—Students will demonstrate the ability to access valid information and products and services to enhance health.

Health Education Standard 4—Students will demonstrate the ability to use inter-personal communication skills to enhance health and avoid or reduce health risks.

Health Education Standard 5—Students will demonstrate the ability to use decision-making skills to enhance health.

Health Education Standard 6—Students will demonstrate the ability to use goal-setting skills to enhance health.

Health Education Standard 7—Students will demonstrate the ability to practice health-enhancing behaviors and avoid or reduce health risks.

Health Education Standard 8—Students will demonstrate the ability to advocate for personal, family, and community health.

*Source:* Reprinted with permission from the American Cancer Society. *National Health Education Standards Achieving Excellence, Second Edition.* (Atlanta, GA: American Cancer Society; 2007), 8, http://www.cancer.org/bookstore

use the information and services to promote health. The first edition of the National Health Education Standards was issued in 1995. As time passed, the standards needed to be reviewed and updated. The release of the second edition concluded a two-year process of review and revision. This process was conducted by a panel of school health education professionals coordinated by the American Association for Health Education. Other participating groups included the American School Health Association, the American Public Health Association, and the Society of Directors of Health, Physical Education and Recreation. These new national standards established the direction and focus of school health education for the foreseeable future. The standards provide a foundation for curriculum development, instruction, and assessment of student performance. A rationale and numerous performance indicators, broken down by grade level groupings, accompany each of the eight standards. The National Health Education Standards also provide an important guide for colleges and universities to enhance preprofessional preparation as well as the continuing education of health education/promotion teachers.

The National Board for Professional Teaching Standards, founded in 1987, recently developed national standards for school health education teachers. These standards go beyond the requirements for state teacher licensure. Since fall 2008, individuals with three years of full-time health education/promotion teaching experience and a valid state teacher's license for those three years may voluntarily complete a rigorous evaluation process to become a National Board Certified Health Education Teacher. This National

Board Certification places school health education on an equal level with other teaching fields and allows highly qualified and dedicated health education teachers to be recognized for their work. Many states and districts provide salary bonuses for these highly qualified teachers who obtain National Board Certification (National Board for Professional Teaching Standards, 2010). It is expected that many exceptional and highly dedicated health education/promotion teachers will seek National Board Certification in the future.

Since 1987, the concept of a coordinated school health program has dominated the school health arena. At first glance, it would seem that schools would be excited to initiate comprehensive school health programs. How could they not embrace a concept that would bring together multiple components of the school in an integrated attempt to improve the health of faculty, staff, students, and the community? A healthy child taught by a healthy teacher in a health-conscious community should forward the school's overall mission to provide each child with the best education possible. Unfortunately, the full potential of coordinated school health programs has never been realized in most school districts. Factors may include the low priority placed on health by many school administrators; a lack of leadership to promote, coordinate, and oversee school health programs; and an overemphasis on competency testing. Another dynamic could be the adverse reactions from conservative groups that perceive coordinated school health as a means of incorporating sex education into the curriculum.

Despite the apparent lack of success with coordinated school health programs, schools still hold tremendous promise for health education/promotion efforts. With 56 million young people attending more than 132,000 schools (CDC, 2010a), health education specialists must remain diligent in their effort to bring health promotion and education programs to this population. Every health education specialist should be advocating for coordinated school health programs with national and state education agencies, federal and state government representatives, and local school boards.

## Patient Protection and Affordable Care Act

On March 23, 2010, amid both fanfare and criticism, President Obama signed into law the Patient Protection and Affordable Care Act. Through a combination of cost controls, subsidies, and mandates, it expands health care coverage to 31 million uninsured Americans (Open Congress, 2010). Another very important feature is the Act's focus on prevention and prevention services (Koh & Sebelius, 2010; SOPHE, 2010). The bill provides better access to clinical prevention services by removing cost barriers. Further, the bill encourages and promotes worksite wellness programs, encourages evidence-based community prevention and wellness programs, and provides strong support for school-based health centers. (See **Table 2.4** for a summary of the Act's prevention provisions.) This bill should create new and expanded opportunities for health education specialists to promote health. More importantly, it is good for the health of Americans. As Koh and Sebelius (2010) state: "In short, to prevent disease and promote health and wellness, the Act breaks new ground . . . Moving prevention toward the mainstream of health may well be one of the most lasting legacies of this landmark legislation" (p. 5).

**Table 2.4**    Wellness and Prevention Provisions in the Patient Protection and Affordable Care Act (H.R. 3590)

**Immediate Effects 2010**

- Establish the National Prevention, Health Promotion and Public Health Council
- Create a Prevention and Public Health Fund—500 million in FY 2010
- Create task forces on prevention services and community preventive services
- Establish a grant program to support the delivery of evidence-based and community-based prevention and wellness services
- Conduct a national worksite health policies and programs survey
- Award grants to support the operation of school-based health centers—50 million in FY 2010
- Eliminate cost sharing for tobacco cessation counseling and prescriptions for pregnant women in Medicaid and Medicare

**2011**

- National strategy to improve nation's health due March 2011
- Prevention & Public Health Fund receives up to 750 million dollars
- School-based health centers receive another 50 million dollars
- Improve access by eliminating cost sharing for prevention services in Medicare and Medicaid
- Provide grants to small employers to establish wellness programs
- Require chain restaurants and food from vending machines to disclose nutritional content

**2012**

- Worksite survey results due
- Prevention & Public Health Fund receives up to one billion dollars
- School based health centers receive up to 50 million dollars

**2013**

- Prevention & Public Health Fund receives up to 1.25 billion dollars
- School-based health centers receive up to 50 million dollars

**2014**

- Permit employers to offer employee rewards in the form of premium discounts, waivers of cost sharing, or other benefits for participating in a wellness program and meeting certain health-related standards
- Establish 10-state pilot program allowing states to apply similar rewards as noted above for employers.
- Prevention & Public Health Fund receives up to 1.5 billion dollars
- School-based health centers receive up to 50 million dollars

**2015 and Beyond**

- Prevention & Public Health Fund receives up to 1.25 billion dollars
- School-based health centers receive up to 50 million dollars

*Source:* From Society for Public Health Education (SOPHE). 2010. What does health care reform do for prevention and wellness? http://www.sophe.org/advocacy_matters.cfm. Reprinted by permission.

## SUMMARY

The history of health and health education/promotion is important to the professional development of health education specialists. By understanding the past, you can appreciate the present and become a leader in this emerging profession.

Today's concept of health education/promotion is relatively new, dating back only to the middle to late 1800s. Since ancient times, however, humans have been searching for ways to keep themselves healthy and free of disease. Without knowledge of disease causation or medical treatment, it was only natural to rely on superstition and spiritualism for answers. The concept of prevention was intriguing, but the knowledge and skills to prevent disease were unknown.

Progress in preventing and treating disease is evident in the early civilizations of Egypt, Greece, and Rome. These cultures recognized a need for humans to maintain sound minds and bodies. Systems of rudimentary pharmacology, better waste disposal, and safer drinking water were among some of the most noteworthy improvements.

During the Middle Ages, much of what had been previously learned was lost. Society took a giant step backward. Science and knowledge were shunned, while religion gained new favor as the preferred means of preventing and treating disease. Great epidemics struck the European continent, and millions of people lost their lives.

The Renaissance witnessed a rebirth of interest in knowledge. Science again flourished, and health care advancements were made. Understanding of disease, however, was still rudimentary, and the effects of treatments were often worse than the diseases. Sanitary conditions were deplorable and would remain so through the 1800s. The emergence of health education/promotion as a profession was still more than a century away.

The Age of Enlightenment saw tremendous growth in cities as the Industrial Revolution got under way in both England and the United States. Unfortunately, this population growth compounded sanitation problems related to overcrowding. Epidemics were still prevalent. In addition, employment conditions of the working class were frequently unsafe and unhealthy.

By the mid-1850s, conditions were ripe for the birth of public health in the United States. The contagion theory of disease emerged, and early reformers called for the government to take control of environmental conditions that led to disease. Health departments at city, state, and county levels were established and began to monitor and regulate food safety, water safety, and waste disposal. Professional organizations for health personnel were created, and voluntary agencies were formed. Major pieces of legislation were passed as government sought to improve working conditions and took greater responsibility for the poor and infirm. During the mid-1900s, emphasis was placed on building new medical facilities and enhancing the technology required to treat disease.

By the 1970s, the cost of medical treatment had escalated, and concern had shifted to prevention. This set the stage for the development of national health objectives for the decades of the 1980s, 1990s, and 2000s. Health education/promotion made great strides as an emerging profession.

In the mid-1800s, as public health was starting to make important strides, school health education was also budding. In addition to reading, writing, and arithmetic, early pioneers saw the need to educate students about health-related matters. In the early 1900s, groups such as the National Tuberculosis Association, the American Cancer

Society, and the Women's Christian Temperance Union strongly supported educating school children about health. Both World War I and World War II provided important impetus for health-related instruction and physical training in the schools.

During the 1960s and 1970s, several important studies supported the need for school health education and documented its effectiveness. Coordinated school health programs, created in the 1980s, are still important for today's schools. School Health Program Guidelines, national health education standards, and identifying the six leading causes of death and disability helped promote health education/promotion.

While health and school health education have made great strides since the first humans contemplated how to treat and prevent disease, there is still a long way to go. Both in the United States and worldwide there are many people who do not have access to medical care or the important information and skills of professionally trained health education specialists. Heart disease, cancers, diabetes, obesity, and HIV are prevalent in developed countries, while traditional infectious diseases, parasitic infections, and malnutrition continue to affect people in developing countries.

As in the past, health professionals must envision what *can* be and strive to make that vision a reality. Turner, Sellery, and Smith (1957) noted,

> As society looks ahead, it can conceive the hope that some day almost every human being will be well, intelligent, physically vigorous, mentally alert, emotionally stable, socially reasonable and ethically sound. At least, society must concern itself with progress toward that goal. (p. 18)

Health education specialists must be important players in this process. The recent Affordable Health Care Act should expand opportunities for health education specialists to impact Americans' health through community, worksite, and school-based programs.

## REVIEW QUESTIONS

1. Describe the earliest efforts at health care and informal health education/promotion.
2. Compare and contrast the great societies of ancient Egypt, Greece, and Rome. How are these cultures similar in relation to health? How are they different?
3. What were the major epidemics of the Middle Ages? Why were they so feared? What factors contributed to their spread? What were some strategies people used to prevent these diseases?
4. Discuss the Renaissance and why it is important to the history of health and health care.
5. Who wrote the *Report of the Sanitary Commission of Massachusetts* (1850)? Explain how this report was important to the history of both school health and public health.
6. Identify at least five major groups or events that forwarded school health programs.
7. What Canadian publication and its U.S. counterpart helped focus attention on the importance of disease prevention and health promotion?
8. What are *national health objectives?* Where can they be found? Why are they so important?

9. Describe the initiatives that have shaped school health education programs over the past ten years.

10. Explain how the Affordable Health Care Act may serve to improve the public's health and advance the health education/promotion profession in the United States.

## CASE STUDY

Angelita is a health education professor employed by a state university. The local newspaper wants to interview her about the Affordable Health Care Act's prevention aspects, including how the Act may enhance the health of their readers. The newspaper reporter also wants her to talk about previous governmental initiatives designed to prevent disease and improve the public's health. In preparation for the interview, Angelita wants to develop an outline of important points she would like to make. Your task, as Angelita's graduate assistant, is to develop the first draft of these important points.

## CRITICAL THINKING QUESTIONS

1. If a health educator is simply considered as someone who educates others about health, who would be considered humanity's first health educators? Defend your answer.

2. If a health education specialist trained in the year 2010 could time-travel back to the Middle Ages, what impact could that person have on the health problems of that era? What positive factors would work in the health education specialist's favor? What negative factors would work against the health education specialist?

3. When the very first schools were being started in Massachusetts, do you believe health education/promotion would have been accepted as an academic subject? Why or why not? Do you believe health education/promotion is accepted as an academic subject at the present time? Why or why not?

4. Go online and find a copy of the new *Healthy People 2020 objectives*. Read the introduction and overview. Find the objectives for one of the topic areas and review them. Next, select one objective in that topic area that you feel strongly about, and explain why you feel it will or will not be met by the year 2020. What role might a health education specialist have in meeting the objective you selected?

## ACTIVITIES

1. Develop a timeline using 100-year increments from the early Egyptians to the current year. Mark all of the important health-related events as they occurred along the timeline. Next, continue your timeline 100 years into the future. Predict and mark important health-related events. Explain why you believe these predictions will come true.

2. Imagine what it would have been like to live through an outbreak of the Black Death in the Middle Ages. Write a thirty-day personal diary, with daily entries depicting what you might have seen or heard and how you might have felt.

3. Interview several individuals who are at least eighty years old concerning the health care they received as young children. Ask them to describe any health education/promotion they can remember. When was it? Where did it take place? Who provided the education? Was it effective?

4. Contact your high school health teacher. Ask if he/she is aware of the new National Standards for Health Education and to what extent the curriculum in the school district has been based on these standards. Ask if the school district has a coordinated school health program. If so, how does the program function? Who coordinates the program? What programs/initiatives are a result of the program? If no program exists, ask why? Try to determine the barriers to initiating a coordinated school health program in the district.

## WEBLINKS

1. **http://www.csctulsa.org/images/CDC%20Fact%20Book%202000%202001.pdf**

   Centers for Disease Control and Prevention

   This CDC Web site contains the *CDC Fact Book 2000/2001*. On page 135 of this document, you will find the brief history of the CDC. This is a concise but informative overview of the most important events in the illustrious history of this organization.

2. **http://history.nih.gov/exhibits/history/**

   National Institutes of Health

   This National Institutes of Health (NIH) Web site provides a brief history of this organization, highlighting some of its more important accomplishments.

3. **http://www.relfe.com/history_1.html**

   Health, Wealth, Happiness

   This is a very interesting history of health, beginning in the year 540. It chronicles many of the epidemics that plagued mankind as well as other health-related issues such as sugar production, chocolate, and tobacco.

4. **http://www.library.vcu.edu/tml/speccoll/musstateco.html**

   Virginia Commonwealth University

   This site provides a list of "History of Health" science museums in the United States and around the world. These are fascinating places to visit, and they provide useful information for understanding how health knowledge has developed and been disseminated throughout history.

5. **http://www.healthypeople.gov/hp2020/**

   Healthy People 2020

This is the home page for the *Healthy People 2020* goals and objectives. From this page you should be able to access the actual *Healthy People 2020* documents, as well as information on how the objectives are developed.

6. **http://www2.edc.org/MakingHealthAcademic/cshp.asp**

Education Development Center, Inc.

This site provides additional detail on Coordinated School Health Program components and how they can be integrated into the school environment. This information is important for health education specialists who want to work in schools.

## REFERENCES

Allensworth, D., & Kolbe, L. (1987). The comprehensive school health program: Exploring an expanded concept. *Journal of School Health, 57,* 409–412.

American Public Health Association. (2010). APHA Sections. Retrieved August 31, 2010 from: http://www.apha.org/membergroups/sections/aphasections/

American Youth Commission. (1942). *"Health and fitness," youth and the future.* Washington, DC: American Council on Education.

Andress, M. J., & Bragg, M. C. (1922). *Suggestions for a program for health teaching in the elementary schools.* U.S. Department of the Interior, Bureau of Education, Health Education No. 10, Washington, DC: U.S. Government Printing Office.

Auld, E. (Winter 1997/1998). Executive edge. *SOPHE News&Views, 24* (4), 4.

Bates, I. J., & Winder, A. F. (1984). *Introduction to health education.* San Francisco: Mayfield.

Bernstein, N. R. (1972). *APHA: The first one hundred years.* Washington, DC: American Public Health Association.

Butler, M., Thornton, F., & Stoltz, D. (1994). *The Battle Creek idea.* Battle Creek, MI: Heritage Publications.

Centers for Disease Control and Prevention (CDC). (2010a). *About Us: Division of Adolescent and School Health.* Retrieved August 31, 2010 from: http://www.cdc.gov/HealthyYouth/about/index.htm

Centers for Disease Control and Prevention (CDC). (2010b). *Coordinated School health Program.* Retrieved August 31, 2010 from: http://www.cdc.gov/HealthyYouth/CSHP/#model

Centers for Disease Control and Prevention (CDC). (2010c). *Healthy Youth! Health topics.* Retrieved August 31, 2010 from: http://www.cdc.gov/HealthyYouth/healthtopics/index.htm

Centers for Disease Control and Prevention (CDC). (2010d). *The National Public Health Performance Standards Program.* Retrieved August 31, 2010 from: http://www.cdc.gov/od/ocphp/nphpsp/

Centers for Disease Control and Prevention (CDC). (2010e). *Recommendations for the framework and format of Healthy People 2020.* Retrieved August 31, 2010 from: http://www.healthypeople.gov/hp2020/advisory/PhaseI/summary.htm

Centers for Disease Control and Prevention (CDC). (2010f). *Vision, mission, core values, and pledge.* Retrieved August 31, 2010, from: http://www.cdc.gov/about/organization/mission.htm

Cipolla, C. M. (1976). *Public health and the medical profession in the Renaissance.* Cambridge, England: Cambridge University Press.

Cortese, P. A. (1993). Accomplishments in comprehensive school health education. *Journal of School Health, 63* (1), 21–23.

De'ath, E. (1995). *The Black Death—1347 AD*. [Film]. (Available from Ambrose Video Publishing Inc., 1290 Avenue of the Americas, Suite 2245, New York, NY 10104)

Donan, C. (1898). *The Dark Ages 476–918*. London: Rivingtons.

Duncan, D. (1988). *Epidemiology: Basis for disease prevention and health promotion*. New York: Macmillan.

Durant, W. (1961). *The Age of Reason begins*. Vol. 7. *The story of civilization*. New York: Simon and Schuster.

Fee, E., & Brown, T. M. (1997). Editorial: Why history? *American Journal of Public Health, 87* (11), 1763–1764.

Goerke, L. S., & Stebbins, E. L. (1968). *Mustard's introduction to public health* (5th ed.). New York: Macmillan.

Gordon, B. (1959). *Medieval and Renaissance medicine*. New York: Philosophical Library.

Green, W. H., & Simons-Morton, B. G. (1990). *Introduction to health education*. Prospect Heights, IL: Waveland Press.

Hansen, M. (1980). *The royal facts of life*. Metuchen, NJ: The Scarecrow Press.

Koh, H. K., & Sebelius, K. G. (2010). Promoting prevention through the Affordable Care Act. *The New England Journal of Medicine*. Retrieved September 3, 2010 from: http://healthpolicyandreform.nejm.org/?p=12171

Lalonde, M. (1974). *A new perspective on the health of Canadians*. Ottawa: Government of Canada.

Libby, W. (1922). *The history of medicine in its salient features*. Boston: Houghton Mifflin.

Marr, J. (1982). Merchants of death: The role of the slave trade in the transmission of disease from Africa to the Americas. *Pharos, 31* (Winter).

McKenzie, J. F., Pinger, R. R., & Kotecki, J. E. (2008). *An introduction to community health* (6th ed.). Boston: Jones and Bartlett.

Means, R. K. (1962). *A history of health education in the United States*. Philadelphia: Lea & Febiger.

Means, R. K. (1975). *Historical perspectives on school health*. Thorofare, NJ: Charles B. Slack.

Moore, H. H. (1923). *Public health in the United States*. New York: Harper & Brothers.

National Board for Professional Teaching Standards. (2010). *Eligibility and policies*. Retrieved September 5, 2010 from: http://www.nbpts.org/become_a_candidate/eligibility_policies

Newsholme, A. (1936). *The last thirty years in public health*. London: Arno Press & *The New York Times*.

Open Congress. (2010). *H.R.3590 - Patient Protection and Affordable Care Act: Open congress summary*. Retrieved September 3, 2010 from: http://www.opencongress.org/bill/111-h3590/show#

Pickett, G., & Hanlon, J. J. (1990). *Public health administration and practice* (9th ed.). St. Louis: Times Mirror/Mosby.

Ravenel, M. P. (Ed.). (1970). *A half century of public health*. New York: Arno Press & *The New York Times*.

Rogers, J. F. (1936). *Training of elementary teachers for school health work*. U.S. Department of the Interior, Office of Education, Pamphlet No. 67. Washington, DC: U.S. Government Printing Office.

Rosen, G. (1958). *A history of public health*. New York: MD Publications.

Rubinson, L., & Alles, W. F. (1984). *Health education foundations for the future*. St. Louis: Times Mirror/Mosby.

Schouten, J. (1967). *The rod and serpent of Asclepius*. Amsterdam: Elsevier.

Shattuck, L. (1850). *Report of the Sanitary Commission of Massachusetts*. Boston: Dutton and Wentworth.

Sliepcevich, E. M. (1964). *School health education study: A summary report.* Washington, DC: SHES.

Society for Public Health Education (SOPHE). (2010). *What does health care reform do for prevention and wellness?* Retrieved September 5, 2010 from: http://www.sophe.org/advocacy_matters.cfm

Turner, C. E., Sellery, C. M., & Smith, S. A. (1957). *School health and health education* (3rd ed.). St. Louis: Mosby.

U.S. Department of Health and Human Services (USDHHS). (1980). *Promoting health/preventing disease: Objectives for the nation.* Washington, DC: U.S. Government Printing Office.

U.S. Department of Health and Human Services (USDHHS). (1999). Changes in the public health system. *Morbidity and Mortality Weekly Report, 48* (50), 1141.

U.S. Department of Health, Education, and Welfare (USDHEW). (1976). *Health in America: 1776–1976.* (DHEW Publication No. (HRA) 76–616). Washington, DC: U.S. Government Printing Office.

U.S. National Center for Health Statistics, National Vital Statistics Reports (NVSR). (2009). *Deaths: Final Data for 2006,* Vol. 57, No. 14, April 17, 2009.

U.S. Public Health Service. (1979). *Healthy people: The surgeon general's report on health promotion and disease prevention.* Washington, DC: U.S. Government Printing Office.

U.S. Public Health Service. (2010). *The mission of the Commissioned Corps.* Retrieved August 31, 2010 from: http://www.usphs.gov/AboutUs/mission.aspx

*Voices From the Past.* (2004). Today's health problems and health education. *American Journal of Public Health, 94*(3), 368–369.

Winslow, C. A. (1944). *The conquest of epidemic disease.* Princeton, NJ: Princeton University Press.

Ziegler, P. (1969). *The Black Death.* New York: Harper & Row.

# 3

# Philosophical Foundations

After reading this chapter and answering the questions at the end, you should be able to:

- Define the terms *philosophy, philodoxy, wellness, holistic,* and *symmetry* and explain the differences between them.
- Discuss the importance of having a personal philosophy about life.
- Compare and contrast the advantages and disadvantages of having a life philosophy and an occupational philosophy that are similar.
- Formulate a statement that describes your personal philosophy of life and identify the influences that account for your philosophy.
- Identify and explain the differences between the following:
  a. behavior change philosophy
  b. cognitive-based philosophy
  c. decision-making philosophy
  d. freeing/functioning philosophy
  e. social change philosophy
  f. eclectic health education/promotion philosophy
- Explain how a health education specialist might use each of the five health education/promotion philosophies to address a situation in a scenario.
- Create and defend your own philosophy of health education/promotion.

Kristy has been exploring health-related careers and is interested in pursuing a major in health education/promotion. Her interest has been partially piqued by the fact that her parents' lives improved when they began to lower cholesterol and increase exercise by incorporating information and strategies presented to them by a health education specialist employed by their physician. The health education specialist worked with Kristy's parents on a regular basis for nearly six months, and they gave rave reviews on that specialist's methodologies. As a result, her parents were able to reduce or eliminate several of the medications they had been taking. Kirsty also had to admit that the entire family's health had benefited from her parents' "new lifestyle."

In thinking about a career as a health education specialist, Kristy formulated several questions in her mind. A few of the questions involved the philosophies, styles, and methods of practice held or used by health education specialists. Others were related to the profession as a whole and how someone decides whether becoming a health education specialist is a good match for her or his philosophy of life.

This chapter addresses some of the same questions that Kristy contemplated in relation to the practice of health education/promotion and possibly becoming a health education specialist. To that end, we will explore questions such as

- What is a philosophy?
- Why does a person need a philosophy?
- What are some of the philosophies or philosophical principles associated with the notion of "health"?
- What philosophical viewpoints related to health education/promotion do some of the past and current leading health education specialists hold?
- How is a philosophy developed?
- What are the predominant philosophies used in the practice of health education/promotion today?
- How will adopting any of the health education/promotion philosophies impact the way health education specialists approach their job?

The purpose of discussing the development of a health education/promotion philosophy is not to provide a treatise on "the nature of the world," so to speak, but to emphasize the importance of a guiding philosophy to the practice of any profession. Smith (2010) notes, "When a health educator identifies and organizes concepts deemed as valuable in relation to health outcomes, he or she can begin to form a philosophical framework for functioning comfortably and effectively" (p. 51).

The term *philosophy* may seem to some to describe an almost ethereal, esoteric academic exercise. In actuality, however, a well-considered philosophy provides the underpinnings that support the bridge between theory and practice.

## What Is a Philosophy?

The word *philosophy* comes from Greek and literally means "the love of wisdom" or "the love of learning." The term **philosophy** in this chapter means a statement summarizing the attitudes, principles, beliefs, values, and concepts held by an individual or a group. In an academic setting, a philosopher studies the topics of ethics, logic, politics, metaphysics, theology, and/or aesthetics. It is certainly not imperative that a person be an academic philosopher to have a philosophy. All of us have convictions, ideas, values, experiences, and attitudes about one or more of the areas listed above as they apply to life. These are the building blocks (sometimes known as principles) that make up any philosophy. Dr. Buzz Pruitt, professor of health education at Texas A&M, has emphasized the difference between having a life guided by a grounded philosophy and one

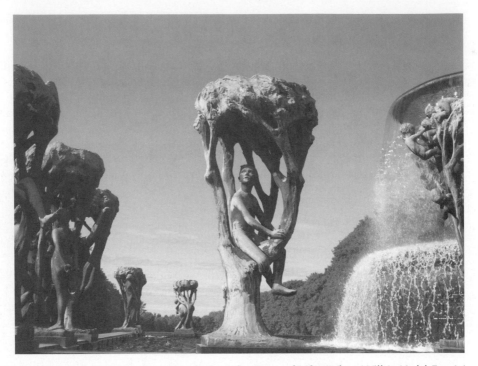

**Figure 3.1** Young Man Contemplating the Tree of Life: What Will It Hold For Me
(James T. Girvan)

shaped by an approach termed **philodoxy** (Pruitt, 2007), literally the love of opinion. The person who has developed a philosophy often asks questions to discover what lies under the surface of issues; thus, the individual seeks answers in a quest for true meaning (reality) and lets that reality define opinion and practice (see **Figure 3.1**). The individual who rejects the possibility of alternative explanations is often practicing philodoxy—letting opinion define reality. Philodoxy presents problems for health education specialists largely because it stifles the incorporation of discovery and new knowledge or insight into the practice of health education/promotion.

Therefore, you most likely have already developed certain philosophical viewpoints or notions about what is real and true in the world as you know it. The manner in which you consistently act toward other people often reflects your philosophy concerning the importance of people in general. That you are studying to become a health education specialist says something about your philosophical leanings in terms of a career. For example, the profession of health education/promotion is considered a helping profession. Those who work in the profession should value helping others.

In today's society there are many examples of the use of a philosophical position. Corporations, for example, create slogans espousing their purported philosophy. (Of course, they are also trying to sell a product or service at the same time.) Many of us recognize certain companies by phrases such as "Just Do It" (Nike), or "When you care enough to send the very best" (Hallmark Cards). The use of caring slogans and catchy phrases is meant to convey to the public that the company is in business solely because it is interested in the welfare of people everywhere and is responsive to their needs. If the company's actions match the slogan, the public is more likely to perceive the slogan as a true representation of the corporate philosophy.

Additionally, many nonprofit and for-profit agencies and companies often have mission statements. A mission statement is meant to convey a philosophy and direction that form a framework for all actions taken by that organization. For example, the mission statement for the Central District Health Department in Boise, Idaho, is as follows:

Healthy People in Healthy Communities

After reading this statement there is little doubt that the overriding philosophy in this department is one of promoting prevention for both individuals and communities. For individuals who have a philosophy that emphasizes prevention and early intervention, this is likely to be a place where they might find employment that is personally rewarding and professionally fulfilling.

Just as often, insight into a person's philosophy can be gained by hearing, reading, or analyzing that person's quotes or sayings. For example, the following quote from actor Michael J. Fox embodies his philosophy of life in the face of an incurable disease: "Parkinson's demanded of me that I be a better man, a better husband, father, and citizen. I often refer to it as a gift. With a nod to those who find this hard to believe, especially my fellow patients who are facing great difficulties, I add this qualifier—it's the gift that keeps on taking . . . but it's a gift" (p. 89). As you will see later and as can be noted from Fox's statement, a philosophy is rarely stagnant, but rather continuous because it is formulated by considering values, beliefs, experiences, and consequences of actions. Composing a philosophy statement allows a person to reflect on what is important to him or her when viewing the world in its many manifestations.

The thoughts stated earlier are well summarized by Loren Bensley (1993), one of the most influential health education specialists of the latter half of the twentieth century:

Philosophy can be defined as a state of mind based on your values and beliefs. This in turn is based on a variety of factors which include culture, religion, education, morals, environment, experiences, and family. It is also determined by people who have influenced you, how you feel about yourself and others, your spirit, your optimism or pessimism, your independence and your family. It is a synthesis of all learning that makes you who you are and what you believe. In other words, a philosophy reflects your values and beliefs which determine your mission and purpose for being, or basic theory, or viewpoint based on logical reasoning. (p. 2)

Please note that a philosophy does not have to be abstract. Pondering the reason for being gives people a chance to integrate their past, present, and future into a coherent whole that guides them through life.

## Why Does One Need a Philosophy?

The answer to the question "Why does one need a philosophy?" is both simple and complex. Each of us already has a view of the world and what is true for us. This image helps shape the way we experience our surroundings and act toward others in our environment. In other words, people's philosophies help form the basis of reality for them.

Of course, some philosophical change is probably inevitable. New experiences, new insights, and new learnings create the possibility that some of the tenets comprising the philosophy might need retooling. This is a normal part of growth. Most people's philosophical views are altered somewhat as they study and experience the world in different ways.

Usually a person's philosophy (e.g., determining how to treat others, what actions are right or wrong, and what is important in life) needs to be synchronous in all aspects of life. This means that a person's philosophical viewpoint holds at home, at school, in the workplace, and at play. If an incongruency develops between a person's philosophy and the philosophy of the leaders in the workplace, problems can occur.

As an example, consider the career of a public health education specialist working in HIV/AIDS prevention education who is employed by a state department of education. Assume that this individual has a philosophical view that all human life is sacred and education is the best source of prevention. Also assume that the person's work both on and off the job reflects consistency and a commitment to those ideals. In other words, the person's actions are synchronous with the aforementioned philosophy. As long as the administration in the state department of education, and family and friends remain supportive of this health education specialist's role and philosophy, chances are that this person will do well. If, however, the state department leadership changes and the new superintendent is opposed to the idea that individuals infected with HIV are worth saving (because they chose their behaviors) or refuses to allow condoms to be mentioned as a secondary source of prevention, the specialist may have a difficult time remaining in that environment. The reason is that this educator is now not allowed to act according to her beliefs, ideals, and knowledge. There is a disharmony between the philosophical stance and the ability to act in concert with that stance.

Certainly, there are exceptions to this rule. Health education specialists might hold philosophies on how they personally live, yet they might have to educate those who have made choices that are opposed to their belief system. This situation begins to cross the bounds of a general philosophy and get into ethics (right behavior—see Chapter 5). Although a possible moral-philosophical conflict seems apparent in this situation, health education specialists need to remember that their primary concern is to protect and enhance the health of those within their jurisdiction. Health is not a moral issue. The health of any one of us affects the health of all of us in some manner (legally, monetarily, physically, or emotionally). At the very least, the health education specialist should refer this situation to another trained individual who can fulfill the obligation to the public.

Former Surgeon General C. Everett Koop (**Figure 3.2**) was confronted with the same dilemma when he was in office. Although he was a strong conservative Christian leader and against the use of drugs and premarital sex, he championed the cause of HIV/AIDS education by stressing that the epidemic is a health problem that requires a health-based prevention message. Through the power of his office, he insisted that HIV/AIDS prevention education include the merits of abstinence, the dissemination of needles to inner-city addicts, and the increased availability of condoms to individuals who choose to be sexually active or promiscuous.

A further example that illustrates the impact of a philosophy on the practice of a profession comes from an article by Governali, Hodges, and Videto (2005) in which they state, "philosophical thought is central to the delivery of health education. For a profession to stay vital and relevant, it is important to assess its activities, regularly evaluate its goals, and assess its philosophical direction" (p. 211). The emphasis the authors place on the influence of activities and goals related to philosophy is a direct reflection of their personal and professional philosophical foundation formed over the

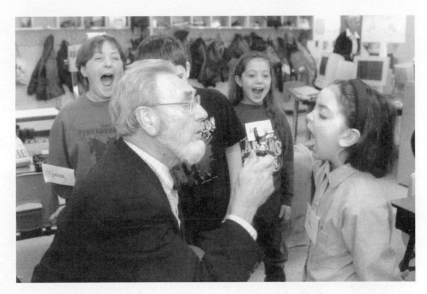

**Figure 3.2** Former Surgeon General C. Everett Koop remains a staunch advocate for the value of health education/promotion as the key to prevention.
(Herbert Medora, Valley News/AP/Wide World)

years. A well-reasoned philosophy often plays an important role in the choice of a career path. A study identifying factors that influence career choices further validates that statement. Tamayose and colleagues (2004) surveyed public health students enrolled at a west coast university to determine what major influences led them to pursue careers in public health. Researchers found that the top two items mentioned by the students were "enjoyment of the profession/commitment to health improvement" and "provide a health/community service to others." Both of these statements reflect a common philosophical thread that permeates the thinking of a majority of individuals currently practicing in the field of health education/promotion with whom we have come in contact.

In summary, the formation of a philosophy is one of the key determining factors behind the choice of an occupation, a spouse, a religious conviction, and friends. A firm philosophical foundation serves as a beacon that lights the way and provides guidance for many of the major decisions in life.

## Principles and Philosophies Associated with Health

In Chapter 1, the meaning of the term *health* was discussed. Recall that, while the term *health* is elusive to define, nearly all definitions include the idea of a multidimensional construct that most people value, particularly when health deteriorates. Over the past thirty to fifty years, educators have identified several philosophies or philosophical principles that tend to be associated with the establishment and maintenance of health. These philosophies provide a set of guiding principles that help create a framework to better understand the depth of the term *health*.

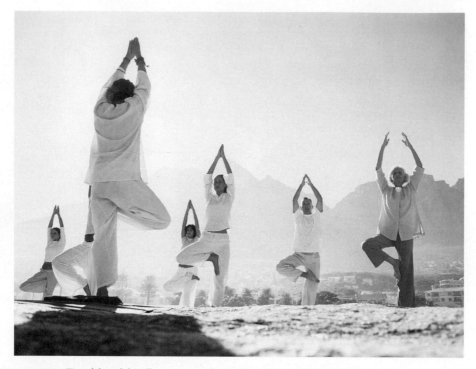

**Figure 3.3** Total health allows people to function at their best.
(Philip North-Coombes/Getty Images)

Rash (1985) mentions that, while health is often not an end in itself, good health does bring a richness and enjoyment to life that will make service to others more possible. He feels that those who seek to enhance the health of others through education should espouse a **philosophy of symmetry;** that is, health has physical, emotional, spiritual, and social components, and each is just as important as the others. Health education specialists should seek to motivate their students or clients toward symmetry (balance) among these components (see **Figure 3.3**).

Oberteufer (1953) rejected the notions of a dualistic (human = mind + body) or a triune (human = mind + body + spirit) nature for humanity. Instead, he embraced the ideal of a **holistic philosophy** of health when he stated, "The mind and body disappear as recognizable realities and in their stead comes the acknowledgment of a whole being . . . man is essentially a unified integrated organism" (p. 105). Thomas (1984) is convinced that the holistic view of health produces health professionals who are more passionate about creating a society in which the promotion of good health is seen as a positive goal.

Greenberg (1992), Donatelle (2011), Edlin and Golanty (2004), and Hales (2004), among others, have elevated the construct of wellness to the level of a philosophy. **Wellness,** always a positive quality (as opposed to illness being always a negative) is visualized as the integration of the spiritual, intellectual, physical, emotional, environmental, and social dimensions of health to form a whole "healthy person." Those who subscribe to this philosophy believe that all people can achieve some measure of wellness,

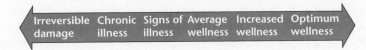

**Figure 3.4** The wellness continuum

*Source:* From Rebecca Donatelle, *Health: The Basics, Green Edition,* 9th ed., Fig 1.3, p. 4. Copyright © 2011. Reproduced by permission of Pearson Education, Inc., Upper Saddle River, NJ.

no matter what limitations they have, and that achieving optimal health is an appropriate journey for everyone. The optimum state of wellness occurs when people have developed all six of the dimensions of health to the maximum of their ability. (See **Figures 3.4** and **3.5**.)

To be sure, there are those who differ in their philosophical view of health. For example, Balog (2005) believes that health must by nature be seen solely as a physical state because "health must reside in the person" (p. 269), and it is not possible for a person to be truly healthy if the systems of the body are not functioning in the way they

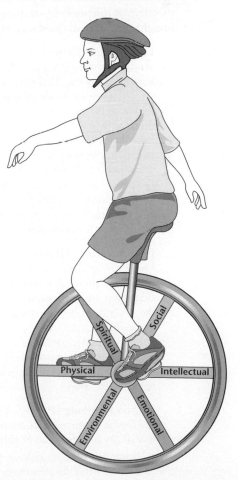

**Figure 3.5** The dimensions of health

*Source:* From Rebecca Donatelle, *Health: The Basics, Green Edition,* 9th ed., Fig 1.4, p. 5. Copyright © 2011. Reproduced by permission of Pearson Education, Inc., Upper Saddle River, NJ.

were intended to operate. He argues that any other view of health is really not objective but introduces subjective views of what others value (the good life). In Balog's view, it is important for health educators to distinguish that which affects health from that which is health. In other words, he cautions against confusing "good life" with "good health."

The philosophies previously mentioned are not meant to be all inclusive. The purpose for discussing them is to help provide a framework to further assist the reader in developing a philosophy about health and, ultimately, health education/promotion.

## Leading Philosophical Viewpoints

Over the past twenty years, several publications and numerous articles have focused on recounting the philosophical positions of past and present leading health education specialists. In order to assist you in formulating your own health education/promotion philosophy, we present here a small sample of the philosophies expressed in these publications. As previously mentioned, one way a philosophical approach is developed is through the influence of role models, or mentors. The viewpoints that follow may help stimulate your thoughts and provide guidance as you consider a career in health education/promotion.

### Becky Smith (2010)
Studying the definitions of health from the perspectives of scholars such as Dubos, Fromm, Maslow, Montagu, Tillich, and Tournier.

. . . helped me develop a personal understanding of how individuals express health and how the potential for health can manifest despite severe limitations in one or more dimension(s). I have come to believe that when internal and external elements that facilitate the development of human potential are available, individuals are more likely to experience optimal health. This has helped me understand my role as a health educator responsible for assisting individuals, communities, and society. It has also led me to believe that nearly everyone expresses some level of health even when they are confronted with the most devastating circumstances. I prefer to look for that expression of health as a starting point for professional interaction, education, and enhancement of health rather than focus on existing debilitation. (p. 52)

### John Allegrante (2006)
I have always believed that the goal of health education is to promote, maintain, and improve individual and community health through the educational process. I believe that there are fundamental conceptual hallmarks and a social agenda that differentiate the practice of health education and that of medicine in achieving this goal. These hallmarks include the use of consensus strategies to identify health needs and problems, voluntary participation as an ethical requirement, and an obligation to foster social and political change. I also believe that our perspective and methodologies require that we enter into a social contract with people that engages them as partners, not merely as patients. (p. 306)

### Marian Hamburg (1993)
Eta Sigma Gamma's invitation to contribute has given me the chance to expound on a few of my beliefs about health education.

1. You can't plan everything. Unexpected opportunities appear and it is important to be ready to take advantage of them. (p. 68)

2. I believe in mentorship. Its power incorporated into health education programming has enormous strength for influencing positive health behaviors. (p. 70)

3. I believe that effective health education programming requires appropriate intersectoral cooperation, and that health educators, regardless of the source of their professional preparation, must be its facilitators. School-community can be one world. (p. 71)

4. I believe that we need to put more of our resources into joint efforts and coalition building. Much of health education's future as a profession depends upon the support that health educators, regardless of their specialized training, provide for the maintenance and expansion of certification. (p. 73)

5. It is not surprising to me that the concept of networking has become an important basis for health education practice. We bring together people with common problems to seek solutions through the sharing of feelings and information. (p. 73)

**John Seffrin (1993)**
I believe the most fundamental outcome of health education is the enabling of individuals to achieve a level of personal freedom not very likely to be obtained otherwise. Freedom means being able to avoid any unnecessary encumbrance on one's ability to make an enlightened choice (p. 110). . . . We need to be resourceful and open to change. In doing so, however, we need to change in ways that do not violate certain basic principles:

1. appreciation for each individual's uniqueness;

2. respect for ethnic and cultural diversity;

3. protection for individual and group autonomy;

4. promotion and preservation of free choice; and

5. intervention strategies based on good science. (p. 114)

Philosophies are as individual as the people themselves, yet some common themes (development of individual potential, learning experiences that help in decision making, free choice, and enhancement of individual uniqueness) seem to emerge and hold true regardless of the health education specialist. Let us now examine how these philosophies are actually applied in the practice of health education/promotion.

## Developing a Philosophy

Now that it is clear that a philosophy is not some abstraction used only by individuals such as the Dalai Lama or Gandhi, let us explore the ways in which a philosophy is formed. In previous sections, it was noted that most practicing professionals and many organizations have developed certain philosophical stances that serve as a road map and guide for living and working in the world. What provides the basis for forming a philosophy?

Suppose you are searching through the Web sites of various health education/promotion programs, trying to determine which one might be best for you. In your search, you come across the Web site for the community health education program at the University of Wisconsin at La Crosse (see the Weblinks section at the end of the chapter for URL references). One of the prominent features of the site is a statement of the mission of the programs.

"The mission of the BS-CHE (Bachelor of Science—Community Health Education) program at the University of Wisconsin-La Crosse (UW-La Crosse) is to prepare professionals using entry-level (BS-CHE) health education competencies and public health core areas who will address quality of life enhancement through health education and health promotion, mindful of the holistic, dynamic and interdependent nature of humans and their interactions with and within the environment."

The process of developing this mission statement most likely involved at least several meetings of faculty, staff, students, and community leaders and administrators. During the meetings the core beliefs and principles regarding health education/promotion of those in attendance were probably assessed. After coupling the list of beliefs with the required list of core competencies, the mission statement was formulated. Notice that the statement concludes with "who will address quality of life enhancement . . . mindful of the holistic, dynamic and interdependent nature of humans and their interactions with and within the environment." This portion of the statement rises to the level of a philosophy.

In drafting your own philosophy statement, you should employ a similar process (without the committee, of course). Think about what a health education specialist does and what the result of his or her work should be. Construct lists of your thoughts under headings such as (1) personal values and beliefs, (2) what "health" means to you, (3) attributes of people you admire and trust, (4) results of health studies and readings that you find meaningful, and (5) outcomes you would like to see from the process of health education/promotion (e.g., better decision making, more community involvement, promotion of positive behaviors). From your lists, some common themes will emerge and the identification of these themes is a key to drafting your own health education/promotion philosophy statement. Exploring why you value the topics represented within these themes should enable you to compose your philosophy statement, or an ultimate product that will reflect a way of thinking, acting, and viewing the world that works for you.

Please note, however, that using this approach to formulate a philosophy is not a guarantee that the philosophy will remain stable. As a matter of fact, there is a strong likelihood that some changes will occur because of new learnings, activities, and experiences (e.g., working in a different culture, experiencing the premature death of a child or spouse, losing a job as a result of downsizing). A philosophy results from the sum of knowledge, experience, and principles from which it was formed.

As a further aid to formulating a philosophy statement about health and health education/promotion, we would like to conclude this section with two short vignettes illustrating several concepts or principles that need to be considered when formulating a philosophy statement about life, health, and health education/promotion practice.

Author and physician, Rachel Naomi Remen (1996), writes a story about her father and his life philosophy. The year Remen's father went bankrupt, he bought her a pair of twenty-four carat gold earrings. Remen recalled:

> I stared at them in silence, bewildered, feeling the weight of my homeliness, my shyness, my hopeless difference from my classmates who easily joked and flirted and laughed. "Aren't you going to try them on?" prompted my father, so I took them into the bathroom, closed the door, and put them on my ears. Cautiously I looked into the mirror. My sallow, pimply face and lank hair, oily before it even dried from a shower, looked much as always. The earrings looked absurd.
>
> Tearing them from my ears, I rushed back into the living room and flung them on the floor. "How could you do this?" I shrieked at my father. "Why are you making fun of me? Take them back. They look stupid. I'm too ugly to wear them. How could you waste all this money?" Then I burst into tears. My father said nothing until I had cried

myself out. Then he passed me his clean, folded handkerchief. "I know they don't look right now," he said quietly. "I bought them because someday they will suit you perfectly." (p. 222)

How things turn out is often a matter of how they are perceived. A personal philosophy is often a reflection of the individual's perspective of the world and how and why it seems to work that way.

The second story, adapted from the book *Kamkwamba and Mealer* (2009), is about the amazing accomplishments of William Kamkwamba of the African nation of Malawi. It goes as follows:

William was curious about how things worked (particularly electricity) and had read a book entitled *Using Energy,* which he accessed in a makeshift library in his town; so he was able to construct a functioning windmill from parts of engines and wrecked automobiles he found in a local junkyard. Most people around him said his dream of supplying his family and his community with reliable electricity for lighting homes and pumping water was "crazy." And like many youths in Africa, William's formal education was cut short by the inability of his family to pay the eighty dollars annual tuition. Yet he maintained the initiative to keep on trying and learning despite his family's suffering through famine, disease, and government graft.

Although rudimentary, the windmill he constructed worked well enough to supply power to light four small light bulbs in his home. Eventually, educators and scientists throughout Africa and beyond learned of the accomplishments of this self-taught scholar. As a result, William has been a featured lecturer at several international conferences; he has completed high school at an international school in South Africa (as a result of a grant); and he began his freshman year at Yale in the fall of 2010. His refusal to abandon his dreams, fueled by his desire to make things better for his village and family, provided a stark contrast to many in his country (and around the world) who take for granted the educational opportunities they have or just give up and settle for the status quo.

All too often, in determining abilities, people set their sights and dreams too low. A personal philosophy needs to incorporate the realization that life sometimes dishes out bumps and bruises. Acknowledging this fact may well prevent any of us from excessively limiting our assessment of our place in the world.

Remember, the formation of a philosophy, whether personal or occupational, requires several steps. First, individuals need to answer the following questions in reference to themselves: What is important? What is most valued? What ideals are held? Second, they need to identify ways the answers to the first questions influence the way they believe and act. Third, after carefully considering and writing down the answers to these questions, a philosophy statement can be formulated. The statement (usually a paragraph or two in length—350–500 words) reflects and identifies the factors, principles, ideals, and influences that help shape reality for those individuals.

As previously mentioned, these steps can be used to formulate any type of philosophy statement. However, for those who are studying health education/promotion, there is one more important question to answer: Is this philosophy statement consistent with being a health education specialist? If the answer is yes, then for that person health education/promotion is a profession worthy of further consideration.

# Predominant Health Education/Promotion Philosophies

Butler (1997) accurately points out that, even though there are several definitions of the phrase *health education/promotion*, recurring themes in many of the definitions allow for a general agreement as to its meaning. He notes, however, that the methods used to accomplish health education/promotion are less clear. The manner in which a person chooses to conduct health education/promotion can be demonstrated to be a direct reflection of that person's philosophy of health education/promotion. With that in mind, have any predominant philosophies of health education/promotion emerged? If so, what are they?

Welle, Russell, and Kittleson (1995) conducted a study to determine the philosophies favored by health education specialists. As part of the background for their study, they conducted a literature review and identified five dominant philosophies of health education/promotion that have emerged during the last 50–60 years. The philosophies identified were behavior change, cognitive-based, decision-making, freeing/functioning, and social change.

1. The **behavior change philosophy** involves a health education specialist using behavioral contracts, goal setting, and self-monitoring to try to foster a modification in an unhealthy habit in an individual with whom he is working. The nature of this approach allows for the establishment of easily measurable objectives, thus enhancing the ability to evaluate outcomes. (Example: setting up a contract to increase the number of hours of study each week)

2. A health education specialist who uses a **cognitive-based philosophy** focuses on the acquisition of content and factual information. The goal is to increase the knowledge of the individuals or groups so that they are better armed to make decisions about their health. (Example: simply posting statistics about the number of people killed or injured in automobile accidents who were not wearing seat belts)

3. In using the **decision-making philosophy**, a health education specialist presents simulated problems, case studies, or scenarios to students or clients. Each problem, case, or scenario requires decisions to be made in seeking a "best approach or answer." By creating and analyzing potential solutions, the students develop skills needed to address many health-related decisions they might face. An advantage of this approach is the emphasis on critical thinking and lifelong learning. (Example: using a variety of case study examples of the Atkins Diet to see competing perspectives of effectiveness)

4. The **freeing/functioning philosophy** was proposed by Greenberg (1978) as a reaction to traditional approaches of health education/promotion that he felt ran the risk of blaming victims for practicing health behaviors that were often either out of their control or not seen as in their best interests. The health education specialist who uses this philosophical approach has the ultimate goal of freeing people to make the best health decisions possible based on their needs and interests—not necessarily the interests of society. Some health education specialists classify this as a subset of the decision-making philosophy discussed above. (Example: lessons on the responsible use of alcohol)

5. The **social change philosophy** emphasizes the role of health education specialists in creating social, economic, and political change that benefits the health of individuals and groups. Health education specialists espousing this philosophy are often at

the forefront of the adoption of policies or laws that will enhance the health of all. (Example: no smoking allowed in restaurants, or new housing developments with pedestrian-friendly areas such as sidewalks and parks)

The previously listed philosophies of health education/promotion are the products of over fifty years of study, experimentation, and dialogue within the profession. The research conducted by Welle, Russell, and Kittleson (1995) alluded to earlier found that the philosophy most preferred by both health education/promotion practitioners and academicians was decision making. Both groups listed behavior change as a second choice, and both agreed that their least favorite was cognitive based. The fact that health education specialists who are employed in the academic setting and those who are employed as practitioners in the field agreed on these choices as predominant philosophies speaks well for the interface between preparation programs and practice.

Another interesting finding from the study occurred when, as a part of the survey, the health education specialists were given health education/promotion vignettes to address or solve. In many cases, the respondents changed the philosophical approach they used depending on the setting (school, community, worksite, medical). The responding health education specialists had earlier identified a specific health education/promotion philosophy they favored. These results indicate that health education specialists are adaptable and resourceful, and they will use any health education/promotion approach that seems appropriate to the situation. The possibility exists that, in practice, health education specialists use an **eclectic health education/promotion philosophy.**

In a thought-provoking essay, Buchanan (2006) introduces a different philosophical paradigm calling for health education specialists to "return to their roots" and reconsider the meaning of the word "education" in the practice of health education/promotion. He feels that the practice of health education/promotion buys into the medical model so often that health education specialists have lost their bearings and are now more often purveyors who almost demand that persons or the public adopt behaviors that "we know" will lead to a healthier life.

Instead he suggests that health education specialists should be "disseminators of factual information and facilitators of rational choice" (p. 301). Using this philosophy,

> The quality of a health educator's work would be evaluated not by its effectiveness in changing people's behavior but by whether their audiences find the dialogue valuable in helping them think about how they want to live their lives, the impact of their behaviors on the pursuit of their life goals, and the kinds of environmental conditions that community members find most conducive to living healthy and fulfilling lives. (p. 301)

In actuality, Buchanan's views seem to incorporate the use of the cognitive-based, the decision-making, and the freeing/functioning health education/promotion philosophies outlined above. This is not surprising, because in any list of philosophies there is always the possibility of one philosophy overlapping with another, so in practice not all is as clean as it might seem. In making a similar argument as Buchanan, Governali, Hodges, and Videto (2005) call for an integrated behavioral ecological philosophy so that health education specialists utilize the multidimensional nature of the interaction of the individual and the environment. This approach also resembles the eclectic philosophical model.

## Box 3.1 Practitioner's Perspective  Philosophy of Health Education/Promotion

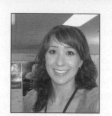

(Reprinted by permission of Heidi Henson)

NAME: Heidi Henson, BS

CURRENT POSITION/TITLE: Health Promotion Coordinator

EMPLOYER: North Central District Health Department, Lewiston, ID

DEGREE/INSTITUTION/YEAR: Bachelor of Science, Boise State University, Boise, 2005

MAJOR: Health Promotion

MINOR: Communication

**Job responsibilities:** North Central District Health Department negotiates health promotion contracts for specific health programs. These funds usually come from federal contracts that are managed at the state level. My job is to make sure the contract goals, objectives, and activities are planned, implemented, and evaluated. My current programs include tobacco prevention and control, tobacco cessation, asthma prevention and control, and comprehensive cancer control. Examples of current contract objectives include: implementing the Teens Against Tobacco Use (TATU) program in local high schools, encouraging health care providers to use Asthma Action Plans in their practices, organizing an Asthma Awareness Walk, facilitating a colorectal cancer coalition, and encouraging businesses to change their tobacco policies. I also attend community health fairs and research and design materials as needed.

**How I obtained my job:** While hoping to relocate to my hometown, my dad told me about a job posting in the local newspaper. In order to make it to the final pool of applicants, I had to pass an online test that asked me to detail my experience and education in the field of public health. After three hours of typing, I was fortunate enough to pass the exam. During the interview, I made sure to express my excitement about the position. I also brought in my portfolio to show samples of my work. But perhaps the most influential reason I obtained my job was having the support of my former employer; I couldn't have asked for a better reference!

**What I like most about my job:** The best thing about my job is the variety. I can honestly say that no two days have been exactly the same.

One day I might attend a health fair, the next day I might teach a class, and the following day might be spent preparing for a coalition meeting. The wide array of job responsibilities keeps my job interesting and exciting.

**What I like least about my job:** The programs I work with are funded on a year-to-year basis. This means a program could be cut at the end of the year if funding is no longer available or if the program is not producing results. It can be a little nerve wracking knowing that the future of your program is uncertain.

**How I utilize my philosophy of health education/promotion in my job:** I am guided by the belief that an individual's behavior is determined by his or her own beliefs. If a woman believes colorectal cancer screening is useless and unnecessary, I will respect her belief. However, I will also try to change her way of thinking by providing education. At this point she has an understanding of why screening is important, but she still has the freedom to make her own choice. In the end, I want to make sure the people I work with have the right tools to make an educated decision about their health behaviors.

Respect is another important part of my health education/promotion philosophy. I try very hard not to demean individuals regarding their current health behaviors. Working with a smoker, I might say, "I understand that quitting smoking is very difficult and at this time you may not be ready to quit. But when you are, here are some resources that can help." Instead of being forceful with my message, I try to be supportive of the person. If I demonstrate an understanding of the difficulty of making a behavior change, I believe the individual will

**Box 3.1 Practitioner's Perspective**    Continued

be more likely to respect me and more likely to listen to my message.

**Recommendations for those preparing to be health education specialists:** I think it is important to ask yourself why you want to be a health education specialist. Whatever the reasons may

be, these will ultimately determine your philosophy of health education/promotion. Understanding yourself and what drives you will make it easier for you to help others and become a successful health education specialist.

## Impacting the Delivery of Health Education/Promotion

This section uses scenarios to help focus on the methods health education specialists might use, depending on their philosophical stance. The decision to use any philosophy involves understanding and accepting the foundation that helped create the philosophy in the first place. To this end, Welle, Russell, and Kittleson (1995) state,

> Health educators must remember that every single educational choice carries with it a philosophical principle or belief. Educational choices carry important philosophical assumptions about the purpose of health education, the teacher, and also the learner. Thus, health educators should take the time necessary for individual philosophical inquiry, in order to be able to clearly articulate what principles guide them professionally. . . . Different settings may produce the need for different philosophies. Every health educator should be aware of which elements of their individual philosophies they are willing to compromise. (p. 331)

At the outset, it is important to remember that one of the overriding goals of any health education/promotion intervention is the betterment of health for the person or the group involved. All of the philosophies have that goal. They differ, however, in how to approach that objective.

Consider the case of Amarosa, a forty-year-old mother of two, who smokes, does not exercise regularly, and has a family history of heart disease. Amarosa is enrolled in a required health education course at a local university. She is going back to school to become an elementary school teacher. Because a health appraisal is a required part of the class, she has come in to visit the health education office. Three health education specialists (Felipe, Nokomis, and Li Ming) are employed in the center. Each one has a different philosophy of health education/promotion. How will their approaches differ? Here is a possible intervention scenario.

Felipe has adopted the philosophy of behavior change. As a proponent of this approach, he believes that all people are capable of adapting their health behavior if they can be shown the steps to success. He would use a behavior change contract method to get Amarosa to try to eliminate one or two of her negative health behaviors. As a part of this process, some preliminary analysis would be done in an attempt to identify the triggers that cause her to practice the negative health behaviors. He would help her identify short-term and long-term goals. Together they would establish objectives to reach those goals, and strategies to reach the objectives. He would also try to ensure that she receives some appropriate reward for every objective and goal she accomplishes.

Nokomis, on the other hand, is an advocate of the health education/promotion philosophy known as decision making. This means that she believes in equipping her clients with problem-solving and coping skills, so that they make the best possible health choices. Initially, she might sit down with Amarosa and hypothesize some situations that would necessitate Amarosa thinking through the rationale behind the negative health behaviors she practices. Nokomis also would most likely try to encourage Amarosa to see that some of her behaviors affect more people than just herself. The main goal is to move Amarosa to a point where she admits that some of her health behaviors need to be changed and to help her identify the reasons that changing them would make her life better.

Finally, Li Ming advocates a freeing/functioning philosophy of health education/promotion. She feels that, too often, health education specialists fail to find out the needs and desires of the client. They simply "barge in" and either overtly or covertly blame the client for any negative health behaviors. Li Ming would advocate change only if the behavior were infringing on the rights of others. In the beginning, Li Ming would confer with Amarosa and find out "how her life was going." She would ask Amarosa to identify any behaviors she wanted to change, making certain that Amarosa had all of the information necessary to make an informed decision. Although Li Ming might believe that Amarosa should stop smoking and start exercising, she would help Amarosa change only those behaviors Amarosa wanted to change.

One sidelight needs to be mentioned at this time. The fact that Amarosa was required to take a health education course in her teacher preparation program and that the instructor required a health assessment illustrates at a microlevel the social change philosophy at work. If health were not a state requirement (legislation) in the first place, she might not have considered changing any of her negative health behaviors.

Amarosa's situation demonstrates a point made earlier—in practice, there often is a natural mixing of some of the philosophies. For example, all of the approaches mentioned used portions of the cognitive-based health education/promotion philosophy. To reiterate, this philosophy is based on the premise that persons need to be provided with the most current information that impacts their health behaviors, and the acquisition of that information should create a dissonance and cause change.

The fifth philosophy, social change, is probably not as well suited to addressing the health behaviors of individuals one on one. Proponents stress changes in social, economic, and political arenas to impact the health of populations. Of course, populations are made up of individuals, so changing the environment of an inner-city neighborhood to be healthier (for example, creating jobs, assuring adequate and safe housing and safe schools, providing health care coverage for all) ultimately impacts the health of people at the individual level as well.

## SUMMARY

The term *philosophy* means a statement summarizing the attitudes, principles, beliefs, and concepts held by an individual or a group. Forming both a personal and an occupational philosophy requires reflection and the ability to identify the factors, principles, ideals, and influences that help shape your reality. The decision to use any philosophy involves understanding and accepting the foundation that helped create the philosophy in the first place. A sound philosophical foundation serves as a guidepost for many of the major decisions in life.

The five predominant philosophies of health education/promotion that were identified in the chapter are (1) behavior change, (2) cognitive based, (3) decision making, (4) freeing/functioning, and (5) social change. Health education specialists might disagree on which philosophy works best. They might even use an eclectic or multidimensional philosophical approach, depending on the setting or situation. However, it is important to remember that one of the overriding goals of any health education/promotion intervention is the betterment of health for the person or group involved. All of the philosophies have that goal. They simply differ in how to attain it.

## REVIEW QUESTIONS

1. Define each of the following and explain their relationship to one another.
   - Philosophy
   - Wellness
   - Holistic
   - Symmetry
2. Why is it important to have a personal philosophy about life?
3. Compare and contrast the value of having a personal life philosophy and an occupational life philosophy that are similar.
4. Define and explain the differences between:
   - A behavior change philosophy and a cognitive-based philosophy
   - A decision-making philosophy and a social change philosophy
   - A freeing/functioning philosophy and an eclectic health education/promotion philosophy
5. Explain how a person might use each of the five major health education/promotion philosophies and the eclectic philosophy to address a societal problem that can be addressed by health education/promotion (e.g., smoking, seat belt use, air pollution, exercise, diet, medication compliance, cancer risk reduction).

## CASE STUDY

You are entering the final semester of your senior year of study with a major in public health education. The health education/ promotion program at your university requires seniors in their last semester to intern a minimum of 25 hours per week at a state or nonprofit agency. For this capstone experience, you have been assigned to the mayor's office in a medium-size city near the campus.

During an orientation on the first day, you overhear that one of the tasks you will be assigned will involve meeting with the leaders of several community groups with the goal of creating smoke-free public parks in the city. The smoke-free park concept represents one of the mayor's main objectives in her second term in office. You also hear that the mayor is very excited to have a health education student intern since she greatly respects the skills that a health education specialist possesses.

The second day you have the opportunity to meet with the mayor, and, in fact, she does introduce to you the idea of a smoke-free public park system. During this meeting you discover that she is quite knowledgeable about the negative health effects of second- and third-hand smoke in part because her son, a lifetime nonsmoker who worked in a pub in town (smoking was allowed in pubs), died last year from lung cancer at the age of 36. At the close of the meeting, the mayor asks you to submit to her your philosophy of health education/promotion so that she can see what approach you might take with the community groups.

Using the model outlined in this chapter, write out your health education/promotion philosophy. Based on your philosophy statement and given the project that you will be assigned, is the mayor's office a good place for you to intern in order to hone your skills? Why or why not?

## CRITICAL THINKING QUESTIONS

1. Of the five basic health education/promotion philosophies identified by Welle, Russell, and Kittleson (1995), why do you think that the least favorite among health education specialists was the cognitive philosophy? Why do you think decision making was viewed as most popular?

2. What is the purpose of health education/promotion? How might the formulation of a purpose statement be reflected in your philosophy of health education/promotion?

3. You have been hired by a local pharmacy to provide health education/promotion services to customers and employees. Shortly after you begin work, however, you discover that much of your job is marketing nutritional supplements and nonpharmaceutical health-related services provided by the pharmacy and not the health education/promotion you had envisioned. How might this apparent conflict of interest have been avoided?

4. Suppose that you are a proponent of the social change health education/promotion philosophy. What advantage does this philosophy have for the health education specialist that might be a disadvantage for the consumer of health services and education? Defend your answer.

5. An article by Bruess (2003) in the *American Journal of Health Education* discusses the notion of "role modeling" for health education specialists. (The reference for the article can be found at the end of this chapter.) After reading the article, summarize Dr. Bruess' main points, and use your answer to determine which philosophical viewpoint(s) a health education specialist must hold to feel as Dr. Bruess does on the issue of role modeling. Finally, assess how you feel about the issue. Do you agree or disagree with him? Provide a rationale for your answer.

## ACTIVITIES

1. Take a survey of your classmates to assess what predominant health education/promotion philosophy each of them might employ. Compare the results with those from the study by Welle, Russell, and Kittleson (1995) described in this chapter. What were the reasons for any differences? Similarities?

2. After reexamining the philosophies of health, write a paragraph that could be used to explain your philosophy of health to a friend or colleague.

3. Interview a school or community health educator in your city. Ask what his or her philosophy of health education/promotion is. Then ask about the influences that helped the educator form his or her philosophy. Summarize the interview in a one-page paper.

4. Use any three of the five philosophical approaches to health education/promotion discussed in the chapter and address the following situation: In the past week in your community, two teenagers have been killed in separate incidents while riding bicycles. In neither case was the teenager wearing a helmet. A local citizens group has asked you and two of your health education specialist colleagues to attend a meeting concerning what to do about this issue.

## WEBLINKS

1. http://www.uwlax.edu/sah/hehp/ug_che/html/description.htm

   Mission statement of the Department of Health Education and Health Promotion program at the University of Wisconsin, La Crosse (retrieved August 10, 2010).

   The site provides a fine example of a mission/philosophy statement for health education and health promotion based on the seven responsibilities of community health educators.

2. http://www.aahperd.org/aahe/advocacy/positionStatements/upload/Philosophy-2009-2.pdf

   American Association of Health Education Philosophy Statement (retrieved August 12, 2010).

   This site provides a working model of a health education philosophy statement from one of the world's leading health education organizations.

3. http://www.ux1.eiu.edu/~jcdietz/HST%203700/3700%20Philosophy%20of%20Health%20Education%20Statement.doc.

   Weblink to the community health education philosophy assignment from Dr Julie Dietz of Eastern Illinois University detailing some key areas to be included and thought questions to be considered in crafting a philosophy statement (retrieved August 12, 2010). This is an excellent resource.

## REFERENCES

Allegrante, J. P. (2006). Commentary: In search of the new ethics for health promotion. *Health Education and Behavior, 33* (3), 305–307.

Balog, J. E. (2005). The meaning of health. *American Journal of Health Education, 36* (5), 266–271.

Bensley, L. B. (1993). This I believe: A philosophy of health education. *The Eta Sigma Gamma Monograph Series, 11* (2), 1–7.

Bruess, C. E. (2003). This I believe: A philosophy of health education. *American Journal of Health Education, 34* (4), 237–239.

Buchanan, D. R. (2006). Perspective: A new ethic for health promotion: Reflections on a philosophy of health education for the 21st century. *Health Education and Behavior, 33* (3), 290–304.

Butler, J. T. (1997). *The principles and practices of health education and health promotion.* Englewood, CO: Morton.

Donatelle, R. J. (2011). *Health: The basics, green edition.* San Francisco, CA: Pearson Education. .

Edlin, G., & Golanty, E. (2004). *Health and wellness* (8th ed.). Sudbury, MA: Jones and Bartlett.

Governali, J. F., Hodges, B. C., & Videto, D. M. (2005). *American Journal of Health Education, 36* (4), 210–214.

Greenberg, J. S. (1978). Health education as freeing. *Health Education, 9* (2), 20–21.

Greenberg, J. S. (1992). *Health education: Learner centered instructional strategies* (2nd ed.). Dubuque, IA: William C. Brown.

Hales, D. (2004). *An invitation to health* (3rd ed.). Belmont, CA: Thomson-Wadsworth.

Hamburg, M. V. (1993). Would I do it all over! *The Eta Sigma Gamma Monograph Series, 11* (2), 67–74.

Kamkwamba, W., & Mealer, B. (2009). *The boy who harnessed the wind.* New York, NY: Harper-Collins.

Oberteufer, D. (1953). Philosophy and principles of school health education. *Journal of School Health, 23* (4), 103–109.

Pruitt, B. E. (2007). Paper presented for the annual American Association for Health Education Scholar Address, March 16, Baltimore, MD.

Rash, J. K. (1985). Philosophical bases for health education. *Health Education, 16* (3), 48–49.

Seffrin, J. R. (1993). Health education and the pursuit of personal freedom. *The Eta Sigma Gamma Monograph Series, 11* (2), 109–118.

Smith, B. J. (2010). Connecting a personal philosophy of health to the practice of health education. In Black, J. M., Furney, S., Graf, H. M., & Nolte, A. E., *Philosophical foundations of health education* (pp. 49–54), San Francisco, CA: Jossey-Bass.

Tamayose, T. S., et al. (2004). Important issues when choosing a career in public health. *Californian Journal of Health Promotion, 2* (1), 65–73.

Thomas, S. B. (1984). The holistic philosophy and perspective of selected health educators. *Health Education, 15* (1), 15–20.

Welle, H. M., Russell, R. D., & Kittleson, M. J. (1995). Philosophical trends in health education: Implications for the 21st century. *Journal of Health Education, 26* (6), 326–333.

# Theories and Planning Models

After reading this chapter and answering the questions at the end, you should be able to:

- Define and explain the difference among *theory, concept, construct, variable*, and *model*.
- Explain the importance of theory to health education/promotion.
- Explain what is meant by behavior change theories and planning models.
- Describe how the concept of socio-ecological approach applies to using theories.
- Explain the difference between continuum theories and stage theories.
- Identify and briefly explain the behavior change theories, and their components, used in health education/promotion:
  - Health Belief Model
  - Theory of Planned Behavior
  - Elaboration Likelihood Model of Persuasion
  - Information-Motivation-Behavioral Skills Model
  - Transtheoretical Model
  - Precaution Adoption Process Model
  - Health Action Process Approach
  - Social Cognitive Theory
  - Social Network Theory
  - Social Capital Theory
  - Diffusion Theory
  - Community Readiness Model
- Identify and briefly explain the planning models, and their components, used in health education/promotion:
  - PRECEDE-PROCEED
  - Multilevel Approach To Community Health (MATCH)
  - Intervention Mapping

- ◆ CDCynergy
- ◆ Social Marketing Assessment and Response Tool (SMART)
- ◆ Mobilizing for Action through Planning and Partnerships (MAPP)
- ◆ Generalized Model for Program Planning (GMPP)

As noted in Chapter 1, the profession of health education/promotion evolved from other biological, behavioral, psychological, sociological, and health science disciplines. As this profession has grown, so has the number of theories and models used by health education specialists in their work. This chapter introduces the terms *theory*, *concept*, *construct*, *variable*, and *model*. It explains why theory is used in health education/promotion. It also presents an overview of theories that focus on behavior change, as well as the models associated with program planning. However, space does not permit comprehensive coverage of all theories and models used by health education specialists. For example, theories and models associated with implementation and evaluation processes are not covered in this chapter.

Because theories and models are dynamic, they change and evolve (Crosby, Kegler, & DiClemente, 2009). As a result, you will continually deal with both revised and new theories and models. Future courses and their books will likely expose you to more complete coverage of health education/promotion's theoretical base (e.g., DiClemente, Crosby, & Kegler, 2009; Edberg, 2007; Glanz, Rimer, & Viswanath, 2008a; Goodson, 2010; Green & Kreuter, 2005; Hayden, 2009; IOM, 2001; Sharma & Romas, 2012).

## Definitions

In order to understand the theoretical foundations presented in this chapter, you must be familiar with some key related terms. Let us begin with **theory.** One of the most frequently quoted definitions of this term was provided by Glanz, Lewis, and Viswanath (2008b), who modified an earlier definition by Kerlinger (1986). It states: "A *theory* is a set of interrelated concepts, definitions, and propositions that presents a *systematic* view of events or situations by specifying relations among variables in order to *explain* and *predict* the events of the situations" (p. 26). Stated a little differently, "a theory is a systematic arrangement of fundamental principles that provide a basis for explaining certain happenings of life" (McKenzie, Neiger, & Thackeray, 2009, p. 160). Thus, "the role of theory is to untangle and simplify for human comprehension the complexities of nature" (Green et al., 1994, p. 398).

As applied to the profession of health education/promotion, a theory is a general explanation of why people act, or do not act, to maintain and/or promote the health of themselves, their families, organizations, and communities. The primary elements of theories are known as **concepts** (Glanz et al., 2008b). When a concept has been developed, created, or adopted for use with a specific theory, it is referred to as a **construct** (Kerlinger, 1986). In other words, "the key concepts of a theory are its constructs" (Rimer & Glanz, 2005, p. 4). The operational form (practical use) of a construct is known as a **variable.** Variables "specify how a construct is to be measured in a specific situation" (Glanz et al., 2008b, p. 28).

A **model** "is a composite, a mixture of ideas or concepts taken from any number of theories and used together" (Hayden, 2009, p. 1). Stated a bit differently, "Models draw on a number of theories to help people understand a specific problem in a particular setting or context. They are not always as specific as theory" (Rimer & Glanz, 2005, p. 4). Models provide health education specialists with a framework for creating program plans. Unlike theories, models do "not attempt to explain the processes underlying learning, but only to represent them" (Chaplin & Krawiec, 1979, p. 68).

Consider how these terms are used in practical application. A personal belief is a *concept* related to various health behaviors. For example, people are more likely to behave in a healthy way—such as, exercise regularly—if they feel confident in their ability to actually engage in a healthy form of exercise. Such a concept is captured in a *construct* of the Social Cognitive Theory (SCT) called self-efficacy. (See the discussion of the SCT later in this chapter.) If health education specialists want to develop an intervention to assist people in exercising, the ability to measure the peoples' self-efficacy toward exercise will help create the intervention. The measurement may consist of a few questions that ask people to rate their confidence in their ability to exercise. This measurement, or operational form, of the self-efficacy construct is a *variable*. However, because of the complexity of getting a nonexerciser to become an exerciser, the health education specialist may need to use a *model*, composed of constructs from several theories, to plan the intervention.

In the health education/promotion profession, the adjective *theory-based* (as in theory-based planning, theory-based practice, or theory-based research) commonly refers to both theories and models. In fact, some of the best known and often used theories use "model" in their title (e.g., Health Belief Model). Goodson (2010) explains why "model" and "theory" are used inconsistently. She indicates that when some models were created, they were properly titled as models. They were created using constructs from several theories to explain specific phenomena. They had little empirical testing to prove their worth. Over time, these models were tested and refined, gaining theory status. Goodson (2010) concludes, "because we tend to borrow the theories we employ from other disciplines and fields and because our concern usually centers in applying these theories (or models) to practice or research, it seems to matter little to us whether we deal with theories or with models; it seems to matter even less what labels we attach to them" (p. 228).

## The Importance of Using Theory in Health Education/Promotion

Using theory is important in all professions, not just in health education/promotion. "It provides direction and organizes knowledge into a pattern so that facts, information, data, observed activities, and learnings are interconnected in a manner which takes on meaning that would not exist in isolation. Thus interconnected learnings provide the basis, foundation, reason, and direction for process activities and research endeavors" (Timmreck, Cole, James, & Butterworth, 2010, p. 75).

Theory helps health education specialists plan, implement, and evaluate programs. More specifically, it: (1) indicates reasons why people are not behaving in healthy ways, (2) identifies information needed before developing an intervention, (3) provides a conceptual framework for selecting constructs to develop the intervention, (4) gives insights into how best to deliver the intervention, and (5) identifies measurements needed to evaluate the intervention's impact (Crosby, Kegler, & DiClemente, 2009; Glanz et al.,

2008b). Theory also "provides a useful reference point to help keep research and implementation activities clearly focused" (Crosby et al., 2009, p. 11), and it infuses ethics and social justice into practice (Goodson, 2010). In addition, "using theory as a foundation for program planning and development is consistent with the current emphasis on using evidence-based interventions in public health, behavioral medicine, and medicine" (Rimer & Glanz, 2005, p. 5).

In the rest of this chapter, some of the theories and models used by health education specialists are presented in two main groups. The first group contains theories that focus on behavior change. Through their constructs, these theories help explain how change might take place. The second group contains planning models, which give structure and organization to the program planning process. These models provide health education specialists with step-by-step procedures, "integrating multiple theories to explain and address health problems," (Rimer & Glanz, 2005, p. 36) as they plan, implement, and evaluate health education/promotion programs.

## Behavior Change Theories

Health education specialists can use multiple theories to design interventions to encourage behavior change. Each theory works better in some situations than in others, depending on which level of influence is used to plan a health education/promotion program.

"Levels of influence" are at the heart of the **socio-ecological approach** (also called the ecological perspective). This multilevel, interactive approach examines how physical, social, political, economic, and cultural dimensions influence behaviors and conditions. The socio-ecological approach "emphasizes the interaction between, and the interdependence of factors within and across all levels of a health problem" (Rimer & Glanz, 2005, p. 10). In other words, changes in health behavior do not take place in a vacuum. "Individuals influence and are influenced by their families, social networks, the organizations in which they participate (workplaces, schools, religious organizations), the communities of which they are a part, and the society in which they live" (IOM, 2001, p. 26).

As noted in Chapter 1, McLeroy, Bibeau, Steckler, and Glanz (1988) identified five levels of influence: (1) intrapersonal or individual factors, (2) interpersonal factors, (3) institutional or organizational factors, (4) community factors, and (5) public policy factors. **Table 4.1** lists and defines each of the five levels. **Figure 4.1**, created by Eng (1997), provides a visual representation of the socio-ecological framework. By examining a health problem using this multilevel approach health education specialists can get a better understanding of how to "attack" the problem.

Consider how the levels of influence can be applied to cigarette smoking in the United States. At the *intrapersonal* (or *individual*) *level*, a large majority of smokers know that smoking is bad for them, and a slightly smaller majority have indicated they would like to quit. Many have tried to quit—some have tried on many occasions. At the *interpersonal level*, many smokers are encouraged to quit by those in their social networks, such as their physician and/or family and friends. Some smokers may attempt to quit on their own, or they may join a formal smoking cessation group.

At the *institutional* (or *organizational*) *level*, institutions, such as churches and businesses, often have policies that regulate smoking. These institutions may offer smoking cessation classes or support groups to assist those who "belong" to the organization, to quit smoking. At the *community level,* some towns, cities, and counties have ordinances

**Table 4.1**   An ecological perspective: levels of influence

| Concept | Definition |
| --- | --- |
| Intrapersonal Level | Individual characteristics that influence behavior, such as knowledge, attitudes, beliefs, and personality traits |
| Interpersonal Level | Interpersonal processes and primary groups, including family, friends, and peers that provide social identity, support, and role definition |
| Community Level | |
|   Institutional Factors | Rules, regulations, policies, and informal structures, which may constrain or promote recommended behaviors |
|   Community Factors | Social networks and norms, or standards, which exist as formal or informal among individuals, groups, and organizations |
|   Public Policy | Local, state, and federal policies and laws that regulate or support healthy actions and practices for disease prevention, early detection, control, and management |

*Source:* Rimer, B. K. & Glanz, K. (2005). *Theory at a Glance: A Guide for Health Promotion Practice,* 2nd ed. (NIH Pub. No. 05-3896). Washington, DC: National Cancer Institute.

that prohibit smoking in public places. At the *public policy or population level,* many states have higher cigarette taxes and/or laws that limit smoking. Also at this level, the federal government spends many dollars for public service announcements (PSAs) and other forms of media advertising the dangers of tobacco use.

In addition to the levels shown in Figure 4.1, there are four terms in bold print: *theory, practice, environments,* and *research.* Eng (1997) noted that for a socio-ecological approach to be successful, the theory must be put into practice in multiple environments where research can be conducted to determine its effectiveness.

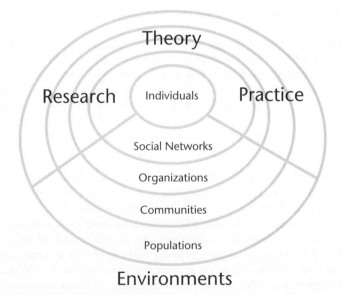

**Figure 4.1** Socio-ecological framework

*Source:* From Eng, E. "Room with a View for a Change." Keynote address to the 1997 Annual Meeting of the Society for Public Health Education, Indianapolis, IN. Used by permission of the author.

The following sections describe some of the theories and models that focus on behavior change. These theories/models are grouped according to the levels of influence where they may be most effective. The last three levels—institutional, community, and public policy factors—are combined into a single "community" level. This modification of the socio-ecological approach was used by Glanz and Rimer (1995).

## Intrapersonal (Individual) Theories

Intrapersonal theories focus on factors within individuals such as knowledge, attitudes, beliefs, self-concept, developmental history, past experiences, motivation, skills, and behavior (Rimer & Glanz, 2005). Several of the theories used by health education specialists to develop interventions at the intrapersonal level are the Health Belief Model (HBM), the Theory of Planned Behavior (TPB), the Elaboration Likelihood Model of Persuasion (ELM), the Information-Motivation-Behavioral Skills Model (IMB), the Transtheoretical Model (TTM), the Precaution Adoption Process Model (PAPM), and the Health Action Process Approach (HAPA).

Although all of the theories listed above fall into the intrapersonal theories category, they can be divided further into continuum theories or stage theories. A **continuum theory** identifies variables that influence actions (i.e., beliefs, attitudes), and combines those variables into a single equation that predicts the likelihood of action (Weinstein, Rothman, & Sutton, 1998; Weinstein, Sandman, & Blalock, 2008). These theories "acknowledge *quantitative* differences among people in their positions on different variables" (Weinstein et al., 2008, p. 122) and "thus, each person is placed along a continuum of action likelihood" (Weinstein et al., 1998, p. 291). The HBM (Rosenstock, 1966), TPB (Ajzen, 2006), ELM (Petty & Cacioppo, 1986), and IMB (Fisher & Fisher, 1992) are examples of continuum theories that are appropriate for use at the intrapersonal level.

A **stage theory** consists of an ordered set of categories into which people can be classified. It identifies factors that could induce movement from one category to the next (Weinstein & Sandman, 2002). More specifically, stage theories have four principal elements: (1) a category system to define the stages, (2) an ordering of stages, (3) barriers to change that are common to people in the same stage, and (4) different barriers to change, facing people in different stages (Weinstein et al., 1998). Advocates of stage theories "claim that there are *qualitative* differences among people and question whether changes in health behaviors can be described by a single prediction equation" (Weinstein et al., 2008, pp. 124–125). Some of the most commonly reported stage theories are the TTM (Prochaska, 1979; Prochaska & DiClemente, 1983), PAPM (Weinstein, 1988; Weinstein et al., 1998), and HAPA (Schwarzer, 2001).

**Health Belief Model (HBM)**    The Health Belief Model (HBM) was developed in the 1950s by a group of psychologists to help explain why people would or would not use health services (Rosenstock, 1966). The HBM "addresses the individual's perceptions of the threat posed by a health problem (susceptibility, severity), the benefits of avoiding the threat, and factors influencing the decision to act (barriers, cues to action, and self-efficacy)" (Rimer & Glanz, 2005, p. 12). As you read the following example of why a person may or may not do self-screening for cancer, refer to the graphic representation of the HBM in **Figure 4.2**.

Suppose a person sees an advertisement about self-screening for cancer, while reading a weekly news magazine. This is a **cue to action** that gets the person thinking about his possibility of getting cancer (see **Figure 4.3**). There may be some variables (demographic, sociopsychological, and structural) that cause the person to think

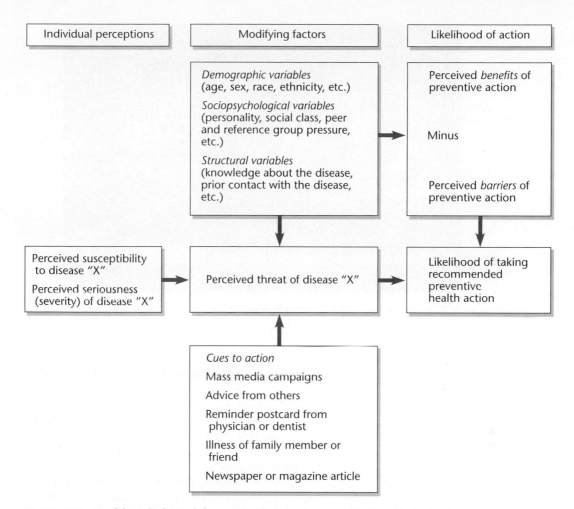

**Figure 4.2** Health Belief Model as a predictor of preventive health behavior

*Source:* Becker, M.H. et al., from "A New Approach to Explaining Sick-Role Behavior in Low Income Populations," *American Journal of Public Health* 64, March 1974: 205–216, Fig 1. Used by permission of Sheridan Press.

about it a little more. The person remembers his college health course, which included information about self-screenings and cancer. This person knows he is at a higher than normal risk for cancer because of family history, age, and less than desirable health behavior. Therefore, he comes to the conclusion that he is susceptible to cancer (**perceived susceptibility**). The person also believes that, if he develops cancer, it can be very serious (**perceived seriousness/severity**).

Based on these factors, the person thinks that there is reason to be concerned about cancer (**perceived threat**). This person knows that self-screening can help detect cancer earlier and thus reduce the severity (**perceived benefits**). But self-screening takes time, and this person does not always remember to do it (**perceived barriers**). He must now analyze the difference between the benefits of self-screening and the barriers to self-screening (**reduction of threat**). For this person, the **likelihood of taking action**

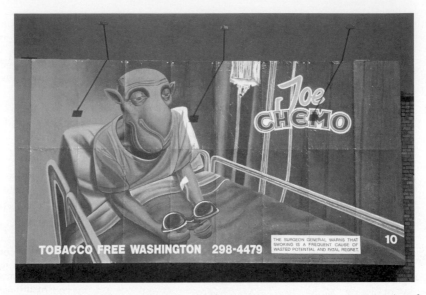

**Figure 4.3** A single billboard along a highway can serve as a cue to action for many people.
(Kevin Schafer/Photo Library)

(self-screening) will be determined by weighing the perceived threat against the reduction of threat.

When the HBM was first conceived, **self-efficacy** (confidence in one's own ability to perform a certain task or function) was not part of the model. However, because evidence showed self-efficacy was a meaningful concept in the perceived barriers construct, it was recommended that self-efficacy be added to the HBM (Rosenstock, Strecher, & Becker, 1988). "For behavior change to succeed, people must (as the original HBM theorizes) feel threatened by their current behavioral patterns (perceived susceptibility and severity) and believe that change of a specific kind will result in a valued outcome at an acceptable cost (perceived benefit). They also must feel themselves competent (self-efficacious) to overcome perceived barriers to take action" (Champion & Skinner, 2008, p. 50).

**Theory of Planned Behavior (TPB)**    The Theory of Planned Behavior (TPB) (see **Figure 4.4**) is an extension of the Theory of Reasoned Action (Fishbein & Ajzen, 1975). According to the TPB, individuals' intention to perform a given behavior is a function of their attitude toward performing the behavior, their beliefs about what relevant others think they should do, and their perception of the ease or difficulty of performing the behavior. **Intention** "is an indication of a person's readiness to perform a given behavior, and it is considered to be the immediate antecedent of behavior" (Ajzen, 2006). Unlike the Theory of Reasoned Action, the TPB was developed to explain not just health behavior but all volitional behaviors ("behaviors that can be performed at will" [Luszczynski & Sutton, 2005, p. 73]). Using the example of the use of spit tobacco as a behavior not fully under volitional control, the TPB predicts that people intend to give up its use if they

- have a positive attitude toward quitting (**attitude toward the behavior**),
- think that others whom they value believe it would be good for them to quit (**subjective norm**) (see **Figure 4.5**),

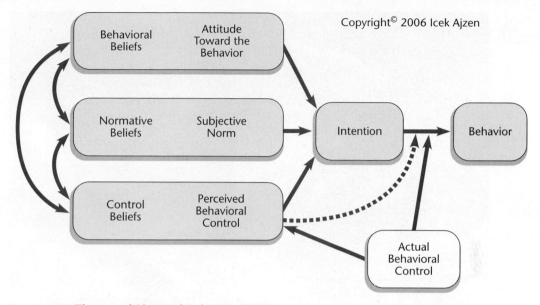

**Figure 4.4** Theory of Planned Behavior (TPB)

*Source:* "Theory of Planned Behavior Diagram" (TPB Diagram) by Dr. Icek Ajzen, http://www.people.umass.edu/aizen/tpb.diag. html. Reprinted by permission.

- perceive that they have control over whether or not they quit (**perceived behavioral control**), and

- have the skills, resources, and other prerequisites needed to quit (**actual behavioral control**).

**Elaboration Likelihood Model of Persuasion (ELM)**   The Elaboration Likelihood Model of Persuasion, or the Elaboration Likelihood Model (ELM) for short, was initially developed to help explain inconsistencies in research results from the study of attitudes (Petty, Barden, & Wheeler, 2009). Specifically, the ELM was designed to help explain how persuasion messages (communication), aimed at changing attitudes, are received and processed by people. Though not created specifically for health communication, the ELM has been used to interpret and predict the impact of health messages.

The ELM does three things. First, it proposes that attitudes can be formed via two different types of routes to persuasion: peripheral routes and central routes (Petty et al., 2009). The distinction between the two routes is the amount of elaboration. **Elaboration** refers to the amount of cognitive processing (i.e., thought) that a person puts into receiving messages. Peripheral route processing involves minimal thought and relies on superficial cues or mental shortcuts (called *heuristics*) about issue-relevant information, as the primary means for attitude change (Petty et al., 2009). For example, people may form an attitude after hearing a persuasive message simply because the person delivering the message is someone they admire.

On the other hand, central route processing involves thoughtful consideration (or effortful cognitive elaboration) of issue-relevant information and one's own cognitive responses as the primary bases for attitude change: "Two conditions are necessary for effortful processing to occur—the recipient of the message must be both *motivated* and

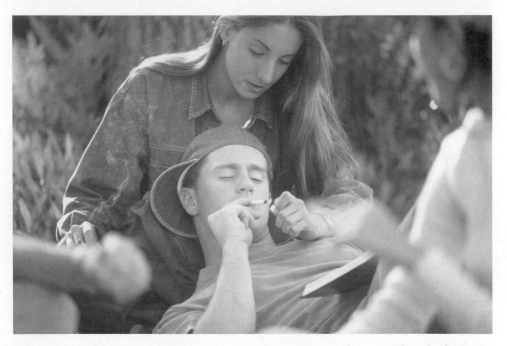

**Figure 4.5** Subjective norm is an important construct to be considered when planning programs for adolescents and young adults.

(Tom & DeeAnn McCarthy/The Stock Market)

*able* to think carefully" (Petty et al., 2009, p. 188). An example of central route processing is a motorcyclist's formation of an attitude about wearing a helmet. Processing is based on thoughtful consideration of a message about the pros/cons of helmet use, recalling knowledge learned in a motorcycle safety class, and possibly the outcomes of a motorcycle crash in which a relative was involved.

Second, when using the ELM, the results of the two routes can be similar. However, the two routes usually lead to attitudes with different consequences. "High effort central route processes are more likely to lead to attitudes that are persistent over time, resistant to counterattack, and influential in guiding thought and behavior than are peripheral processes" (Petty et al., 2009, pp. 207–208).

Third, "the model specifies how variables have an impact on persuasion" (Petty et al., 2009, p. 197). The variable can have an influence on people's motivation to think or ability to think, as well as the valence of people's thought or the confidence in the thoughts generated (Petty et al., 2009). For example, variables that have an impact on how a message is processed include the source of the message (e.g., friend, expert), the message itself (e.g., funny, serious), the context (e.g., delivered person-to-person, on the Internet), and various characteristics of the recipient (e.g., intelligence, age, attentiveness).

Keeping in mind these three things that the ELM provides, health education specialists can create health messages that are more meaningful to a priority population, and in turn, can be more successful in reaching program goals. **Figure 4.6** provides a diagram of the ELM as presented by Petty and colleagues (2009).

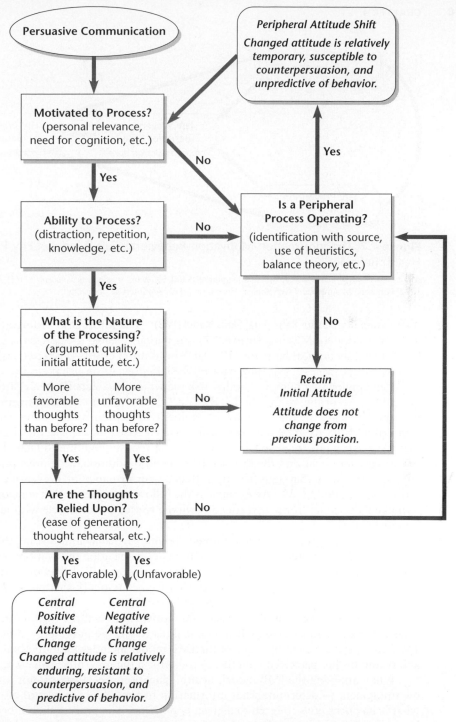

**Figure 4.6** The Elaboration Likelihood Model of Persuasion (ELM)

*Source:* From Petty, R.E., Barden J., & Wheeler, S.C., "The Elaboration Likelihood Model of Persuasion: Developing Health Promotions for Sustained Behavioral Change" in *Emerging Theories in Health Promotion Practice and Research*, 2nd ed., DiClemente, R.J., Crosby, R.A., & Kegler, M. (Eds.), p. 196. Copyright © 2009 John Wiley & Sons, Inc. Reproduced with permission of John Wiley & Sons, Inc.

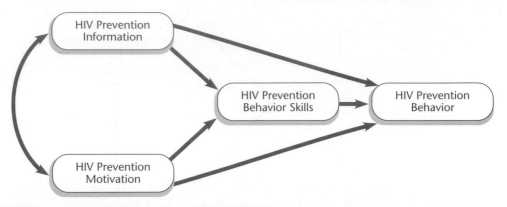

**Figure 4.7** The Information-Motivation-Behavioral Skills Model of HIV Prevention Health Behavior

*Source:* From Fisher, J.D. & Fisher, W.A., "Changing AIDS Risk Behavior," *Psychological Bulletin 111*(3), 455–474, 1992. Published by American Psychological Association (APA). Reprinted by permission.

**Information-Motivation-Behavioral Skills Model (IMB)**    The Information-Motivation-Behavioral Skills Model (IMB) (see **Figure 4.7**) was initially created to address the critical need for a strong theoretical basis for HIV/AIDS prevention efforts (Fisher & Fisher, 1992). Because of its success in dealing with HIV/AIDS prevention behavior, the IMB model has been applied to a number of other risk reduction behaviors (Fisher, Fisher, and Shuper, 2009). According to this model, the constructs of information, motivation, and behavioral skills are the fundamental determinants of preventive behavior. The information provided needs to be relevant, easily enacted based on the specific circumstances, and serve as a guide to personal preventive behavior. "In addition to facts that are easy to translate into behavior, the IMB model recognizes additional cognitive processes and content categories that significantly influence performance of preventive behavior" (Fisher et al., 2009, p. 27). An example is the following guideline that someone may use to make a decision: "If my best friend is willing to ride a motorcycle without a helmet, it must be okay."

Even though people are well informed about a particular health issue, they may not be motivated to act. According to the IMB model, prevention motivation includes both personal motivation to act (i.e., one's attitude toward a specific behavior) and social motivation to act (social support for the preventive behavior) (Fisher et al., 2009). Both types of motivation are necessary to act.

In addition to being well informed and motivated to act, the IMB model also indicates that people must possess behavioral skills to engage in the preventive behavior. The behavioral skills component of the IMB model includes an individual's objective ability and his/her perceived self-efficacy to perform the preventive behavior.

When applying the IMB model, health education specialists cannot just use their own judgment to determine what information to provide, how best to motivate, and what behavioral skills to teach to a given population. The process should begin by eliciting information from a subsample of the priority population to identify deficits in their health-relevant information, motivation, and behavioral skills. Next, health education specialists need to design and implement "*conceptually-based, empirically-targeted, population-specific*" (p. 29) interventions, constructed on the bases of the elicited findings

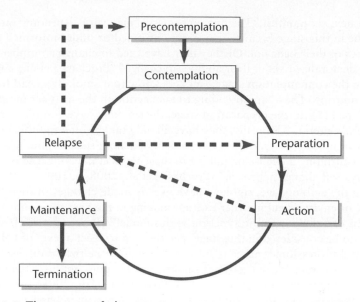

**Figure 4.8** The stages of change

*Source:* From Goldstein et al., "Models for Provider-Patient Interaction: Application to Health Behavior Change," in *The Handbook of Health Behavior Change,* 2nd ed., S.A. Shumaker et al. (Eds.), p. 98. Copyright © 1998 by Springer Publishing Company, Inc. Reproduced with permission of Springer Publishing Company, Inc. and by permission of the author.

(Fisher et al., 2009). Then, after the implementation of the intervention, health education specialists must evaluate the intervention to determine if it had significant and sustained effects on the information, motivation, and behavioral skill determinants of the preventive behavior and on the preventive behavior itself (Fisher et al., 2009).

**Transtheoretical Model (TTM)**    "The Transtheoretical Model is an integrative framework for understanding how individuals and populations progress toward adopting and maintaining health behavior change for optimal health. The Transtheoretical Model uses stages of change to integrate processes and principles of change from across major theories of intervention, hence the name 'Transtheoretical'" (Prochaska, Johnson, & Lee, 1998, p. 59). The core constructs of TTM include the stages of change, the processes of change, the pros and cons of changing, and self-efficacy.

Although each TTM construct is important, this model is best known for its stages of change. (See **Figure 4.8**.) TTM suggests that "people move from *precontemplation,* not intending to change, to *contemplation,* intending to change within 6 months, to *preparation,* actively planning change, to *action,* overtly making changes, and into *maintenance,* taking steps to sustain change and resist temptation to relapse" (Prochaska, Redding, Harlow, Rossi, & Velicer, 1994, p. 473).

TTM was first used in psychotherapy. It was developed by Prochaska (1979) after he completed a comparative analysis of various therapy systems and many therapy studies. Since then, program planners have used TTM with a wide variety of topics ranging from alcohol abuse to weight control (Prochaska, Redding, & Evers, 2008; Spencer, Adams, Malone, Roy, & Yost, 2006).

Following is an example of TTM's stage construct applied to smoking cessation. In the **precontemplation stage,** smokers are not seriously thinking about stopping smoking in the next six months. "The outcome interval may vary, depending on behavior. People may be in this stage because they are uninformed or under-informed about the consequences of their behavior. Or they may have tried to change a number of times and become demoralized about their abilities to change" (Prochaska et al., 2008, p. 100).

In the **contemplation stage,** smokers know that smoking is bad for them and consider quitting. They "are intending to take action in the next six months" (Prochaska, 2005, p. 111). In the **preparation stage,** the smokers have combined intention and behavioral criteria. "Typically, they have already taken some significant step toward the behavior in the past year. They have a plan of action, such as joining a health education class, consulting a counselor, talking to their physician, buying a self-help book, or relying on a self-change approach" (Prochaska et al., 2008, p. 100).

In the **action stage,** smokers have overtly made changes in their behavior, experiences, or environment in order to stop smoking in the past six months. "Not all modifications of behavior count as action in this model" (Prochaska et al., 2008, p. 100). In order to be considered in this stage, people need to meet a level of behavior that scientists and professionals agree is sufficient to reduce the risk of disease. In our example, reducing the number of cigarettes smoked per day does not meet the necessary level for action; only total abstinence qualifies (Prochaska et al., 2008). As the smokers make these changes, they are moving toward the next stage, maintenance.

The focus of the **maintenance stage** is to prevent relapse. Thus, individuals who have quit smoking are working not to smoke again. People in this stage have changed their problem behavior for at least six months and are increasingly more confident that they can continue their change (Prochaska et al., 1998; Redding, Rossi, Rossi, Velicer, & Prochaska, 1999). In other words, their change is more of a habit, and their chance of relapse is lower, but their new behavior still requires some attention (Redding et al., 1999).

The final stage is **termination.** This stage is defined as the time when individuals who made a change now have zero temptation to return to their old behavior. They have 100 percent self-efficacy (a lifetime of maintenance). In our example, smokers have become nonsmokers. No matter what their mood, they will not return to their old behavior (Prochaska et al., 2008). This is a stage that few people reach with certain behaviors (e.g., alcoholism).

**Precaution Adoption Process Model (PAPM)**   The Precaution Adoption Process Model (PAPM) "attempts to explain how a person comes to decisions to take action, and how he or she translates that decision into action" (Weinstein et al., 2008, p. 126). Although the Transtheoretical Model and the PAPM are both stage models that appear similar, they are applied quite differently. The PAPM is most applicable for the adoption of a new precaution (e.g., getting a mammogram or a hepatitis B vaccination), or the abandonment of a risky behavior that requires a deliberate action (e.g., not wearing a safety belt). It can also be used to explain why and how people make deliberate changes in habitual patterns (e.g., flossing one's teeth two times a day instead of one). The PAPM is not applicable for actions that require the gradual development of habitual patterns of behavior, such as exercise and diet (Weinstein et al., 2008).

In the following example, the seven stages of the PAPM (see **Figure 4.9**) are applied to participating in a medical screening program. In Stage 1, Unaware of Issue, people are totally unaware of the need to be screened. When people first learn something about the screening, they are no longer unaware, but they are not necessarily engaged by it, either. This is Stage 2, Unengaged.

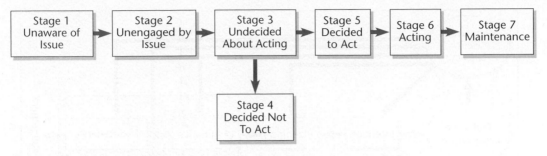

**Figure 4.9** Stages of the Precaution Adoption Process Model (PAPM)

*Source:* From Weinstin, N.D., Sandman, P.M., & Blalock, S.J., "The Precaution Adoption Process Model" in *Health Behavior and Health Education: Theory, Research, and Practice,* 4th ed., K. Glanz, B. K. Rimer, and K. Viswanath, (Eds.), p. 127. Copyright © 2008 John Wiley & Sons, Inc. Reproduced with permission of John Wiley & Sons, Inc.

In Stage 3, Undecided About Acting, people have become engaged in thinking about the screening, and they are considering participation. "This decision-making process can result in one of three outcomes: they may suspend judgment, remaining in Stage 3 for the moment; they may decide to take no action, moving to Stage 4 and halting the precaution adoption process, at least for the time being; or they may decide to adopt the precaution, moving to Stage 5" (Weinstein, et al., 2008, p. 126).

Once the people participate in the screening, they have initiated the behavior, and they are in Stage 6, Acting. Finally, if the people participate in the screening at the medically recommended intervals, they are in Stage 7, Maintenance. Note that this last stage of the PAPM is not applicable to some decision-making processes, for example, actions required only once in a lifetime, such as a vaccination that immunizes a person for life (Weinstein et al., 2008).

**Health Action Process Approach (HAPA)**   The Health Action Process Approach (HAPA) (Schwarzer, 2001) is another stage model that applies to all health-compromising and health-enhancing behaviors (Luszczynska & Sutton, 2005). Like the other stage theories discussed earlier in this chapter, this model provides a concise description of behavior change over time. The HAPA is divided into two distinct phases: motivation to change and self-regulatory processes. It also has five stages: (1) intention, (2) planning, (3) initiative, (4) maintenance, and (5) recovery (see **Figure 4.10**).

The *motivation to change phase* includes the preintentional processes that lead to the development of behavioral intention (Luszczynska & Sutton, 2005). These processes revolve around the interaction of the variables of risk perception, outcome expectancies, and perceived self-efficacy.

Although HAPA's motivation to change phase is important, this model emphasizes the *self-regulatory phase* that leads to actual health behavior. "The pursuit of a goal of behavior change can be subdivided into a sequence of activities, such as planning, initiation, maintenance, relapse management, and disengagement" (Schwarzer, 2001, p. 48). Planning deals with determining the when, where, and how a behavior takes place. Trying behavior change is one thing, but maintaining it takes a lot of work. Schwarzer (2001) states:

A health-related behavior is adopted and then maintained not through an act of will, but rather through the development of self-regulatory skills and strategies. In other

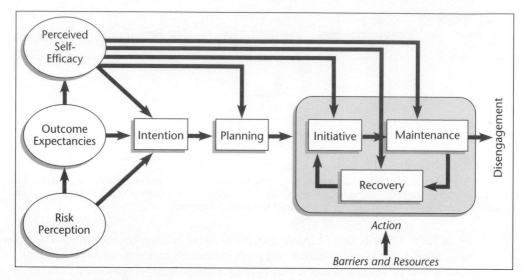

**Figure 4.10** The Health Action Process Approach

*Source:* From Schwarzer, R., "Social-Cognitive Factors in Changing Health Related Behaviors." *Current Directions in Psychological Science 10*(2), p. 50, Fig 1. Copyright © 2001 by Association for Psychological Science. Reprinted by permission of Sage Publications.

words, individuals embrace a variety of means to influence their own motivation and behaviors. For example, they set attainable sub-goals, create incentives for themselves, draw from an array of options for coping with difficulties, and mobilize support from other people. (p. 49)

Maintaining a behavior is difficult, and many people go back to their old, health-compromising ways. If they do not have the skills and strategies needed to deal with a relapse, they may completely disengage from the change. The real keys to the self-regulatory phase are the successful completion of the previous stage and the optimistic sense of control over the next one (Schwarzer, 2001).

## Interpersonal Theories

The category of interpersonal theories contains theories that "assume individuals exist within, and are influenced by, a social environment. The opinions, thoughts, behavior, advice, and support of the people surrounding an individual influence his or her feelings and behavior, and the individual has a reciprocal effect on those people" (Rimer & Glanz, 2005, p. 19). Research shows that social relationships can be a powerful influence on health and health behaviors (Heaney & Israel, 2008). As such, a number of theories have been created to explain concepts such as

- *Social learning*—learning that occurs in a social context
- *Social power*—ability to influence others or resist activities of others
- *Social integration*—structure and quality of relationships
- *Social networks*—"web of social relationships that surround individuals" (Heaney & Israel, 2008, p. 190)

- *Social support*—"aid and assistance exchanged through social relationships and interpersonal transactions" (Heaney & Israel, 2008, p. 191)
- *Social capital*—"relationships between community members including trust, reciprocity, and civic engagement" (Minkler, Wallerstein, & Wilson, 2008, p. 294)
- *Interpersonal communication*

Because of space limitations, only three interpersonal theories are overviewed in this chapter, one that is well-established (Social Cognitive Theory) and two newer theories (Social Network Theory and Social Capital Theory). The latter two may be theories in name only. As stated earlier in this chapter, some theories have the term "model" in their title because that is the way they were initially identified. Even though there is now empirical evidence to call them theories, the "model title" has remained. The social network and social capital theories may have been called theories prematurely; they are probably more in the model stage. However, you should be aware of the main concepts in each one.

**Social Cognitive Theory (SCT)**    The Social Cognitive Theory (SCT) (Bandura, 1986) dates back to the 1950s (Bandura, 1977; Rotter, 1954), when it was known as the Social Learning Theory (SLT). Some still refer to it as the SLT. In brief, the SCT describes learning as a shared interaction among an individual's environment, cognitive processes, and behavior (Parcel, 1983). Those who advocate the SCT believe that reinforcement contributes to learning. But, the combination of reinforcement with an individual's expectations of the behavior's consequences is what determines the behavior. The SCT explains learning through its constructs. Those constructs most often used in health education/promotion are presented in **Table 4.2**, along with an example of each.

**Social Network Theory (SNT)**    The term **social network** refers to the "web of social relationships that surround people" (Heaney & Israel, 2008, p. 190). Barnes, a sociologist who studied Norwegian villages (Barnes, 1954), created the term in the 1950s. He used it to describe villagers' social relationships and characteristics that were not traditional social units like families (Edberg, 2007; Heaney & Israel, 2008). Since that time, sociologists and professionals in various disciplines, including health education/promotion, have continued to study and use the social network concept.

Social epidemiological observational studies clearly document the beneficial effects of supportive networks on health status (Heaney & Israel, 2008). But some people question whether there is enough evidence to suggest a Social Network Theory (SNT). Heaney and Israel (2008) feel that the social network concept, and the closely related one of social support, "do not connote theories per se. Rather, they are concepts that describe the structure, processes, and functions of social relationships" (p. 193). They feel that intervention studies are "needed to identify the most potent causal agents and critical time periods for social network enhancement" (p. 197). For example, it is not known how much social networking is needed to enhance health, or how much is too much. Also unknown are the characteristics of "good networks" that result in positive health behavior (i.e., regular exercise) versus characteristics of "bad networks" that lead to negative health behavior (i.e., smoking). We do know, however, that people who are part of social networks are healthier, as a whole, than those who are not involved in social networks.

**Table 4.2**    Often-used constructs of the Social Cognitive Theory and examples
of their application

| Construct | Definition | Example |
|---|---|---|
| **Behavioral capability** | Knowledge and skills necessary to perform a behavior | If people are going to exercise aerobically, they need to know what it is and how to do it. |
| **Expectations** | Beliefs about the likely outcomes of certain behaviors | If people enroll in a weight-loss program, they expect to lose weight. |
| **Expectancies** | Values people place on expected outcomes | How important is it to people that they become physically fit? |
| **Locus of control** | Perception of the center of control over reinforcement | Those who feel they have control over reinforcement are said to have internal locus of control. Those who perceive reinforcement under the control of an external force are said to have external locus of control. |
| **Reciprocal determinism** | "Environmental factors influence individuals and groups, but individuals and groups can also influence their environments and regulate their own behavior" (McAlister, Perry, & Parcel, 2008, p. 171) | Lack of use of vending machines could be a result of the choices within the machine. Notes about the selections from the nonusing consumers to the machine's owners could change the selections and change the behavior of the nonusing consumers to that of users. |
| **Reinforcement** (directly, vicariously, self-management) | Responses to behaviors that increase the chances of recurrence | Giving verbal encouragement to those who have acted in a healthy manner |
| **Self-control**, or **self-regulation** | Gaining control over own behavior through monitoring and adjusting it | If clients want to change their eating habits, have them monitor their current eating habits for seven days. |
| **Self-efficacy** | People's confidence in their ability to perform a certain desired task or function | If people are going to engage in a regular exercise program, they must feel they can do it. |
| **Collective efficacy** | Beliefs about the ability of the group to perform concerted actions that bring desired outcomes (McAlister et al., 2008, p. 171) | If a group of people is going to work to change a community's cultural toward healthy behavior, they must feel that they can do it. |
| **Emotional-coping response** | For people to learn, they must be able to deal with the sources of anxiety that surround a behavior. | Fear is an emotion that can be involved in learning, and people would have to deal with it before they could learn a behavior. |

*Source:* From Created from Baranowski, T. Perry, C.L., & Parcel, G.S., (2002). "How Individuals, Environments, and Health Behavior Interact: Social Cognitive Theory," in K. Glanz, B.K. Riner & F.M. Lewis (Eds.), *Health behavior and health education: Theory, research, and practice,* 3rd ed., 165–184; McAlister, A.L., Perry, C.L. & Parcel, G.S. (2008). "How Individuals, Environments, and Health Behavior Interact: Social Cognitive Theory," in K. Glanz, B.K. Rimer, & K. Viswanath (Eds.), *Health behavior and health education: Theory, research, and practice,* 4th ed., 169-188;  McKenzie, J.F., Neiger, B.L. & Thackery, R. (2009). *Planning, implementing, and evaluating health promotion programs: A primer,* 5th ed., Pearson Education, Inc., Upper Saddle River, NJ.

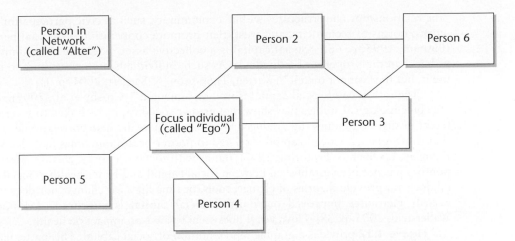

**Figure 4.11**  A simple sociogram, centered on a "focus individual" or ego

*Source:* From Edberg, M., *Essentials of Health Behavior: Social and Behavioral Theory in Public Health,* 1st ed., Fig. 5-1, p. 56. Copyright © 2007, Jones and Bartlett Publishers, Sudbury, MA. http://www.jblearning.com. Reprinted by permission.

Edberg (2007) described different types of social networks such as ego-centered networks and full relational networks (see **Figure 4.11**). He indicated that the key component to Social Network Theory is the relationships between and among individuals, including how those relationships influence beliefs and behaviors. He further stated that those using SNT need to consider the following items when assessing a network's role on the health behavior of individuals who are part of the network (Edberg, 2007):

- Centrality vs. marginality of individuals in the network: How involved is the person in the network?

- Reciprocity of relationships: Are relationships one-way or two-way?

- Complexity or intensity of relationships in the network: Do the relationships exist between two people, or are they multiplexed?

- Homogeneity or diversity of people in the network: Do all members of the network have similar characteristics, or are they different from one another?

- Subgroups, cliques, and linkages: Are there concentrations of interactions among some members? If so, do they interact with others, or are they isolated from others?

- Communication patterns in the network: How does information pass between the members in the network?

In summary, we know that social networks can impact health, but the specifics of who is most affected and how best to set up and use social networks are unknown. Even so, health education specialists who are planning interventions need to consider whether social networks should be a part of their strategy to bring about change. With the power of the Internet, the impact of social networks in the work of health education specialists will continue to grow.

**Social Capital Theory**    The term **social capital** got its start in political science and has been used in health education/promotion since the mid-1990s. An often-quoted definition is "the relationships and structures within a community, such as civic participation, networks, norms of reciprocity, and trust, that promote cooperation of mutual benefit" (Putnam, 1995, p. 66). "Social capital is a collective asset, a feature of communities rather than the property of individuals. As such, individuals both contribute to it and use it, but they cannot own it" (Warren, Thompson, & Saegert, 2001, p. 1).

"The influence of social capital is well documented" (Crosby et al., 2009). There are epidemiological studies that show that greater social capital is linked to several different positive outcomes (i.e., reduced mortality). There are also correlational studies that show a lack of social capital is related to poorer health outcomes (e.g., Kawachi, Kennedy, Lochner, & Prothrow, 1997). But as with social networks, a cause-effect relationship has not been established between social capital and better health. "Social capital does not provide theories of change, tools, or time lines for change; nor does it necessarily guarantee improved outcomes if social capital is improved" (Minkler & Wallerstein, 2005, p. 38). However, it does seem to have an impact on health.

**Figure 4.12** provides a graphic representation of social capital. This particular figure includes the key concepts of Putman's (1995) definition of social capital and three different types of network resources: bonding, bridging, and linking social capital. These three types are differentiated based on the strength of the relationships between/among those people in the social network (Hayden, 2009). Originally, *bonding social capital*, sometimes referred to as exclusive social capital, was defined as "the type that brings closer together people who already know each other" (Gittell & Vidal, 1998, p.15). More recently, this concept was expanded to include people who are similar, or people who are members of the same group. Examples of bonding social capital include those who may be members in a service organization (e.g., Lions, Elks, American Legion) or religious community.

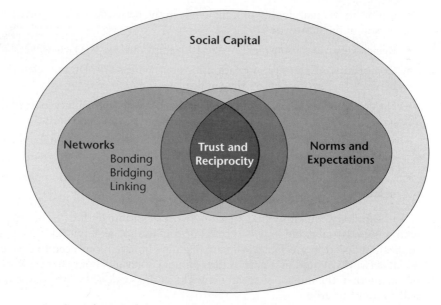

**Figure 4.12** Social capital

*Source:* From Hayden, J., *Introduction to Health Behavior Theory,* 1st ed., Fig 9-3, p. 125. Copyright © 2009, Jones and Bartlett Publishers, Sudbury, MA. http://www.jblearning.com. Reprinted by permission.

*Bridging social capital,* sometimes referred to as inclusive social capital, was originally defined as "the type that brings together people or groups who previously did not know each other" (Gittell & Vidal, 1998, p. 15). Bridging social capital is now seen more as the resources people obtain from their interaction with others outside their group, who often are people with different demographic characteristics. An example is people from different parts of a community who come together to create a community park.

The most recently recognized and weakest (Hayden, 2009) network resource is *linking social capital.* This type of network resource comes from relationships between or among "individuals and groups in different social strata in a hierarchy where power, social status, and wealth are accessed by different groups" (U.K. Office of National Statistics, 2001, p. 11). An example may be where a boss and an employee are working together on a project.

As with social networks, it is important that health education specialists think about the concept of social capital when planning interventions. Although it is not an intervention in itself, it is a concept that needs to be considered and monitored.

## Community Theories

This group of theories includes three categories of factors from the socio-ecological approach—institutional, community, and public policy. Institutional factors include rules, regulations, and policies of an organization that can impact health behavior. Community factors include social norms, while public policy includes legislation that can impact health behavior (see **Figure 4.13**). Theories associated with these three factors include theories of community organizing and community building (see Chapter 1), organizational change, the Diffusion Theory, and the Community Readiness Model (a stage model). The latter two are described in the following sections.

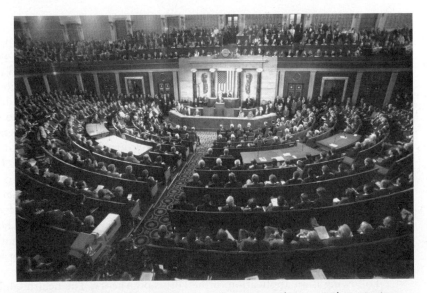

**Figure 4.13** Public policy has become an important intervention strategy for health promotion.

(Ron Edmonds/AP Wide World Photos)

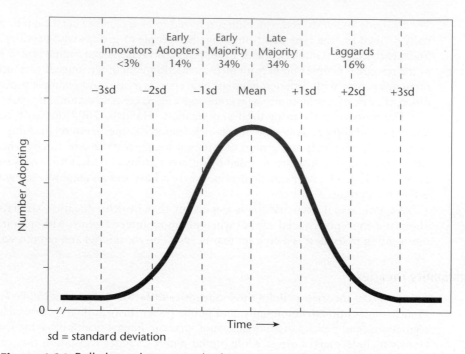

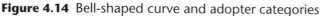

sd = standard deviation

**Figure 4.14** Bell-shaped curve and adopter categories

*Source:* Adapted with the permission of The Free Press, a Division of Simon & Schuster, Inc., from *Diffusion of Innovations,* 4th ed., by Everett M. Rogers. Copyright © 1995 by Everett M. Rogers. Copyright © 1962, 1971, 1983 by The Free Press. All rights reserved.

**Diffusion Theory (DF)**   The Diffusion Theory (DF) provides an explanation for the diffusion of innovations in populations. In health education/promotion, innovations come in the form of new ideas, techniques, behaviors, and programs. When people become "consumers" of an innovation, they are referred to as adopters. Rogers (2003) categorized adopters on the basis of when they adopt innovations. These categories include innovators, early adopters, early or late majority, and laggards. The rate at which people become adopters can be represented by the bell-shaped curve (see **Figure 4.14**).

Innovators are the first to adopt an innovation. They are venturesome, independent, risky, and daring. They want to be the first to do something. **Early adopters** are very interested in innovation, but they do not want to be the first involved. Early adopters are respected by others in the social system and looked at as opinion leaders.

Following the early adopters is the **early majority.** This group of people may be interested in the innovation but need some external motivation to get involved. These people, along with those in the late majority, make up the largest groups. The **late majority** comprises people who are skeptical. They will not adopt an innovation until most people in the social system have done so. The **laggards** are the last ones to get involved in an innovation, if they get involved at all.

Following is an application of the Diffusion Theory. The health education staff at the Walkup Health Maintenance Organization (HMO) is beginning a new series of stress management classes for the HMO members. About 3 percent of the priority population (the innovators) will sign up and attend the classes as soon as they hear about the series. Shortly thereafter, another 14 percent (early adopters) will probably get involved, possibly after reading about the program's merits. At this point, the health education staff must work harder to attract others to the program. It will take constant reminders to get the early majority involved. Buddy, peer, or mentoring programs might be needed to get the late majority involved. The laggards probably will not attend the series at all.

**Community Readiness Model (CRM)**  The Community Readiness Model (CRM) is a stage theory for communities. Communities, like individuals, are in various stages of readiness for change. Yet, the stages of change for communities are not the same as for individuals. "The stages of readiness in a community have to deal with group processes and group organization, characteristics that are not relevant to personal readiness" (Edwards, Jumper-Thurman, Plested, Oetting, & Swanson, 2000, pp. 296–297). Although the CRM was developed initially to deal with alcohol and drug abuse, it also has been used in a variety of health and nutrition areas, environmental issues, and social programs (Edwards et al., 2000). The CRM has nine stages (Edwards et al., 2000):

1. *No Awareness.* The problem is not generally recognized by the community or leaders.

2. *Denial.* There is little or no recognition in the community that there is a problem. If recognition exists, there is a feeling that nothing can be done about the problem.

3. *Vague Awareness.* Some people in the community feel there is a problem and something should be done, but there is no motivation or leadership to do so.

4. *Preplanning.* There is a clear recognition by some that a problem exists and something should be done. There are leaders, but no focused or detailed planning.

5. *Preparation.* Planning is taking place but it is not based on collected data. There is leadership and modest support for efforts. Resources are being sought.

6. *Initiation.* Information is available to justify and begin efforts. Staff is either in training or has just completed training. Leaders are enthusiastic. There is usually little resistance and involvement from the community members.

7. *Stabilization.* The program is running, staffed, and supported by the community and decision makers. The program is perceived as stable with no need for change. This stage may include routine tracking, but no in-depth evaluation.

8. *Confirmation/Expansion.* Standard efforts are in place, which are supported by the community and decision makers. The program has been evaluated and modified, and efforts are in place to seek resources for new efforts. There is ongoing data collection to link risk factors and problems.

9. *Professionalism.* Much is known about prevalence, risk factors, and cause of problems. Highly trained staff members run effective programs aimed at the general population and appropriate subgroups. Programs have been evaluated and modified. The community is supportive but should hold programs accountable.

A community's readiness can be assessed through interviews with key informants. As with other stage theories, once the stage of readiness is known, there are suggested processes for moving a community from one stage to the next. **Table 4.3** presents the nine stages and the goal for each stage.

**Table 4.3**   Community readiness stages and goals

| Stage | Goal |
|---|---|
| (1) *No Awareness* | Raise awareness of the issue. |
| (2) *Denial* | Raise awareness that the problem or issue exists in the community. |
| (3) *Vague Awareness* | Raise awareness that the community can do something. |
| (4) *Preplanning* | Raise awareness with the concrete ideas to combat condition. |
| (5) *Preparation* | Gather existing information to help plan strategies. |
| (6) *Initiation* | Provide community specific information. |
| (7) *Stabilization* | Stabilize efforts/programs. |
| (8) *Confirmation/Expansion* | Expand and enhance service. |
| (9) *Professionalism* | Maintain momentum and continue growth. |

*Source:* Created from Edwards, R.W., Jumper-Thurman, P., Plested, B.A., Oetting, E.R., & Swanson, L. (2000). "Community Readiness: Research to Practice." *Journal of Community Psychology, 28* (3), 291–307.

## Planning Models

Good health education/promotion programs are not created by chance. Well-thought-out and well-conceived models provide health education specialists with "frames" on which to build plans (see **Box 4.1**). Although many planning models have similar principles and common elements, those elements may have different labels. In fact, "there are important differences in sequence, emphasis, and the conceptualization of the major components that make certain models more appealing than others to individual practitioners" (Simons-Morton, Greene, & Gottlieb, 1995, pp. 126–127).

---

**Box 4.1 Practitioner's Perspective**   **Theories and Planning Models**

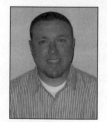

(Reprinted by permission of Trevor W. Newby)

NAME: Trevor W. Newby

CURRENT POSITION/TITLE: Health Education Specialist, Senior

EMPLOYER: Idaho State Tobacco Prevention and Control Program (Project Filter)

MAJOR: Health Promotion

DEGREES: Master of Health Science in Health Promotion and Bachelor of Science in Health Promotion

INSTITUTION: Boise State University

**How I Obtained My Job:** During my graduate assistantship, I was fortunate to align myself with a number of individuals and professors that made me more marketable for employment upon graduation. Knowing I was ready to graduate, a professor forwarded me a job posting for a Senior Health Education Specialist position with the Idaho State Respiratory Health Pro-

gram. While in this capacity, I've been able to work with a number of statewide programs and a variety of different organizations while taking part in a number of collaboration efforts related to Project Filter. My job has allowed me to work a great deal with marketing, evaluation, and reporting, and has provided me with countless networking and educational opportunities.

**Box 4.1 Practitioner's Perspective**    Continued

**How I Use Theory in My Job:** At the state level, we are responsible for reporting progress in relation to tobacco prevention and control efforts to the Centers for Disease Control and Prevention (CDC). Because of this, we use a wide variety of theories, specifically those related to the stages of change, to assist us in achieving our work plan goals. This is very evident in the tobacco cessation services Project Filter offers to the general public through 1-800-QuitNow and Idaho.QuitNet.com. Both of these services utilize the behavior change model to help interested individuals to quit using tobacco.

Every model, strategy, or program that is implemented by Project Filter is evaluated to measure its effectiveness. Logic models are used as the marquee planning tool by CDC and other state programs to help strategize, plan, implement, and evaluate programs in most of the public health disciplines. In addition, Project Filter uses a variety of other methods to supplement the use of logic models in verifying programming effectiveness. These include use of work plans, quarterly and monthly reports from contracted agencies or groups, marketing analysis reports, event debriefing reports, and a variety of data collected from a host of different sources related to tobacco. This variety allows Project Filter to effectively plan, implement, and evaluate all facets of their programming efforts.

**Recommendations for Health Education Specialists:** First, secure internship opportunities. Internship settings will not only provide valuable work experience that will put you ahead of other potential job seekers, but will also allow you to apply classroom learning while offering networking opportunities at the same time. The more internships you secure, the more diverse and enticing your portfolio will become for potential employers. Second, be proficient in grant writing. This is a valuable skill that is necessary in the public health profession. Third, take a number of marketing classes. Marketing plays an imperative role in public health. An agency could have the most dynamic program or resource available, but it won't provide any benefit unless it is effectively marketed to its intended audience. Lastly, don't be afraid to learn. Public health is a constantly evolving field with a wide variety of topics. In order to be a proficient educator, constant research and information gathering are critical.

**Future of the Health Education/Promotion Profession:** I consider the future of health education specialists in public health to be very positive. It's taken many years for businesses, lawmakers, and policy makers to realize the worth of proper prevention methods provided by public health professionals, but now the dynamic is changing. Prevention practices have already been proven to be effective with research surrounding tobacco. Prevention practices have saved millions of dollars in health care costs to tax payers in relation to tobacco use and have begun to change the social norm of tobacco use as a whole. I am certain prevention practices will play a vital role in the new health care reform as the government saves millions of dollars on secondary and tertiary clinical care by implementing effective prevention practices provided by public health professionals. This will provide many jobs to health education specialists in an increasingly changing and meaningful profession.

The following sections provide an overview of seven models used for planning health education/promotion programs. Although many more models exist, these seven have been used successfully, and they represent a wide range of planning approaches. **Box 4.2** lists other planning models that may be just as good from a theoretical perspective, but currently they are not used as often. For more detailed explanations, see the original publications of the models.

| **Box 4.2** | OTHER PLANNING MODELS |
| --- | --- |

- *Comprehensive Health Education Model* (Sullivan, 1973).
- *Model for Health Education Planning* (Ross & Mico, 1980).
- *Model for Health Education Planning and Resource Development* (Bates & Winder, 1984).
- *Planned Approach To Community Health (PATCH)* (CDC, n. d.).
- *Generic Health/Fitness Delivery System* (Patton et al., 1986).
- *Assessment Protocol for Excellence in Public Health* (APEX/PH) (NACHO, 1991).
- *Healthy Plan-It* (CDC, 2000).
- *Healthy People in Healthy Communities* (USDHHS, 2001).
- *The Health Communication Model* (NCI, 2002).
- *The Planning, Program Development, and Evaluation Model* (Timmreck, 2003).

## PRECEDE-PROCEED

Currently, the best known and most frequently used planning model is **PRECEDE-PROCEED.** As its name implies, this model has two components. PRECEDE is an acronym that stands for *p*redisposing, *r*einforcing, and *e*nabling *c*onstructs in *e*ducational/*e*cological *d*iagnosis and *e*valuation. PROCEED stands for *p*olicy, *r*egulatory, and *o*rganizational *c*onstructs in *e*ducational and *e*nvironmental *d*evelopment (Green & Kreuter, 2005).

The PRECEDE-PROCEED model was developed over a period of fifteen to twenty years. The PRECEDE framework was conceived in the early 1970s (Green, 1974) and evolved into a planning model in the late 1970s (Green, 1975, 1976; Green, Levine, & Deeds, 1975; Green et al., 1978; Green et al., 1980). The PROCEED portion was developed in the early to mid-1980s (Green, 1979, 1980, 1981a, 1981b, 1982, 1983a, 1983b, 1984a, 1984b, 1984c, 1984d, 1986a, 1986b, 1986c, 1986d, 1986e, 1987a, 1987b; Green & Allen, 1980; Green & McAlister, 1984; Green, Mullen, & Friedman, 1986; Green, Wilson, & Lovato, 1986; Green, Wilson, & Bauer, 1983).

As shown in **Figure 4.15**, PRECEDE-PROCEED has eight phases. The first four phases, which make up the PRECEDE portion of the model, consist "of a series of planned assessments that generate information that will be used to guide subsequent decisions" (Green & Kreuter, 2005, p. 8). PROCEED also has four phases and "is marked by the strategic implementation of multiple actions based on what was learned from the assessments in the initial phase" (Green & Kreuter, 2005, p. 9).

At first glance, the PRECEDE-PROCEED model appears overly complicated. However, there is a very logical sequence to the eight phases that outlines the health promotion planning process. The underlying approach of this model begins by identifying the desired outcome, then determines what causes it, and finally designs an intervention aimed at reaching the desired outcome. In other words, PRECEDE-PROCEED starts with the final consequences and works backwards to the causes (McKenzie et al., 2009). **Table 4.4** provides an overview of the eight phases of this model.

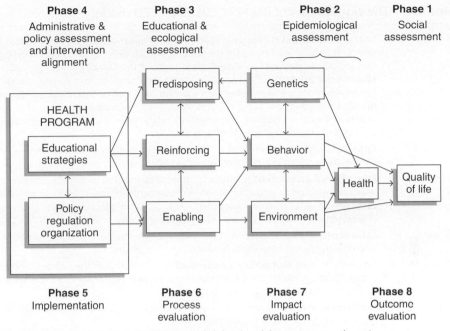

**Figure 4.15** PRECEDE-PROCEED model for health program planning

*Source:* From Green, L.W. & Kreuter, M.W., *Health Program Planning: An Educational and Ecological Approach,* 4th ed., p. 17, Fig 1.5. Copyright © 2005 The McGraw-Hill Companies, Inc. Reprinted by permission.

## MATCH

**MATCH** is an acronym for Multilevel Approach To Community Health. This planning model (see **Figure 4.16**) was developed in the late 1980s (Simons-Morton, Simons-Morton, Parcel, & Bunker, 1988). Like the PRECEDE-PROCEED model, MATCH has also been used in a variety of settings. For example, several intervention handbooks created by the Centers for Disease Control and Prevention utilized MATCH (Simons-Morton et al., 1995).

MATCH is a socio-ecological planning approach. It recognizes that intervention activities can and should be aimed at a variety of objectives and individuals. This approach is illustrated in Figure 4.16 by the various levels of influence. **Table 4.5** presents the phases and steps of MATCH, along with an explanation of each.

The MATCH framework is recognized for emphasizing program implementation (Simons-Morton et al., 1995). "MATCH is designed to be applied when behavioral and environmental risk and protective factors for disease or injury are generally known and when general priorities for action have been determined, thus providing a convenient way to turn the corner from needs assessment and priority setting to the development of effective programs" (Simons-Morton et al., 1995, p. 155).

## Intervention Mapping

Intervention Mapping is a relatively new model for planning health promotion programs (Bartholomew, Parcel, & Kok, 1998). It focuses on planning programs that are

**Table 4.4** The eight phases of the PRECEDE-PROCEED model

| | |
|---|---|
| Phase 1. | **Social assessment** is "the assessment in both objective and subjective terms of high-priority problems or aspirations for the common good, defined for a population by economic and social indicators and by individuals in terms of their quality of life" (p. G-8), **situational analysis** is "the combination of social and epidemiological assessments of conditions, trends, and priorities with a preliminary scan of determinants, relevant policies, resources, organizational support, and regulations that might anticipate or permit action in advance of a more complete assessment of behavioral, environmental, educational, ecological, and administrative factors" (pp. G-7–8). |
| Phase 2. | **Epidemiological assessment** is "the delineation of the extent, distribution, and causes of a health problem in a defined population" (p. G-3). |
| Phase 3. | **Educational assessment** is "the delineation of factors that predispose, enable, and reinforce a specific behavior, or through behavior, environmental changes" (p. G-3), and **ecological assessment** is "a systematic assessment of factors in the social and physical environment that interact with behavior to produce health effects or quality-of-life outcomes" (p. G-3). |
| Phase 4a. | **Intervention alignment** is matching appropriate strategies and interventions with projected changes and outcomes identified in earlier phases. |
| Phase 4b. | **Administrative and policy assessment** is "an analysis of the policies, resources, and circumstances prevailing in an organizational situation to facilitate or hinder the development of the health program" (p. G-1). |
| Phase 5. | **Implementation** is "the act of converting program objectives into actions through policy changes, regulation, and organization" (p. G-5). |
| Phase 6. | **Process evaluation** is "the assessment of policies, materials, personnel, performance, quality of practice or services, and other inputs and implementation experiences" (p. G-6). |
| Phase 7. | **Impact evaluation** is "the assessment of program effects on intermediate objectives including changes in predisposing, enabling, and reinforcing factors, as well as behavioral and environmental changes, and possibly health and social outcomes" (p. G-5). |
| Phase 8. | **Outcome evaluation** is an "assessment of the effects of a program on its ultimate objectives, including changes in health and social benefits or quality of life" (p. G-6). |

*Source:* From Green, L.W. & Kreuter, M.W., *Health Program Planning: An Educational and Ecological Approach,* 4th ed. Copyright © 2005 The McGraw-Hill Companies, Inc. Reprinted by permission.

based on theory and evidence (Bartholomew, Parcel, Kok, & Gottlieb, 2006). It also draws on multiple principles used in the PRECEDE-PROCEED and MATCH models.

Intervention mapping has six steps. The first step, *needs assessment,* includes two major components: (1) scientific, epidemiologic, behavioral, and social analysis of a priority population or community; and (2) an effort to get to know and understand the character of the priority population (Bartholomew et al., 2006).

Step 2, *matrices of change objectives,* specifies who and what will change as a result of the intervention (Bartholomew et al., 2006). Although the identification of goals and objectives is included in all planning models, intervention mapping makes a unique contribution in how this is carried out. In this step, planners create a matrix of change objectives for the intervention. By doing so, planners can more clearly see who and what will change as a result of the intervention.

In Step 3, *theory-based methods and practical strategies,* planners work to identify theory-based interventions and strategies that hold the greatest promise to change the health behavior(s) of individuals in the priority population. While planners seek theory-based methods, they also ensure that practical strategies are selected and that final strategies match the change objectives from the matrices.

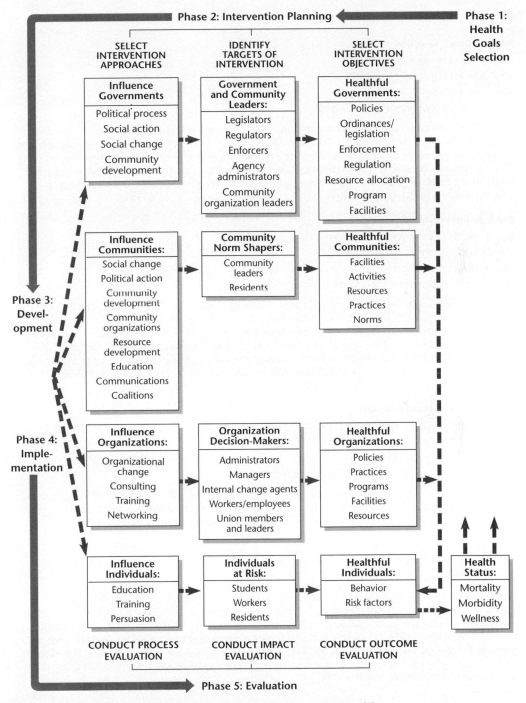

**Figure 4.16** MATCH: Multilevel Approach To Community Health

*Source:* Reprinted by permission of Waveland Press, Inc., from Simons-Morton, B.G., Greene, W.H. & Gottlieb, N.H., *Introduction to Health Education and Promotion,* 2nd ed. Long Grove, IL: Waveland Press, Inc., 1995. All rights reserved.

**Table 4.5**    MATCH phases and steps

**PHASE I: GOALS SELECTION**

Step 1: Select health status goals

Step 2: Select high-priority population(s)

Step 3: Identify health behavior goals

Step 4: Identify environmental factor goals

Explanation of Phase I: Planners select health status goals based upon several different factors including the prevalence of the health problem, the relative importance of the health problem, the changeability of the problem, and other considerations unique to the program. Also, planners need to select the high-priority populations, identify the health behaviors most associated with the health status goals in order to create health behavior goals, and identify the environmental factors such as access, availability of resources, enabling practices, and barriers so that environmental goals can be created.

**PHASE II: INTERVENTION PLANNING**

Step 1: Identify the targets of the intervention

Step 2: Select intervention objectives

Step 3: Identify mediators of the intervention objectives

Step 4: Select intervention approaches

Explanation of Phase II: This phase begins with the matching of objectives with the intervention targets and intervention actions. Targets of the intervention actions are those individuals that exert influence or control over the personal or environmental conditions that are related to the target health and behavior goals. After identifying the TIAs, they are matched with the health behavioral and environmental factors identified in Phase I. Once this match is made, planners select an intervention action(s) to be used. Intervention actions commonly used by health educators include teaching, training, counseling, policy advocacy, consulting, community organization, social marketing, and social action.

**PHASE III: PROGRAM DEVELOPMENT**

Step 1: Create program units or components

Step 2: Select or develop curricula and create intervention guides

Step 3: Develop session plans

Step 4: Create or acquire instructional materials, products, and resources

Explanation of Phase III: After the creation of the program components, planners either select from already developed curricula or develop their own guides. This would include the development of individual session or lesson plans, and the acquisition or creation of instructional materials, products, and resources.

**PHASE IV: IMPLEMENTATION PREPARATIONS**

Step 1: Facilitate adoption, implementation, and maintenance

Step 2: Select and train implementers

Explanation of Phase IV: Planners prepare for implementation and conduct the interventions. To achieve effective implementation planners must (a) develop a specific proposal and advocate for the adoption of change, (b) develop the need, readiness, and environmental supports for change, (c) provide evidence that the intervention works, (d) identify and select change agents and opinion leaders and sell them on the need for change, and (e) establish good working relationships with the decision makers. In addition, depending on who will implement the program, there may be a need to select, train, support, and monitor those who do the implementation.

(Table 4.5 continues)

**Table 4.5**    (*continued*)

**PHASE V: EVALUATION**
Step 1: Conduct process evaluation
Step 2: Measure impact
Step 3: Monitor outcomes

Explanation of Phase V: Planners carry out three different types of evaluation—process (utility, extent, quality, and effects of implementation on immediate learning outcomes), impact (assessing target mediators such as knowledge, attitudes, and practices), and outcome (long-term effects of the program, usually health behaviors, or environmental factors).

In Step 4, *program,* planners create the intervention details and materials needed for the program's implementation. This step is based on the methods and strategies identified in Step 3.

Step 5, *adoption and implementation,* is like Step 2 in that it includes the development of matrices. However, these matrices focus on adoption and implementation performance objectives (Bartholomew et al., 2006). In other words, instead of concentrating on who and what will change within the priority population, the focus is on what will be done by whom among planners or program partners.

The sixth, and last, step of this model is *evaluation planning.* In this step, planners decide if determinants were well specified, if strategies were appropriately matched to methods, what proportion of the priority population was reached, and whether or not implementation was complete and executed as planned (Bartholomew et al., 2006).

## CDCynergy

**CDCynergy,** or **Cynergy** for short, is a health communication planning model developed in 1997 by the Office of Communication at the Centers for Disease Control and Prevention (CDC). It was first issued in July 1998 (Parvanta & Freimuth, 2000). Cynergy was developed primarily for the CDC public health professionals who had responsibilities for health communication. However, because of widespread interest in the model, the CDC made it available to other health professionals in a variety of health education/promotion settings. Currently, CDCynergy is considered public domain, which means restrictions are not placed on copying or general use. A copy of CDCynergy can be obtained via training by the Society for Public Health Education (SOPHE), or directly from the Public Health Foundation (see Weblinks at the end of this chapter).

The basic edition of Cynergy presents a general methodology for health communication planning, a step-by-step guide, a reference library, and links to templates that allow tailored plans to be created (CDC, 2003). Cynergy uses six phases involving multiple steps to help planners: acquire a thorough understanding of a health problem and whom it affects; explore a wide range of possible intervention strategies for influencing the problem; systematically select the intervention strategies that show the most promise; understand the role communication can play in planning, implementing, and evaluating selected strategies; and develop a comprehensive communication plan (CDC, 2003). **Table 4.6** displays the six sequential, yet interrelated, phases, which are designed to build upon the previous phases and prepare program planners for subsequent phases.

**Table 4.6**   *CDCynergy lite* (an abridged version of the CDCynergy health communication model)

**PHASE 1: DESCRIBE PROBLEM**

- Identify and define health problems that may be addressed by your program interventions.
- Examine and/or conduct necessary research to describe the problems.
- Assess factors and variables that can affect the project's direction, including strengths, weaknesses, opportunities, and threats (SWOT).

**PHASE 2: ANALYZE PROBLEM**

- List causes of each problem you plan to address.
- Develop goals for each problem.
- Consider strengths, weaknesses, opportunities, threats, and ethics of health 1) engineering, 2) communication/education, 3) policy/enforcement, and 4) community service intervention options.
- Select the types of intervention(s) that should be used to address the problem(s).

**PHASE 3: PLAN INTERVENTION**

- Decide whether communication is needed as a dominant intervention and/or as support for other intervention(s).
  - If communication is used as a dominant intervention, list possible audiences.
  - If communication is to be used to support Community Services, Engineering, and/or Policy/Enforcement interventions, list possible audiences to be reached in support of each selected intervention.
- Conduct necessary audience research to segment intended audiences.
- Select audience segment(s) and write communication objectives for each audience segment.
- Write a creative brief to provide guidance in selecting appropriate concepts/messages, settings, activities, and materials.

**PHASE 4: DEVELOP INTERVENTION**

- Develop and test concepts, messages, settings, channel-specific activities, and materials with intended audiences.
- Finalize and briefly summarize a communication implementation plan. The plan should include:
  - Background and justification, including SWOT and ethics analyses
  - Audiences
  - Communication objectives
  - Messages
  - Settings and channels for conveying your messages
  - Activities (including tactics, materials, and other methods)
  - Available partners and resources
  - Tasks and timeline (including persons responsible for each task, date for completion of each task, resources required to deliver each task, and points at which progress will be checked)
  - Internal and external communication plan
  - Budget
- Produce materials for dissemination.

(Table 4.6 continues)

**Table 4.6**   *(continued)*

---

**PHASE 5: PLAN EVALUATION**

- Determine stakeholder information needs.
  - ◆ Decide which types of evaluation (e.g., implementation, reach, effects) are needed to satisfy stakeholder information needs.
  - ◆ Identify sources of information and select data collection methods.
  - ◆ Formulate an evaluation design that illustrates how methods will be applied to gather credible information.
  - ◆ Develop a data analysis and reporting plan.
  - ◆ Finalize and briefly summarize an evaluation implementation plan. The plan should include:
    - Stakeholder questions
    - Intervention standards
    - Evaluation methods and design
    - D ata analysis and reporting
    - Tasks and timeline (including persons responsible for each task, date for completion of each task, resources required to deliver each task, and points at which progress will be checked)
    - Internal and external communication plan
    - Budget

**PHASE 6: IMPLEMENT PLAN**

- Integrate, execute, and manage communication and evaluation plans.
- Document feedback and lessons learned.
- Modify program components based on feedback.
- Disseminate lessons learned and evaluation findings.

---

*Source.* Centers for Disease Control and Prevention (CDC), U.S. Department of Health and Human Services (USD-HHS). 2003. *CDCynergy 3.0: Your Guide to Effective Health Communication (CD-ROM Version 3.0).* Atlanta: Author.

Completion of these phases will lead to a strategic communication plan that is both science and audience based.

In addition to the basic edition of Cynergy, CDC and its partners have produced content-specific editions of Cynergy to meet the particular needs of health education specialists addressing various health problems. There are content-specific editions for American Indian/Alaska Native Diabetes, Cardiovascular Disease, Diabetes, Emergency Risk Communication, Immunizations, Micronutrients, Social Marketing, STD Prevention, Tobacco Prevention and Control, and Violence Prevention. Several other content-specific editions were being developed at the time this book was written.

## SMART

**Social marketing** has been defined as "the application of commercial marketing technologies to the analysis, planning, execution, and evaluation of programs designed to influence the voluntary behavior of target audiences in order to improve their personal welfare and that of their society" (Andreasen, 1995, p. 7). This process offers benefits the audience wants, reduces barriers the audience faces, and uses persuasion to influence intentions to act favorably (Albrecht, 1997). The concept of social marketing is more than thirty years old, but its application to health education/promotion is much more recent (McDermott, 2000).

Even though the use of social marketing is relatively new in health education/ promotion, several different authors (Andreasen, 1995; Bryant, 1998; Walsh, Rudd, Moeykens, & Moloney, 1993) have presented planning processes, models, or frameworks based upon social marketing. The Social Marketing Assessment and Response Tool (**SMART**) is a social marketing planning framework developed by Neiger and Thackeray (1998). It is presented here because it provides a composite of other social marketing models, and because it has been used from start to finish on multiple occasions in several social marketing interventions (Neiger & Thackeray, 2002). This model also provides an excellent overview of social marketing in general (McKenzie et al., 2009).

SMART is composed of seven phases (see **Table 4.7**). "Like other social marketing planning frameworks, the central focus of SMART is consumers. The heart of this model, composed of Phases 2 through 4, pertains to acquiring a broad understanding of the consumers who will be the recipients of a program and its interventions. These three phases seek to understand consumers before interventions are even developed or implemented. Though these phases (2–4) are displayed in linear fashion... they are typically performed simultaneously with members of the priority population" (McKenzie et al., 2009, p. 39).

## MAPP

**MAPP** is an acronym for Mobilizing for Action through Planning and Partnerships. It is a relatively new planning model created by the National Association of County and City Health Officials (NACCHO) to assist local health departments (LHDs) at the city or county level with planning. This model blends many of the strengths of the five planning models already presented in this chapter. The MAPP approach is designed to improve health and quality of life by mobilizing partnerships and taking strategic action (NACCHO, 2001).

MAPP is composed of multiple steps within six phases (see **Figure 4.17**). In the first phase of MAPP, Organizing for Success and Partnership Development, planners assess whether or not the MAPP process is timely, appropriate, and even possible. This involves assessing resources, including funding, personnel, and general interest of community members. If resources are not in place, the process is delayed. If resources are sufficient, the following work groups are created: (1) a core support team, which prepares most, if not all, of the material needed for the process; (2) the MAPP Committee, composed of key sponsors from the community who provide legitimacy and resources, and stakeholders who guide and oversee the process; and (3) the community itself, which provides input, representation, and decision making.

In Phase 2, Visioning, the community is guided through a process that results in a shared vision—what the ideal future looks like—and common values—principles and beliefs that will guide the remainder of the planning process (NACCHO, 2001). This phase is usually handled by a facilitator and involves anywhere from 50–100 participants, including the advisory committee, the MAPP committee, and key community leaders.

The strength and defining characteristic of MAPP are found in Phase 3, the Four MAPP Assessments. The four assessments include (1) the community themes and strengths assessment (community or consumer opinion); (2) the local public health system assessment (general capacity of the local public health system); (3) the community

**Table 4.7**   The SMART model

---

**PHASE 1: PRELIMINARY PLANNING**

- Identify a health problem and name it in terms of behavior.
- Develop general goals.
- Outline preliminary plans for evaluation.
- Project program costs

**PHASE 2: CONSUMER ANALYSIS**

- Segment and identify the priority population.
- Identify formative research methods.
- Identify consumer wants, needs, and preferences.
- Develop preliminary ideas for preferred interventions.

**PHASE 3: MARKET ANALYSIS**

- Establish and define the market mix (4Ps).
- Assess the market to identify competitors (behaviors, messages, programs, etc.), allies (support systems, resources, etc.), and partners.

**PHASE 4: CHANNEL ANALYSIS**

- Identify appropriate communication messages, strategies, and channels.
- Assess options for program distribution. Determine how channels should be used.
- Assess options for program distribution.
- Identify communication roles for program partners.

**PHASE 5: DEVELOP INTERVENTIONS, MATERIALS, AND PRETEST**

- Develop program interventions and materials using information collected in consumer, market, and channel analyses.
- Interpret the marketing mix into a strategy that represents exchange and societal good.
- Pretest and refine the program.

**PHASE 6: IMPLEMENTATION**

- Communicate with partners and clarify involvement.
- Activate communication and distribution strategies.
- Document procedures and compare progress to timelines.
- Refine the program.

**PHASE 7: EVALUATION**

- Assess the degree to which the priority population is receiving the program.
- Assess the immediate impact on the priority population and refine the program as necessary.
- Ensure that program delivery is consistent with established protocol.
- Analyze changes in the priority population.

---

*Source:* Adapted from Walsh, R.E., et al. (1993). "Social Marketing for Public Health," *Health Affairs 12*(2), 104–119 ; and adapted from Neiger, B.L., & Thackeray, R. (1998). "Social Marketing: Making Public Health Sense." Paper presented at the annual meeting of the Utah Public Health Association, Provo, UT.

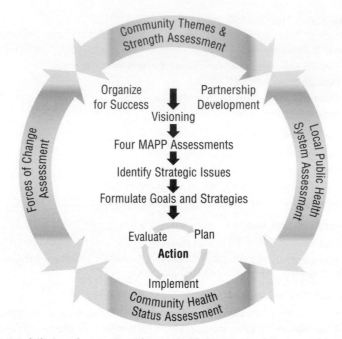

**Figure 4.17** Mobilizing for Action through Planning and Partnerships (MAPP) model

*Source:* National Association of County and City Health Officials, "Mobilizing for Action through Planning and Part-nerships (MAPP) Model" from http://www.naccho.org/topics/infrastructure/mapp/upload/MAPP_Handbook_fnl.pdf. Reprinted by permission.

health status assessment (measurement of the health of the community by use of epidemiological data); and (4) the forces of change assessment (forces such as legislation, technology, and other environmental or social phenomena that do or will impact the community) (McKenzie et al., 2009). The four assessments help identify the gaps that exist between current status in the community and the vision identified in Phase 2, as well as strategic direction for goals and strategies (NACCHO, 2001).

In Phase 4, Identify Strategic Issues, a prioritized list of the issues facing the health of the community is developed. Only issues that jeopardize the vision and values of the community are considered. Important tasks in this phase include considering what would happen if certain issues are not addressed, understanding why an issue is strategic, consolidating overlapping issues, and identifying a prioritized list (McKenzie et al., 2009).

In Phase 5, Formulate Goals and Strategies, the goals and strategies to reach the vision are created. Finally, Phase 6, The Action Cycle, is similar to implementation and evaluation phases in other planning models. In this phase, implementation details are considered, evaluation plans are developed, and plans for disseminating results are made (NACCHO, 2001).

## Generalized Model for Program Planning (GMPP)

As seen in the planning models presented so far, there are various approaches and frameworks on which to develop a program. Each model seems to have its own characteristics,

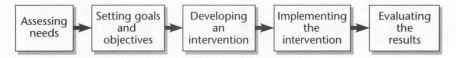

**Figure 4.18** Generalized Model for Program Planning

*Source:* From McKenzie, J.F., Neiger, B.L. & Thackery, R., *Planning, Implementing and Evaluating Health Promotion Programs: A Primer*, 5th ed., p. 17, Fig 2.1. Copyright © 2009. Reproduced by permission of Pearson Education, Inc., Upper Saddle River, NJ.

whether it is the terminology used (e.g., predisposing, enabling, and reinforcing or analyze problem or consumer analysis), the number of components (e.g., eight phases versus six steps), or the progression through the phases or steps (e.g., circular, linear, or starting with the desired end and working backward). In other words, there are many ways to get from point A to point B. However, each of the models previously presented revolves around the five primary tasks incorporated in the Generalized Model for Program Planning (McKenzie et al., 2009). These five tasks are:

1. Assessing the needs of the priority population
2. Developing appropriate goals and objectives
3. Creating an intervention that considers the peculiarities of the setting
4. Implementing the intervention
5. Evaluating the results (see **Figure 4.18**)

To better understand the planning process in health education/promotion and the various models presented, consider the following scenario. A health education specialist was hired to develop health education/promotion programs in a corporate setting. She began her work by trying to find out as much as possible about the "community" of this corporate setting and get those in the priority population involved in the program planning process. She did this by reading all the material she could find about the company. She also spent time talking with various individuals and subgroups in the company (i.e., new employees, longtime employees, management, clerical staff, labor representatives, etc.) to find out what they wanted from a health education/promotion program. In addition, she reviewed old documents of the company (i.e., health insurance records, labor agreements, written history of the company, etc.). As part of this background work, she formed a program planning committee with representation from the various subgroups of the work force.

With the help of the planning committee, the health education/promotion specialist was ready to assess the needs of the priority population. She did this by reviewing the relevant literature, examining company health insurance claims, conducting a survey of employees, and holding focus groups with selected employees. As a result of the needs assessment, she was able to identify a target health problem. In this company, the problem was a higher than expected number of breast cancer cases in the priority population. This was due in part to (1) the limited knowledge of employees about breast cancer, (2) the limited number of employees conducting breast self-examination (BSE), and (3) the low number of employees having mammograms on a regular basis.

With an understanding of the needs of the priority population, the health education specialist created specific objectives to increase the (1) employees' knowledge of breast cancer from baseline to after program participation, (2) number of women receiving mammograms by 30 percent, and (3) number of women reporting monthly breast self-examination by 50 percent. Using these objectives, she planned multiple intervention activities:

1. An information sheet on the importance of BSE and mammography, for distribution with employee paychecks

2. A mobile mammography van on-site every other month

3. Plastic BSE reminder cards, suitable for hanging from a showerhead, for distribution to all female employees

4. An article in the company newsletter covering the company's high rate of breast cancer and the new program to help women reduce their risk

5. Posters and pamphlets from the American Cancer Society in the company's lunchroom

Next, all of the listed intervention activities were carried out. Last, the health education specialist completed an evaluation to determine if there was an increase in knowledge, mammograms, and monthly BSE. As can be seen from this scenario, health education/promotion involves careful, systematic planning to achieve successful programs.

## SUMMARY

Health education/promotion is a multidisciplinary profession that has evolved from the theory and practice of other biological, behavioral, sociological, and health science disciplines. Many of the theories and models used in health education/promotion also have evolved from these other disciplines. This chapter presented an overview of the theoretical foundations and planning models of health education/promotion. Readers were introduced to the definitions of *theory, concept, construct, variable,* and *model.* A rationale was also provided to explain why it is important that health education specialists use theory in their work. Readers were then introduced to twelve of the behavior change theories that health education specialists use in their work. These theories were presented within the socio-ecological approach, which incorporates the five levels of influence. There was also a distinction made between continuum theories and stage theories. And finally, overviews of seven planning models were provided.

## REVIEW QUESTIONS

1. Define each of the following and explain how they relate to each other.
   - *Theory*
   - *Concept*
   - *Construct*
   - *Variable*
   - *Model*

2. Why is it important to use theory in the practice of health education/promotion?

3. What are behavior change theories?

4. What are the five levels of influence within the socio-ecological approach? How do they relate to behavior change theories?

5. Identify the twelve theories presented in this chapter that focus on health behavior change. Briefly describe each of the theories and name their components.

6. What is the difference between continuum theories and stage theories?

7. Explain why it might be important that health education specialists have a good understanding of stage models.

8. Name the seven planning models presented in this chapter, and list one distinguishing characteristic of each.

9. Of the seven planning models presented in this chapter, which one is most commonly used? Name the phases of this model.

10. What five components seem to be common to the planning models presented in this chapter?

## CASE STUDY

Mike graduated a year ago with a bachelor's degree in health education. He felt extremely lucky to "beat out" fifteen interviewees for the health education specialist position at the Lancaster County Health Department. Though the health department has a good reputation throughout the state, Mike is the only person on the staff hired to do health education.

Mike's supervisor, Dan Santoro, is Coordinator of Chronic and Infectious Disease for the health department. Mr. Santoro has worked for the department for about thirty years. He also holds a bachelor's degree from the same university Mike graduated from. However, Mr. Santoro received his degree in health and physical education prior to the implementation of the current community health education major.

Throughout Mike's tenure with the health department, he and Mr. Santoro have had a good working relationship. However, while planning a weight-loss program for a group of teenagers in the county, Mike ran into a situation that caused him some concern. After conducting a needs assessment and writing the program goals and objectives, he could not decide which behavior change theory to use to plan his intervention. He decided to seek Mr. Santoro's advice. When he asked Mr. Santoro what theory or model he would recommend, Mr. Santoro responded, "Theory-shmeary, you don't need to use that stuff, just skip the theory part and plan the intervention. This program needs to be up and running by the end of the month."

Based on this short conversation with Mr. Santoro, Mike was not sure how to proceed. During his undergraduate preparation at the university, Mike was told to "never plan an intervention that was not based on theory." Mike does not want to upset his supervisor, but he also knows that his program should be grounded in theory. What do you see as Mike's options at this point? What do you think Mike should do next? How would you solve this dilemma?

## CRITICAL THINKING QUESTIONS

1. This chapter presented a number of different theories focusing on health behavior change. If you were trying to help a friend stop smoking, at the friend's request, what behavior change theory would you use to develop the intervention to help your friend? Defend why you selected this theory and explain how you would apply each of the constructs.

2. You have been invited by the Garber Corporation to interview for a newly created position in the company as a health education specialist. The position has been described as one that will focus on helping employees change their health behavior. As a part of the interview, the director of human resources asks you this question: "Of all the theories related to health education/promotion you studied in your college courses, which one do you think will have the greatest application to your work here at the Garber Corporation?" Defend your response.

3. You have been given an assignment by one of your college professors to conduct an in-depth study of one of the theories presented in this chapter. Which one would you select? Why?

## ACTIVITIES

1. Interview a practicing health education specialist, asking about the theories and models the person has used in planning and implementing health education/promotion programs. Ask why those theories and models were used. Also, find out if the health education specialist has run into any problems trying to use the theories and models. Summarize the interview in a one-page paper.

2. Choosing and selecting from the components found in the planning models, create your own model. Draw a diagram of your model and, in two paragraphs, explain why you have included the components you did.

3. Pick one of the behavior change theories. Then choose a health behavior. In a one-page paper, explain how the theory can be applied to the health behavior you chose.

## WEBLINKS

1. http://www.naccho.org/topics/infrastructure/mapp/index.cfm

   National Association of County and City Health Officials

   At this Web site, the MAPP model is comprehensively presented and explained. In order to get access to the specifics you have to register. There is no cost to do so.

2. http://www.cdc.gov/healthmarketing/cdcynergy

   Health Marketing at the Centers for Disease Control and Prevention

   This Web site provides an overview of *CDCynergy*, news and updates, information on all editions, current campaigns, practice areas, and resources.

3. http://www.uri.edu/research/cprc/

   Cancer Prevention Research Center (CPRC), University of Rhode Island

   This is the Web site of the CPRC, which is the home of the Transtheoretical Model. Information about the model as well as measures that can be used to "stage" a person can be found at this site.

4. http://people.umass.edu/aizen/tpb.html

   Theory of Planned Behavior

   This is a Web page of Icek Ajzen, creator of the Theory of Planned Behavior. Information about the theory as well as example measures that can be used to measure the constructs of the theory can be found at this site.

5. http://deeps.cancer.gov/cr-reports.html

   National Cancer Institute (NCI), Reports and Reviews

   This is a page at the NCI Web site that presents a number of different reports and reviews. One such publication is the primer *Theory at a Glance: A Guide for Health Promotion Practice*. This volume explains why theories and models are important. It also describes how to use theory. Explanations of several behavior change theories, as well as a couple of program planning models, are included.

6. http://des.emory.edu/mfp/self-efficacy.html#bandura

   Information on Self-Efficacy: A Community of Scholars

   This is a Web page that includes a lot of information about self-efficacy. The information ranges from a definition of self-efficacy to a listing of many publications about self-efficacy.

## REFERENCES

Ajzen, I. (2006). *Theory of planned behavior diagram.* Retrieved August 23, 2010, from: http://www.people.umass.edu/aizen/index.html

Albrecht, T. L. (1997). Defining social marketing: Twenty five years later. *Social Marketing Quarterly, 3,* 21–23.

Andreasen, A. (1995). *Marketing sound change: Changing behavior to promote health, social development, and the environment.* San Francisco: Jossey-Bass.

Bandura, A. (1977). *Social learning theory.* Englewood Cliffs, NJ: Prentice-Hall.

Bandura, A. (1986). *Social foundations of thought and action.* Englewood Cliffs, NJ: Prentice-Hall.

Barnes, J. A. (1954). Class and committees in a Norwegian island parish. *Human Relations, 7,* 39–58.

Bartholomew, L. K., Parcel, G. S., & Kok, G. (1998). Intervention mapping: A process for developing theory- and evidence-based health education programs. *Health Education & Behavior, 25*(5), 545–563.

Bartholomew, L. K., Parcel, G. S., Kok, G., & Gottlieb, N. H. (2006). *Planning health promotion programs: An intervention mapping approach* (2nd ed.). San Francisco: Jossey-Bass.

Bates, I. J., & Winder, A. E. (1984). *Introduction to health education.* Palo Alto, CA: Mayfield.

Bryant, C. (1998). *Social marketing: A tool for excellence.* Eighth annual conference on social marketing in public health. Clearwater Beach, FL.

Centers for Disease Control and Prevention (CDC), U.S. Department of Health and Human Services (USDHHS). (2003). *CDCynergy 3.0: Your Guide to Effective Health Communication* (CD-ROM Version 3.0). Atlanta, GA: Author.

Centers for Disease Control and Prevention. (2000). *Healthy plan-it: A tool for planning and managing public health programs. Sustainable Management Development Program.* Atlanta, GA: Author.

Centers for Disease Control and Prevention (CDC), U.S. Department of Health and Human Services (USDHHS). (n.d.). *Planned approach to community health: Guide for local coordinators.* Atlanta, GA: Author.

Chaplin, J. P., & Krawiec, T. S. (1979). *Systems and theories of psychology* (4th ed.). New York: Holt, Rinehart & Winston.

Champion, V. L., & Skinner, C. S. (2008). The health belief model. In K. Glanz, B. K. Rimer, & K. Viswanath (Eds.), *Health behavior and health education: Theory, research, and practice* (4th ed.) (pp. 45–65). San Francisco, CA: Jossey-Bass.

Crosby, R. A., Kegler, M. C., & DiClemente, R. J. (2009). Theory in health promotion practice and research. In R. J. DiClemente, R. A. Crosby, & M. C. Kegler (Eds.). *Emerging theories in health promotion practice and research* (2nd ed.) (pp. 4–17). San Francisco, CA: Jossey-Bass.

DiClemente, R. J., Crosby, R. A., & Kegler, M. (2009). *Emerging theories in health promotion practice and research* (2nd ed.). San Francisco, CA: Jossey-Bass.

Edberg, M. (2007). *Essentials of health behavior: Social and behavioral theory in public health.* Sudbury, MA: Jones & Bartlett.

Edwards, R. W., Jumper-Thurman, P., Plested, B. A., Oetting, E. R., & Swanson, L. (2000). Community readiness: Research to practice. *Journal of Community Psychology, 28*(3), 291–307.

Eng, E. (1997). *Room with a view for a change.* Keynote address to the annual meeting of the Society for Public Health Education, Indianapolis, IN.

Fishbein, M., & Ajzen, I. (1975). *Belief, attitude, intention and behavior: An introduction to theory and research.* Reading, MA: Addison-Wesley.

Fisher, J. D., & Fisher, W. A. (1992). Changing AIDS risk behavior. *Psychological Bulletin, 111,* 455–474.

Fisher, J. D., Fisher, W. A., & Shuper, P. A. (2009). The informational-motivation-behavioral skills model of HIV preventive behavior. In R. J. DiClemente, R. A. Crosby, & M. C. Kegler (Eds.). *Emerging theories in health promotion practice and research* (2nd ed.) (pp. 21–63). San Francisco, CA: Jossey-Bass.

Gittell, R., & Vidal, A. (1998). *Community organizing: Building social capital as a development strategy.* Thousand Oaks, CA: Sage.

Glanz, K., & Rimer, B. K. (1995). *Theory at a glance: A guide for health promotion practice* (NIH publication no. 95–3896). Bethesda, MD: National Institutes of Health, National Cancer Institute.

Glanz, K., Rimer, B. K., & Viswanath, K. (Eds.). (2008a). *Health behavior and health education: Theory, research, and practice* (4th ed.). San Francisco, CA: Jossey-Bass.

Glanz, K., Rimer, B. K., & Viswanath, K. (2008b). Theory, research, and practice in health behavior and health education. In K. Glanz, B. K. Rimer, & K. Viswanath (Eds.), *Health behavior and health education: Theory, research, and practice* (4th ed.) (pp. 23–40). San Francisco, CA: Jossey-Bass.

Goodson, P. (2010). *Theory in health promotion research and practice: Thinking outside the box.* Sudbury, MA: Jones & Bartlett.

Green, L. W. (1974). Toward cost-benefit evaluations of health education: Some concepts, methods, and examples. *Health Education Monographs, 2*(Suppl. 1), 34–64.

Green, L. W. (1975). Evaluation of patient education programs. Criteria and measurement techniques. *In Rx: Education for the patient: Proceedings of the Continuing Education Institution, Southern Illinois University* (pp. 89–98). Carbondale, IL: Southern Illinois University Press.

Green, L. W. (1976). Methods available to evaluate the health education components of preventive health programs. In *Preventive Medicine, USA* (pp. 162–171). New York: Prodist.

Green, L. W. (1979). National policy on the promotion of health. *International Journal of Health Education, 22*, 161–168.

Green, L. W. (1980). Healthy people: The surgeon general's report and the prospects. In W. J. McNervey (Ed.), *Working for a healthier America* (pp. 95–110). Cambridge, MA: Ballinger.

Green, L. W. (1981a). Emerging federal perspectives on health promotion. In J. P. Allegrante (Ed.), *Health promotion monographs.* New York: Teachers College, Columbia University.

Green, L. W. (1981b). The objectives for the nation in disease prevention and health promotion: A challenge to health education training. In *Proceedings of the National Conference for Institutions Preparing Health Educators* (DHHS Publication No. 81–50171) (pp. 61–73). Washington, DC: U.S. Office of Health Information and Health Promotion.

Green, L. W. (1982). Reconciling policy in health education and primary care. *International Journal of Health Education, 24* (Suppl. 3), 1–11.

Green, L. W. (1983a). New policies in education for health. *World Health* (April/May), 13–17.

Green, L. W. (1983b). *New policies for health education in primary health care* (Background document for the technical discussions of the 36th World Health Assembly, May 1983). Geneva: World Health Organization.

Green, L. W. (1984a). La educación para la salud en el medio urbano. In *Conferencia InterAmericana de Educación Para La Salud* (pp. 80–82). Mexico City: Sector Salud, SEP, and International Union for Health Education and World Health Organization.

Green, L. W. (1984b). Health education models. In J. D. Matarazzo, S. M. Weiss, & J. A. Herd (Eds.), *Behavioral health: A handbook of health enhancement and disease prevention* (pp. 181–198). New York: Wiley.

Green, L. W. (1984c). Modifying and developing health behavior. *Annual Review of Public Health, 5*, 215–236.

Green, L. W. (1984d). A triage and stepped approach to self-care education. *Medical Times, 111*, 75–80.

Green, L. W. (1986a, October). *Applications and trials of the PRECEDE framework for planning and evaluation of health programs.* Paper presented at the meeting of the American Public Health Association, Las Vegas, NV.

Green, L. W. (1986b). Evaluation model: A framework for the design of rigorous evaluation of efforts in health promotion. *American Journal of Health Promotion, 1*(1), 77–79.

Green, L. W. (1986c). *New policies for health education in primary health care.* Geneva: World Health Organization.

Green, L. W. (1986d). Research agenda: Building a consensus on research questions. *American Journal of Health Promotion, 1*(2), 70–72.

Green, L. W. (1986e). The theory of participation: A qualitative analysis of its expression in national and international health policies. In W. B. Ward (Ed.), *Advances in health education and promotion* (pp. 211–236). Greenwich, CT: JAI Press.

Green, L. W. (1987a). How physicians can improve patients' participation and maintenance in self-care. *Western Journal of Medicine, 147*, 346–349.

Green, L. W. (1987b). *Program planning and evaluation guide for lung associations.* New York: American Lung Association.

Green, L. W., & Allen, J. (1980). *Toward a healthy community: Organizing events for community health promotion* (PHS Publication No. 80–50113). Washington, DC: USDHHS, Office of Disease Prevention and Health Promotion.

Green, L. W., Glanz, K., Hochbaum, G. M., Kok, G., Kreuter, M. W., Lewis, F. M., Lorig, K., Morisky, D., Rimer, B. K., & Rosenstock, I. M. (1994). Can we build on, or must we replace, the theories and models in health education? *Health Education Research, 9*(3), 397–404.

Green, L. W., & Kreuter, M. W. (2005). *Health program planning: An educational and ecological approach.* (4th ed.) Boston, MA: McGraw-Hill.

Green, L. W., Kreuter, M. W., Deeds, S. G., & Partridge, K. B. (1980). *Health education planning: A diagnostic approach.* Palo Alto, CA: Mayfield.

Green, L. W., Levine, D. M., & Deeds, S. G. (1975). Clinical trials of health education for hypertensive outpatients: Design and baseline data. *Preventive Medicine, 4*, 417–425.

Green, L. W., & McAlister, A. L. (1984). Macro-intervention to support health behavior: Some theoretical perspectives and practical reflections. *Health Education Quarterly, 11*, 323–339.

Green, L. W., Mullen, P. D., & Friedman, R. (1986). An epidemiological approach to targeting drug information. *Patient Education and Counseling, 8*, 255–268.

Green, L. W., Wang, V. L., Deeds, S. G., Fisher, A. A., Windsor, R., & Rogers, C. (1978). Guidelines for health education in maternal and child health programs. *International Journal of Health Education, 21*(suppl.), 1–33.

Green, L. W., Wilson, A. L., & Lovato, C. Y. (1986). What changes can health promotion achieve and how long do these changes last? The tradeoffs between expediency and durability. *Preventive Medicine, 15*, 508–521.

Green, L. W., Wilson, R. W., & Bauer, K. G. (1983). Data required to measure progress on the objectives for the nation in disease prevention and health promotion. *American Journal of Public Health, 73*, 18–24.

Hayden, J. (2009). *Introduction to health behavior theory.* Sudbury, MA: Jones & Bartlett.

Heaney, C. A., & Israel, B. A. (2008). Social networks and social support. In K. Glanz, B. K. Rimer, & K. Viswanath (Eds.), *Health behavior and health education: Theory, research, and practice* (4th ed.) (pp. 189–210). San Francisco, CA: Jossey-Bass.

Institute of Medicine (IOM). (2001). *Health and behavior: The interplay of biological, behavioral, and societal influences.* Washington, DC: National Academy of Sciences.

Kawachi, I., Kennedy, B. P., Lochner, K., & Prothrow-Stith, D. (1997). Social capital, oncome, equality, and mortality. *American Journal of Public Health, 87*(9), 1491–1497.

Kerlinger, F. N. (1986). *Foundations of behavioral research* (3rd ed.). Austin, TX: Holt, Rinehart & Winston.

Luszczynska, A., & Sutton, S. (2005). Attitudes and expectations. In J. Kerr, R. Weitkunat, & M. Moretti (Eds.), *ABC of behavior change: A guide to successful disease prevention and health promotion* (pp. 71–84). Edinburgh: Elsevier.

McAlister, A. L., Perry, C. L., & Parcel, G. S. (2008). How individual, environments, and health behaviors interact: Social cognitive theory. In K. Glanz, B. K. Rimer, & K. Viswanath (Eds.),

*Health behavior and health education: Theory, research, and practice* (4th ed.) (pp. 169–188). San Francisco, CA: Jossey-Bass.

McDermott, R. J. (2000). Social marketing: A tool for health education. *American Journal of Health Behavior, 24*(1), 6–10.

McKenzie, J. F., Neiger, B. L., & Thackeray, R. (2009). *Planning, implementing, and evaluating health promotion programs: A primer* (5th ed.). San Francisco: Benjamin Cummings.

McLeroy, K. R., Bibeau, D., Steckler, A., & Glanz, K. (1988). An ecological perspective for health promotion programs. *Health Education Quarterly, 15*(4), 351–378.

Minkler, M., & Wallerstein, N. (2005). Improving health through community organization and community building: A health education perspective. In M. Minkler (Ed.), *Community organizing and community building for health* (2nd ed.) (pp. 26–50). New Brunswick, NJ: Rutgers University Press.

Minkler, M., Wallerstein, N., & Wilson, N. (2008). Improving health through community organization and community building. In K. Glanz, B. K. Rimer, & K. Viswanath (Eds.), *Health behavior and health education: Theory, research, and practice* (4th ed.) (pp. 287–312). San Francisco, CA: Jossey-Bass.

National Association of County and City Health Officials (NACCHO). (2001). *Mobilizing for action through planning and partnerships (MAPP)*. Washington, DC: Author.

National Association of County Health Officials (NACHO). (1991). *APEX/PH, Assessment protocol for excellence in public health*. Washington, DC: Author.

National Cancer Institute (NCI). (2002). *Making health communication programs work* (NIH Publication No. 02-5145). Washington, DC: U.S. Department of Health and Human Services (USDHHS).

Neiger, B. L., & Thackeray R. (1998). *Social marketing: Making public health sense*. Paper presented at the annual meeting of the Utah Public Health Association. Provo, UT.

Neiger, B. L., & Thackeray, R. (2002). Application of the SMART model in two successful social marketing campaigns. *American Journal of Health Education, 33*, 291–293.

Parcel, G. S. (1983). Theoretical models for application in school health research. *Health Education, 15*(4), 39–49.

Parvanta, C. F., & Freimuth, V. (2000). Health communication at the Centers for Disease Control and Prevention. *American Journal of Health Behavior, 24*(1), 18–25.

Patton, R. P., Corry, J. M., Gettman, L. R., & Graff, J. S. (1986). *Implementing health/ fitness programs*. Champaign, IL: Human Kinetics.

Petty, R. E., Barden, J., & Wheeler, S. C. (2009). The elaboration likelihood model of persuasion: Developing health promotions for sustained behavioral change. In R. J. DiClemente, R. A. Crosby, & M. C. Kegler (Eds.). *Emerging theories in health promotion practice and research* (2nd ed.) (pp. 185–214). San Francisco, CA: Jossey-Bass.

Petty, R. E., & Cacioppo, J. T. (1986). The elaboration likelihood model of persuasion. In L. Berkowitz (Ed.). *Advances in experimental social psychology* (Vol. 19, pp. 123–205). New York, NY: Academic Press.

Prochaska, J. (2005). Stages of change, readiness, and motivation. In J. Kerr, R. Weitkunat, & M. Moretti (Eds.), *ABC of behavior change: A guide to successful disease prevention and health promotion* (pp. 111–123). Edinburgh: Elsevier.

Prochaska, J. O. (1979). *Systems of psychotherapy: A transtheoretical analysis*. Homewood, IL: Dorsey Press.

Prochaska, J. O., & DiClemente, C. C. (1983). Stages and processes of self-change of smoking: Toward an integrative model of change. *Journal of Consulting and Clinical Psychology, 51*(3), 390–395.

Prochaska, J. O., Johnson, S., & Lee, P. (1998). The transtheoretical model of behavior change. In S. A. Shumaker, E. B. Schron, J. K. Ockene, & W. L. McBee (Eds.), *The handbook of health behavior change* (2nd ed.) (pp. 59–84). New York: Springer Publishing Company.

Prochaska, J. O, Redding, C. A., & Evers, K. E. (2008). The transtheoretical model and stages of change. In K. Glanz, B. K. Rimer, & K. Viswanath (Eds.), *Health behavior and health education: Theory, research, and practice* (4th ed.) (pp. 97–121). San Francisco, CA: Jossey-Bass.

Prochaska, J. O., Redding, C. A., Harlow, L. L., Rossi, J. S., & Velicer, W. F. (1994). The transtheoretical model of change and HIV prevention: A review. *Health Education Quarterly, 24*(4), 471–486.

Putman, R. D. (1995). Bowling alone: America's declining social capital. *Journal of Democracy, 6*(1), 65–78.

Redding, C. A., Rossi, J. S., Rossi, S. R., Velicer, W. F., & Prochaska, J. O. (1999). Health behavior models. In G. C. Hyner, K. W. Peterson, J. W. Travis, J. E. Dewey, J. J. Foerster, & E. M. Framer (Eds.), *SPM handbook of health assessment tools* (pp. 83–93). Pittsburgh, PA: The Society of Prospective Medicine.

Rimer, B. K., & Glanz, K. (2005). *Theory at a glance: A guide for health promotion practice* (2nd ed.). [NIH Pub. No. 05-3896]. Washington, DC: National Cancer Institute.

Rogers, E. M. (2003). *Diffusion of innovations* (5th ed.). New York: Free Press.

Rosenstock, I. M. (1966). Why people use health services. *Milbank Memorial Fund Quarterly, 44,* 94–124.

Rosenstock, I. M., Strecher, V. J., & Becker, M. H. (1988). Social learning theory and the health belief model. *Health Education Quarterly, 15*(2), 175–183.

Ross, H. S., & Mico, P. R. (1980). *Theory and practice in health education.* San Francisco: Mayfield.

Rotter, J. B. (1954). *Social learning and clinical psychology.* New York: Prentice-Hall.

Schwarzer, R. (2001). Social-cognitive factors in changing health-related behaviors. *Current Directions in Psychological Science, 10,* 47–51.

Sharma, M., & Romas, J. A. (2012). *Theoretical foundations of health education and health promotion* (2nd ed.). Sudbury, MA: Jones & Bartlett.Simons-Morton, B. G., Greene, W. H., & Gottlieb, N. H. (1995). *Introduction to health education and health promotion* (2nd ed.). Prospect Hts., IL: Waveland Press, Inc.

Simons-Morton, D. G., Simons-Morton, B. G., Parcel, G. S., & Bunker, J. F. (1988). Influencing personal and environmental conditions for community health: A multilevel intervention model. *Family and Community Health, 1*(2), 25–35.

Spencer, L., Adams, T. B., Malone, S., Roy, L., & Yost, E. (2006). Applying the transtheoretical model to exercise: A systematic and comprehensive review of the literature. *Health Promotion Practice, 7*(4), 428–443.

Sullivan, D. (1973). Model for comprehensive, systematic program development in health education. *Health Education Report, 1*(1), (November/December), 4–5.

Timmreck, T. C. (2003). *Planning, program development, and evaluation* (2nd ed.). Boston: Jones & Bartlett.

Timmreck, T. C., Cole, G. E., James, G., & Butterworth, D. D. (2010). Health education and health promotion: A look at the jungle of supportive fields. Philosophies, and theoretical foundations. In J. M. Black, S. Furney, H. M. Graf, & A. E. Nolt (Eds.), *Philosophical foundations of health education* (pp. 67–78). San Francisco, CA: Jossey-Bass.

U.K. Office of National Statistics, Social Analysis and Reporting Division. (2001). Social capital: A review of the literature. Retrieved August 26, 2010, from http://www.statistics.gov.uk

U.S. Department of Health and Human Services (USDHHS). (2001). *Healthy people in health communities: A community planning guide using Healthy People 2010.* Washington, DC: Author.

Walsh, D. C., Rudd, R. E., Moeykens, B. A., & Moloney, T. W. (1993). Social marketing for public health. *Health Affairs, 12,* 104–119.

Warren, M. R., Thompson, J. P., & Saegert, S. (2001). The role of social capital in combating poverty. In S. Saegert, J. P. Thompson, & M. R. Warren (Eds.). *Social capital and poor communities* (pp. 1–28). New York, NY: Sage Foundation.

Weinstein, N. D. (1988). The precaution adoption process. *Health Psychology, 7,* 355–386.

Weinstein, N. D., Rothman, A. J., & Sutton, S. R. (1998). Stage theories of health behavior: Conceptual and methodological issues. *Health Psychology, 17,* 290–299.

Weinstein, N. D., & Sandman, P. M. (2002). The precaution adoption process model and its application. In R. J. DiClemente, R. A. Crosby, & M. C. Kegler (Eds.), *Emerging theories in health promotion practice and research: Strategies for improving public health* (pp. 16–39). San Francisco: Jossey-Bass.

Weinstein, N. D., Sandman, P. M., & Blalock, S. J. (2008). The precaution adoption process model. In K. Glanz, B. K. Rimer, & K. Viswanath (Eds.), *Health behavior and health education: Theory, research, and practice* (4th ed.) (pp. 123–147). San Francisco, CA: Jossey-Bass.

## CHAPTER 5

# Ethics and Health Education/Promotion

After reading this chapter and answering the questions at the end, you should be able to:

- Identify and define the three major areas of philosophy.
- Define *ethics*.
- Explain the difference between ethics and morality.
- Explain why it is important to act ethically.
- Define *professional ethics*.
- Explain and briefly describe the two major categories of ethical theories.
- Identify principles that create a common ground for all ethical theories.
- Outline a guide for making ethical decisions.
- Identify ethical issues associated with the profession of health education/promotion.
- Explain how a profession can ensure that its professionals will act ethically.
- Define *code of ethics* and identify the source of the code available for health education specialists.

In recent years, there has been an increasing interest in ethical questions in all walks of life. The interest has become so great that it is difficult to avoid the topic of ethics in everyday living. Newspapers and television networks are constantly covering stories that involve ethical issues, many of which are related to health. Examples include genetic engineering, abortion, the right to die, nuclear waste storage, the marketing of harmful products such as tobacco in developing countries, the reduction of welfare benefits, health research, appropriate sexual behavior, and professional behavior, to name a few.

How is it that we determine what is ethical or unethical? By whose standards do we make such judgments? To answer these questions requires some background and perspective. In this chapter, we will provide the background and perspective to understand how ethics relates to the profession of health education/promotion. First, we will present key terms that relate to the study of ethics and examine the origin of ethics. Next we look at reasons why people should work from an ethical base. We will then briefly look at the theories used to create ethical "yardsticks" and how these theories can be used to make ethical decisions. Within this context, a sampling of ethical issues facing health education specialists today will be presented. Finally, we conclude with a discussion on how a profession, or an emerging profession, can ensure that its professionals will act ethically.

## Key Terms and Origin

**Ethics,** the study of morality (Morrison, 2006), is one of the three major areas of philosophy. The other two are **epistemology,** the study of knowledge, and **metaphysics,** the study of the nature of reality (Thiroux, 1995). Ethics, or **moral philosophy** as it is often stated, dates back two thousand plus years to Socrates (470–399 B.C.), "the ancient Greek philosopher, who spent his days in the Athenian marketplace challenging people to think about how they lived" (White, 1988, p. 7). Though philosophers do not sit in the marketplace (or malls) today to challenge people, the behavior, actions, and values of people are constantly being examined for their appropriateness.

You will note that the word *ethics* was described using the words *moral* and *morality*. "'Ethics' and 'morals' come to us from two words in ancient Greek and Latin, *ethos* and *mores;* both mean 'character.' When we ask if an action is ethical, we can think, 'Is it the sort of thing somebody with a 'good character' would do?'" (White, 1988, p. 8.). Sperry (2007) has made a distinction between morality and ethics saying that morality "is the activity of making choices and of deciding, judging, justifying, and defending those actions or behaviors called moral," whereas ethics is "the science of how choices are made or should be made" (p. 38). Pigg (2010) has stated that "*ethics* defines acceptable and unacceptable behavior within the norms of a particular group" (pp. 11–12), while "*morality* sets standards for right and wrong in human behavior" (p. 12). Nevertheless, to avoid confusion throughout the rest of this chapter, we will use **ethical** and **moral** to mean the same thing. "The important thing to remember here is that moral, ethical, immoral, and unethical, essentially mean, good, right, bad, and wrong, often depending on whether one is referring to people themselves or to their actions" (Thiroux, 1995, p. 3).

White (1988) refers to the words *good, right, bad,* and *wrong* as the labels people use when making ethical judgments about human actions. Some authors have used these words to define ethics. Feeney and Freeman (1999) state, "Ethics is the study of right and wrong, duty and obligation" (p. 5). "It is a discipline practiced by everyone who ever wondered, 'why should I do this rather than that?'" (Mellert, 1995, p. 2). Penland and Beyrer (1981, p. 6) defined ethics as "the study of rightness and wrongness in human conduct." "Acting 'ethically' is connected *with* what a person is doing and *how* he or she is doing it" (White, 1988, p. 8).

## Why Should People Act Ethically?

Because ethics is one of the three major areas of philosophy, a philosophical answer to the question of why people should act ethically is that to act ethically brings meaning or purpose to the life of an individual (McGrath, 1994). It provides a standard by which to live. Ethical living, in turn, provides for a better society for all. It is the right thing to do for society and self.

From a more personal viewpoint, observation has shown "that those who are ethical tend to lead healthier (both physically and psychologically), more emotionally satisfying lives" (McGrath, 1994, p. 131). "In fact, the ethical life promises rewards for everyone involved. Your friends and associates will obviously feel better about life and about you if you treat them decently. And they'll probably reciprocate, treating you the same way, which will make your life better" (White, 1988, pp. 84–85). In short, the ethical person is more mature, stronger, healthier, and more advanced and has a more fully developed personality than those who are not ethical (White, 1988).

From a professional viewpoint, those who implement community interventions (including health education specialists) have much to gain from ethical behavior. Rabinowitz (2010) has noted that it makes their programs more effective; it cements their standing in the community; it allows them to occupy the moral high ground when arguing the merits of their programs, and to exercise moral leadership in the community; and it assures that they remain in good standing legally and professionally.

## Professional Ethics

Whereas personal values and morality may guide us in our everyday living, it is important to note that they may not be sufficient to guide our professional behavior. People come to their work with different personal experiences. Because of these different experiences, they do not hold the same values nor have they learned the same moral lessons. Even those who hold the same beliefs may not apply them in the same way in a professional setting (Feeney & Freeman, 1999). Thus, in a work setting, individuals are guided by professional ethics. **Professional ethics** focuses on the "actions that are right and wrong in the workplace and are of public matter. Professional moral principles are not statements of taste or preference; they tell practitioners what they ought to do and what they ought not do" (Feeney & Freeman, 1999, p. 6).

Ethical behavior is expected from professionals. "'Ethics' delineates what we consider acceptable and unacceptable conduct regarding professional practice in Health Science education. Ethical conduct is particularly important to professional health educators, since we belong to a profession with a mission to serve the individual" (Pigg, 1994, p. iii). Health education/promotion is a profession with much human interaction. Dorman (1994) adds, "As writers, reviewers, and scientists we must insist on the highest of ethical practices in publication and research. As practitioners, we must seek to actively practice ethical behavior in our service and teaching. Individually, we must aspire for a reputation which reflects a life of personal integrity. The wisdom of King Solomon probably puts it best: *'A good name is more desirable than great riches; to be esteemed is better than silver or gold'*" (p. 4). Or, as Pigg (2006) stated when he summarized the lesson on integrity he learned from observing his father throughout life, "When fame and fortune fade, only our reputations remain as important but fragile reflections of our true nature" (p. 41).

Within the larger realm of *professional ethics* there may be some subsets of ethical behavior that are specific to certain tasks of the professional. For example, among the seven responsibilities of health education specialists is Responsibility IV "Conduct Evaluation and Research Related to Health Education" (NCHEC, 2010) (see the discussion of the responsibilities in Chapter 6). In order to conduct evaluation and research, health education specialists need to be aware not only of appropriate general professional ethics but also of ethical behavior as it relates to the evaluation and research processes. Such behavior falls under the area of *research ethics*. **Research ethics** "comprises principles and standards that, along with underlying values, guide appropriate conduct relevant to research decisions" (Kimmel, 2007, p. 6). An ethical principle associated with the research process is the concept of voluntary participation. That is, potential research participants should not be forced or coerced into participating in a research study, but rather should do so on a voluntary basis.

## Ethical Theories

Philosophers do not speak with a common voice about the standards of morality. Depending on the ethical theory espoused, one philosopher may see a certain behavior as moral or ethical, while another may see the same behavior as immoral or unethical. For example, one philosopher may see corporal punishment as a moral action to punish a person for murder, while the other sees the taking of another life, for whatever reason, as immoral. The purpose of this section is not to present a detailed description of ethical theories—that has been done elsewhere—but to categorize and summarize the better-known theories (see **Table 5.1**) and to suggest ways by which their content can be applied to health education/promotion practice.

Ethical theories provide frameworks whereby health education specialists and others are able to evaluate whether human actions are acceptable (Shive & Marks, 2006). The primary means by which ethical theories have been categorized has been to place them in the category of deontology (**formalism,** or **nonconsequentialism,** as some refer to it) or teleology (or **consequentialism** as some refer to it) theories. **Deontological theories** (from Greek *deontos,* 'of the obligatory') "are those that claim that certain actions are inherently right or wrong, or good or bad, without regard for their consequences" (Reamer, 2006, p. 65). For example, a deontologist would argue that lying to a client or patient is wrong even if it is done to help that person. According to this theory, the mere act of lying is wrong, regardless of the benefits it may bring. "What is moral or immoral is decided on some standard or standards of morality other than consequences" (Thiroux, 1995, p. 84)—that is to say, the end (the consequences) *does not* justify the means (the act).

**Teleological theories** (from Greek *teleios,* 'brought to its end purpose'), on the other hand, evaluate the moral status of an act by the goodness of the consequences (Reamer, 2006). If the act produces good or happiness, it is morally okay; if it does not, it is

**Table 5.1**    Summary of ethical theories

| Category | Primary Reasoning | Examples of Such Theories |
|---|---|---|
| Deontology (also known as formalism or nonconsequentialism) | The end does not justify the means. | Natural law morality, deontological ethics, existentialism |
| Teleology (also known as consequentialism) | The end does justify the means. | Contractarian ethics, utilitarianism, pragmatism |

immoral. Using the same example of lying to a patient/client, if the consequences turned out okay, the consequentialist would see this act as morally okay. In short, this category of ethical theories states that the end *does* justify the means.

As can be seen from these descriptions of formalism and consequentialism, the primary point of contention is whether or not the means justify the end. "The ethical question in both systems is: 'What is the right thing to do?'" (Tschudin, 2003, p. 47). "Is there a way to reconcile these two approaches to ethics, or must we simply make a choice between them?" (Mellert, 1995, p. 133). Most people would say that neither category of ethical theory can answer all moral questions in their lives. In fact, Summers (2009) has stated, "humans have yet to develop an ethical theory that will satisfactorily handle all issues" (p. 56). There are times when deontology provides guidance for the ethical way to act, while teleology is best in other situations. What this means is that each person must carefully study the ethical theory options, combine what is compatible and resolve what is inconsistent in those options, and attempt to work out a moral consensus for herself and society (Mellert, 1995). This is not an easy process. Many times, philosophical questions and problems are abstract or conceptual in nature. For example, is there ever a time when it is okay for a health education specialist to lie to his supervisor? Such questions are answered through philosophical thought, using reason, logic, and argument. Thus, the most important tool people can use to find these answers is the mind.

When analyzing an ethical problem, people need to depend more on thinking than feeling—using their minds and not their hearts (White, 1988). For example, if a person says, "I feel that abortion, no matter when it occurs, is morally wrong," that person is really saying there is something about abortion that makes her uneasy, unhappy, or distressed. This person is expressing a feeling, not a moral position. This person's feelings would be better stated if she were to say, "Abortion makes me feel upset." However, if a person states that abortion is immoral, then she should be prepared to provide specific reasons for holding this belief (White, 1988). For example, she may hold the belief that life begins at conception, and having an abortion is ending the life of another human being. It is for these reasons that answering ethical questions is a thinking, not a feeling, process. Or, as Penland and Beyrer (1981) have stated, "If ethics is to have personal meaning it demands thoughtful examination. The answers to ethical questions are found by looking within, examining our personal belief systems and values, and using our intelligence to integrate what we have learned and what we have experienced with what we believe and value" (p. 6).

## Basic Principles for Common Moral Ground

As was shown in the previous section, deontoloists and teleologists are not in agreement when it comes to the rationale to be used in making moral decisions. No single ethical theory can answer every ethical question to the satisfaction of all, yet, to live in a moral society, all must be able to work from a common moral ground. "We must search for a larger meeting ground in which the best of all these theories and systems can operate meaningfully with a minimum of conflict and opposition" (Thiroux, 1995, p. 172).

To help us with this common ground, Thiroux (1995) has identified five basic principles that can apply to human morality, regardless of the embraced theory. The principles do not provide the answers to how one should behave, but rather "help to direct the thinking towards achieving a consensus on what ought to be done in difficult circumstances" (Tschudin, 2003, p. 51). The first is the **value of life** principle. This is the most basic of principles. Without living human beings, there can be no ethics. Thiroux (1995) has specifically stated this principle as "human beings should revere life and accept death" (p. 180). This means that no life should be ended without very strong justification. This, for example, is why topics such as abortion, suicide, euthanasia, and capital punishment raise a number of ethical questions.

The second is the principle of **goodness (rightness)**. "Good" and "right" are at the core of every ethical theory. Theorists may disagree on what is good and bad and right and wrong, but they all strive for goodness and rightness. "'Good' should not only be in abstract, but it should be seen in relation to (other) human beings. As an example, a person who is suicidal may no longer value his or her life as 'good,' but that person's mother may have a very different concept of the value of her child's life" (Tschudin, 2003, p. 56).

The principle of goodness includes two parallel principles of ethics: (1) the principle of **nonmaleficence** and (2) the principle of **beneficence**, or **benevolence**. "Briefly, nonmaleficence refers to the non infliction of harm to others. The principle involves a moral obligation to 'above else, do no harm.' It encompasses bringing intentional harm to others as well as the risk of bringing harm that is non-intentional. It also encompasses harm which may result from both action and inaction—acts of omission and commission" (Balog et al., 1985, p. 91). Further, nonmaleficence can "be broken into three components: not inflicting harm, preventing harm, and removing harm when it is present" (Greenberg, 2001, p. 3). Though the concepts presented in this explanation of nonmaleficence are seemingly straightforward, the application of the concepts can be difficult. For example, what is meant by harm? Are there degrees of harm like "a little harm" and "a lot of harm"? Must an action produce no harm to be acceptable from an ethical point of view? These are difficult questions to answer and make some situations difficult to respond to in an ethical way.

"Beneficence means simply doing good. It holds that we have the responsibility for taking positive steps to help others, including acts that involve doing good, removing evil and/or harm, and preventing harm or evil. Beneficence is generally thought to be more altruistic and more far reaching than nonmaleficence because it requires that we take positive steps to help others" (Balog et al., 1985, pp. 91–92). In the bioethical realm, nonmaleficence and beneficence make up the "benefit-harm ratio" in which, ideally, benefits outweigh costs and in which the "minimization of harm" rather than the "maximation of good" is more strongly emphasized (Fox & Swazey, 1997).

Thiroux's third principle is the principle of **justice (fairness)**. This principle deals with people treating other people fairly and justly in distributing goodness (benefits) and badness (burdens) (Summers 2009; Thiroux, 1995). Justice can be examined in two ways— (1) *procedural* and (2) *distributive* (Summers, 2009). **Procedural justice** deals with whether or not fair procedures were in place and whether those procedures were followed, while **distributive justice** deals with the allocation of resources (Summers, 2009). Does this mean that all people will always get their fair share of goodness and badness? No, but it does mean everyone will have an equal chance at obtaining the good (Thiroux, 1995). "The bottom line is that one has indeed acted justly toward a person when that person has been given what she or he is due or owed" (Balog et al., 1985, p. 90).

"The ethical questions are: Who should receive the benefits from good human actions and how should they be distributed?" (Tschudin, 2003, p. 57). For example, should only those who are able to pay for them receive health education/promotion services, or should only the poor shoulder all of the burden?

The fourth principle of this common moral ground is that of **truth telling (honesty)**. At the heart of any moral relationship is communication. A necessary component of any meaningful communication is telling the truth, being honest. This may be the most difficult principle to live by. This is not to say that people will never lie or that lying might be justified, but there is a need for a strong attempt to be truthful. In the end, morality depends on what people say and do (Thiroux, 1995). Health education specialists working in a clinical setting may be faced with this principle when caught in a situation in which an ill child (and a minor by law) asks about his or her health problem, but the child's parent or guardian has strictly forbidden such communication.

The fifth principle is that of **individual freedom (equality principle** or **principle of autonomy)**. (See **Figure 5.1**.) "The word *autonomy* comes from the Greek words *autos* ('self') and *nomos* ('rule,' 'governance,' or 'law') and originally referred to as self-governance in Greek city-states" (Greenberg, 2001, p. 3). "This principle means that people, being individuals with individual differences, must have the freedom to choose their own ways and means of being moral within the framework of the first four basic principles" (Thiroux, 1995, p. 187). This is to say that individual freedom is limited by the other four principles. Underlying the principle "of autonomy is the idea that we are to respect others for who they are" (Summers, 2009, p. 44). This is a principle that health education specialists deal with on a regular basis, specifically as it relates to helping others engage in enhancing health behavior. Health education specialists need to respect the rights of others to deliberate, choose, and act (Balog et al., 1985).

With the grounding of the ethical theories and the establishment of these basic principles, let us examine the process of making ethical decisions.

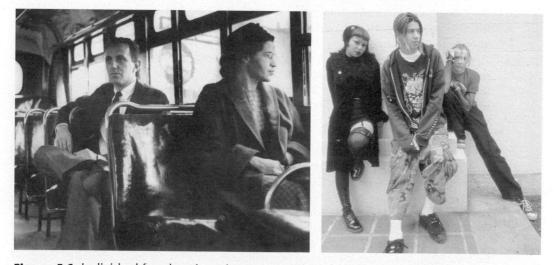

**Figure 5.1** Individual freedom is an important principle of human morality.
(l. Corbis; r. Michael Newman/PhotoEdit)

## Making Ethical Decisions

"Ethical decision making in health education, as in other areas, involves determining right and wrong within situations where clear demarcations do not exist or are not clearly apparent to the decision maker. . . . To be considered a professional health educator, one must possess requisite skill and knowledge in making individual decisions. And, in making decisions it is imperative that one has analyzed his or her decisions in terms of standards of right and wrong, good and bad" (Balog et al., 1985, p. 88). In order to decide and, in turn, act in an ethical manner, people must rely on their values, principles, and ethical thinking. To assist in this process, a number of authors (e.g., Balog et al., 1985; Fisher, 2003; Mellert, 1995; Reamer, 2006; Remley & Herlihy, 2007; Svara, 2007; Thompson, Melia, & Boyd, 2000) have presented guides for applying the concepts presented earlier in this chapter to everyday ethical decision making. Though the number of steps and labels used to identify the steps are different from guide to guide, they "have in common a process of moving from the present problematic to a future more satisfactory situation" (Tschudin, 2003, p. 111). Because of the limitation of space, we are presenting a single approach (see **Figure 5.2**) to ethical decision making that blends the ideas and is representative of these guides.

The ethical decision-making process should begin long before any ethical problems surface. The process begins when a person develops and sustains a professional commitment to doing what is right (Fisher, 2003). Such a commitment will go a long way toward creating a work environment that can prevent many ethical problems. This is not to say that all ethical problems will be avoided. Ethical problems can arise in situations

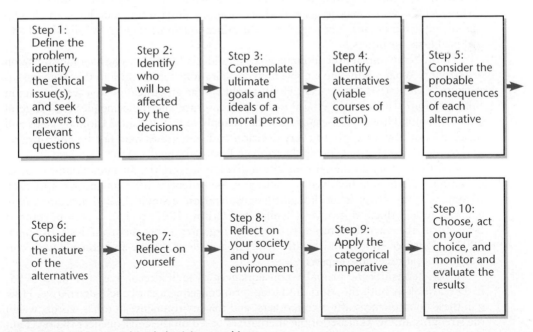

**Figure 5.2** Steps in ethical decision making

*Sources:* Adapted from: Balog et al., (1985); Mellert (1995); Reamer (2006); Remley & Herlihy (2007); Svara, (2007).

in which two or more ethical principles appear to be in conflict, in unforeseen reactions from those with whom health education specialist may work, or in unexpected events (Fisher, 2003). However, having a commitment to doing what is right becomes a form of "primary prevention" for many ethical problems.

Closely aligned with a commitment to doing what is right, is familiarity with what the health education/promotion profession expects of practicing professionals. Stated differently, what are the expected norms for those who practice health education/promotion? Such expectations can be found in the profession's code of ethics. With a commitment to doing what is right and knowing what is expected of a practicing health education specialists are enhancing their *moral sensitivity*. Rest and colleagues (1999) have explained **moral sensitivity** as being aware that an ethical problem exists and having an understanding of what impact different courses of action may have on the people involved.

The first step to take when confronted with an ethical decision is to define the problem/concern, identify the ethical issue(s), clarify the facts, and seek answers to relevant questions (Mellert, 1995; Reamer, 2006; Remley & Herlihy, 2007; Svara, 2007). This first step is one of clarification and gathering relevant information. Several questions need to be answered. What is the problem/concern that makes you believe there is an ethical decision to be made? Is it indeed an ethical dilemma? Is there a legal question that needs to be answered? What do you know? What do you need to find out? Does a decision have to be made? If so, by when, and in what context? Are these decisions within the realm of your authority, or does someone else with other responsibilities/authority/resources determine them?

Second, identify the individuals, groups, and organizations that are likely to be affected by this ethical decision (Reamer, 2006) and what stakes they have in the outcome (Svara, 2007). When making an ethical decision, it is important to understand all who will be impacted because one solution to the ethical dilemma may create additional ethical problems for others.

Third, "contemplate the ultimate goals and ideals for which you as a moral person are striving. What are the most noble human aspirations that pertain to this concrete situation?" (Mellert, 1995, p. 156). How should you as an ethical person want to act in this situation? Consider the ethical theory you embrace and the principles for common ethical ground. How do these goals and ideals apply to this decision? Ultimate goals and ideals do not always apply to every decision and sometimes may not be appropriate, but, to the extent that they do apply, let them help with the decision.

Fourth, identify all the possible alternatives to solving the dilemma (viable courses of action), the people involved in each, and the potential benefits and risks of each (Reamer, 2006). "Even after thoughtful consideration, a single desired outcome rarely emerges in an ethical dilemma" (Remley & Herlihy, 2007, p. 13). It is important to brainstorm the various alternatives to help organize subsequent analysis (Reamer, 2006). Consider ethical and health theories, a code of ethics, and consult with colleagues and, if necessary, experts.

Fifth, "consider the probable consequences of each alternative" (Mellert, 1995, p. 157). Look at both the short- and long-term consequences of each alternative. How will these consequences affect you, others, and the environment? In other words, weigh the strengths and weaknesses of the alternatives based on the consequences (Balog et al., 1985). Maybe the consequences are very different, or maybe they are not and, thus, may not be important in the final decision.

Sixth, "consider the nature of the alternatives" (Mellert, 1995, p. 157). Consider the deontologist approach to the decision-making process in selecting an alternative. Does the alternative lead to an act or a behavior that is wrong, according to the natural law hypothesis? Would you be violating anyone's basic rights? Does it go against basic human ideals and intrinsic moral values? If you answer yes to these questions, you do not need to eliminate the alternative from further consideration but should give greater consideration to alternatives that do not violate this portion of your reflection.

Seventh, "reflect on yourself" (Mellert, 1995, p. 157). What impact will a proposed course of action have on you as a moral person? Will it enhance or detract from your moral stature? If it detracts, then maybe other alternatives should be considered. If you cannot accept a course of action "as part of your inner self and as data for your own moral growth, then there must be something morally questionable about it" (Mellert, 1995, pp. 157–158). Although you may be striving to be objective as you work toward a decision, be aware that your emotions will also play a part. Your emotions will influence your judgment and may help guide you in your decision making (Remley & Herlihy, 2007).

Eighth, "reflect on your society and your environment" (Mellert, 1995, p. 158). Will your action mesh with that of society and the environment? Moral acts are unselfish acts in that they do not prefer one's own interests at the expense of the interests of others (Mellert, 1995). Will society in general see your action as morally correct? (See **Figure 5.3**.)

Ninth, "apply the categorical imperative" (Mellert, 1995, p. 158). Would you want your course of action to be a role model for others? If others were faced with the same decision, is this how you would want them to act?

Tenth, choose the best alternative, provide a reasoned justification for the choice (Svara, 2007), "act courageously and decisively" (Mellert, 1995, p. 158), monitor and

**Figure 5.3** An anti-abortion rally

(Janine Wiedel Photolibrary Alamy)

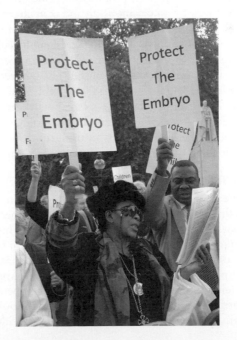

evaluate the results, and if necessary make adjustments (Svara, 2007). "Choosing among conflicting options is difficult, but at least one can feel confident that the choice did not ignore an important alternative" (Svara, 2007, p. 109). Having said this, you still may not feel comfortable after the choice has been made.

In considering the components in this decision-making process, it is important to note that moral decision making does not occur in a vacuum (Mellert, 1995). If it did, every decision would be resolved with the "right" alternative for all. Each decision is surrounded by the context in which it must be made. Mellert feels that, when working through the process, a person must consider and be aware of the context. When making ethical decisions, people must have a sense of the following:

1. **Place.** Be aware of the appropriateness of an action in a particular environment. One action may be appropriate in one setting but not in another.

2. **Time.** Be aware of the history leading up to the decision and other similar decisions. Learn from past decisions.

3. **Identity.** Who am I? How does this moral decision relate to me?

4. **Social relationships.** Be aware that making moral decisions will impact social relationships. There is a good chance that not everyone will agree with your decision and action.

5. **The ideal.** When making a moral decision, aim for the most noble ideals of humanity.

6. **The concrete.** Never lose sight of the fact that choices arise from concrete events.

7. **Seriousness.** When making a moral decision, do so with an attitude that is appropriate to the situation.

Now let us see if we can apply this decision-making process to the profession of health education/promotion. A health education specialist, let's call her Anne, is employed by an organization and is in charge of the organization's employee health promotion program. Based upon the results of the health risk assessments (HRA) taken by employees, Anne is aware that one employee, "high up in the organization" (e.g., school principal, department manager), is a consistent abuser of alcohol. The person's supervisor is aware of the situation but has ignored it. The employee in question is well liked within the organization and is a good employee. To the best of Anne's knowledge, alcohol has not impacted this person's work performance, but she feels it has the potential to do so. Anne is not sure if the alcohol has impacted the employee's personal life. What should Anne do with this information? Let's look at how we might analyze this situation using the ten-step process presented on the previous pages.

**Step 1.** Define the problem, identify the ethical issue, and gather relevant information.

The problem is that the employee is abusing a substance and the health education specialist knows it, as does the employee's supervisor. Is it an ethical problem? Anne knows that an alcohol-impaired person can harm him/herself and others, either intentionally or unintentionally, and thus has an obligation to protect their health (see Article I, Section 4, of Appendix A). Anne also knows she has an obligation to protect the privacy of the employees (see Article I, Section 6, of Appendix A). This appears to be an ethical dilemma to Anne because of the two competing issues. Anne has decided to get more information before acting. She decides to look at the employee handbook to see if anything like this appears there. She also decides to ask her own supervisor for guidance and check with the Human Resources (HR) Department for information. And, last, she looks to see when the employee is scheduled for his/her HRA feedback appointment.

**Step 2.** Identify who will be affected.

Anne is aware that, depending on what actions are taken, the parties impacted by those actions are the employee, his/her supervisor, the organization and its reputation, family members of the employee, and even Anne herself and her supervisor.

**Step 3.** Contemplate the ultimate goals and ideals.

Anne wants to do what is ethically right. From a theoretical point of view, Anne embraces the deontological viewpoint of dealing with ethical dilemmas. In other words, she believes that the ends do not justify the means. She is trying to make sense of how that applies to this situation.

**Step 4.** Identify the alternatives (viable courses of action).

Anne sees the following as viable courses of action: (1) Approach the employee's supervisor and ask him/her to handle it; (2) Talk to the employee about it at his/her scheduled HRA feedback appointment; (3) Turn the information over to the HR Department to let someone there deal with the problem; (4) Turn the information over to the her supervisor so that it can be dealt with at the managers' level; (5) Do nothing until something happens because of the employee's alcohol use; or (6) Do nothing at all.

**Step 5.** Consider the consequences of the alternatives.

Here are the consequences Anne sees with each of the alternatives she identified in Step 4: Alternative 1—The supervisor may do nothing or may now be forced to act because someone else is aware of the situation. This may lead to the employee's dismissal, or the employee may get the help he/she needs, or the supervisor may decide not to act on the information. Alternative 2—This alternative would protect the employee's privacy, bring the problem to the attention of the employee, and let the employee act without others knowing about it. Anne also knows that the employee may not take the feedback session well and "blow up" at Anne. Alternative 3—This alternative places the situation in the hands of those trained to deal with them effectively. Depending on the organization's policy, it may also lead to the employee's dismissal, or the employee may get the help he/she needs. Alternative 4—Similar to Alternatives 2 and 4, it places the problem in someone else's hands and would probably have much the same consequences as those two alternatives. Alternative 5—Nothing may ever come of the employee's alcohol abuse, or some serious harm may come to the employee or someone around him/her. or Alternative 6—Doing nothing at all, which would change nothing. The employee possibly will continue as a good employee with no problem for him/herself or others, or harm could come to the employee, his/her co-workers, or members of the employee's family.

**Step 6.** Consider the nature of the alternatives.

Anne does not feel that by acting she would be violating any human ideals or intrinsic moral rules or values. She does feel, however, that she cannot do "nothing." She doesn't like the alternatives, but she feels an ethical obligation to act.

**Step 7.** Reflect on yourself.

Anne knows that if she does nothing, she will not be able to live with herself, since she sees herself as a moral person. But she is concerned about being seen as the "goody-goody" employee or even a "tattle tale" or an employee that cannot be trusted with confidential information.

**Step 8.** Reflect on society and the environment.

Anne had a hard time reasoning through this step of the process. Because a large percentage of American adults consume alcohol, she feels that society in general may see the employee's situation as "none of her business." But she still sees a need to act.

**Step 9.** Apply the categorical imperative.

Anne feels she needs to act because it is her duty. She wonders what kind of health education specialist she would be if she were not concerned about the health of a co-worker and the possible harm that co-worker could bring to self or others. She feels that she needs to be a role model for others.

**Step 10.** Choose an alternative, provide a rationale, act, and monitor the results.

Anne decided to act by talking to the employee about the alcohol abuse at his/her scheduled HRA feedback appointment. She chose this approach not only because it does not violate the employee's privacy, but it also tries to protect both the employee's health and that of those around him/her. If this approach does not induce the employee to change, Anne feels that she may need to take further action.

As you can see, moral decisions are not easy to make. They are not to be taken lightly, and responsible action is important. Remember, this decision will not occur in a vacuum; the "ideal" decision may not be the best decision. What do you think about Anne's actions?

## Ethical Issues and Health Education/Promotion

As noted at the beginning of this chapter, ethical concerns interface with all aspects of our lives. That includes our professional lives too. "Professional ethics seeks to determine what the role of professions is and what the conduct of professionals should be" (Bayles, 1989, p. 13). "Ethical issues permeate almost every decision and action undertaken in health education" (Goldsmith, 2006, p. 33). Although some of the ethical issues faced by health education specialists are very specific to the profession, such as the ethical issues surrounding getting clients to begin a health-enhancing behavior, the majority of concerns affecting most professions are similar (Hiller, 1987).

Bayles (1989) has organized the substantive obligations of professions and professionals, regardless of the profession, from which most professional ethical dilemmas arise. The following is a list of these obligations, with several questions that relate the obligations to the practice of health education/promotion. [Note: These obligations closely align with the *Code of Ethics for the Health Education Profession* (CNHEO, 1999).]

1. **Obligations and availability of services.** The primary issue related to this obligation is the equality of opportunity for making professional services available to all citizens. Examples of ethical issues associated with this obligation include the right to legal counsel, access to health care, and refusal to accept clients for lack of ability to pay. (Who should receive health education/promotion? What about clients who are hard to reach? In what settings should it be offered? Should clients have to pay

**Figure 5.4** The professional–client relationship is an obligation that is often encountered by health education sepecialists.

(Spencer Grant/PhotoEdit)

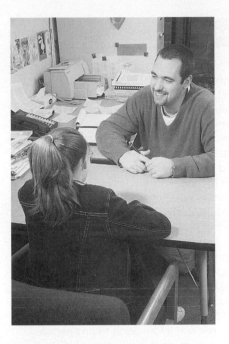

for health education/promotion, or should health education/promotion be denied if a person cannot pay? Should health education specialists ever terminate an intervention before it is complete? Is there ever a time when a health education specialist should use an intervention in which the possible outcomes are questionable?)

2. **Obligations between professionals and clients.** Once the services of a professional have been secured, a number of ethical issues can arise from the professional–client relationship. (See **Figure 5.4**.) "The fiduciary model presents the best ethical ideal for the professional-client relationship" (Bayles, 1989, p. 100). In such a model, the professional is honest, candid, competent, loyal, fair, and discrete. At the same time, the client keeps commitments to the professional, is truthful to the professional, and does not request unethical acts from the professional. (Is there ever a time when health education specialists should not be candid or honest with their clients? How should health education specialists respond when their clients ask them about their personal behavior? Is there ever a time when a health education specialists should not obtain informed consent before proceeding with an intervention?) (See **Box 5.1**.)

3. **Obligations to third parties.** This obligation revolves around what others need to know about the professional–client relationship. Often professionals are confronted with the issue of whether or not to share client information with family members of the client, people in a supervisory capacity (e.g., teachers, employers), legal authorities (e.g., police, lawyers), or peers (e.g., professional colleagues). (What duty does a health education specialist have to share information with a student' s parents when the student has shared the information with the health education specialist in confidence? Is there ever a time when a health education specialist can share confidential information? How about with the insurance company of a client? With the client' s employer?) (See **Box 5.2**.)

| Box 5.1 | INFORMED CONSENT: AN ETHICAL OBLIGATION |

The term **"informed consent"** is often associated with medical procedures or research projects, but it is also important in health education/promotion. The concept behind informed consent is that people—whether patients, research participants, or participants in a health education/promotion program—should be given sufficient information from which to make informed choices about whether or not they want a certain medical procedure, or to participate in a research project or health education/promotion program. From an ethical standpoint, "the idea of consent is based on the principle of respect for the person, and thus on the concept of human rights of life and liberty" (Tschudin, 2003, p. 172).

Valid informed consent requires: a) disclosure of relevant information to prospective participants about the program; b) their comprehension of the information; and c) their voluntary agreement, free from coercion and undue influence, to participate (OHSR, 2006).

Though receiving a medical procedure or participating in a clinical trial often carries more risks than participating in a health education/promotion program, individuals should not be allowed to participate in any health education/promotion program without giving their informed consent (McKenzie, Neiger, & Thackeray, 2009). In practice, the informed consent process should include: 1) the health education specialist discussing the details of the program (i.e., purpose of the program, description of the intervention, risks and benefits associated with participation, alternative programs that will accomplish the same thing, and the freedom to discontinue participation at any time) with the prospective participant; 2) the participant having an opportunity to ask questions about the program; 3) the participant understanding what he/she has been told; and 4) the participant signing a written informed consent document (Cottrell & McKenzie, 2011).

4. **Obligations between professionals and employers.** Employed professionals have obligations to employers that are similar to the obligation they have to their clients (see #2). "However, the obligation to obey employers is stronger than an obligation to clients. It includes acting as, and only as, authorized" (Bayles, 1989, p. 158). On the other hand, "employers' obligations to professional employees are universal, role related, and contractual" (Bayles, 1989, p. 159). Ethical issues related to this obligation often involve due process, confidentiality, and professional support. (Should health education specialists always implement "company" policy when they know it is wrong or could bring harm to a client? What if a health education specialist has a conflict of interest between his personal life and what his employer says he must do? Is there ever a time when health education specialists should publicly speak against their employers?)

5. **Obligations to the profession.** "These obligations rest on the responsibilities of a profession as a whole to further social values" (Bayles, 1989, p. 179). Issues associated with this obligation include conducting research, reforming the profession, and maintaining respect for the profession. (Is there ever a reason why health education specialists should not behave in a professional manner? What duty does a health education specialist have to report the inappropriate behavior of a colleague? What obligations do health education specialists have to keep up-to-date on the content of their fields?)

**Box 5.2**    PRIVACY AND HIPAA

One of the most basic concepts associated with providing a service (e.g., health education) to other people is that of privacy. **Privacy** has been defined as "the claim of individuals, groups, or institutions to determine for themselves when, how, and to what extent information about them is communicated to others" (Westin, 1968, p. 7). Thus, when people have agreed to participate in a health education/promotion program, it becomes the duty of the health education specialist to protect the information provided by participants.

The importance of privacy for health education specialists, and all others associated with health care, was further emphasized with the enactment of the Health Insurance Portability and Accountability Act of 1996 (officially known as Public Law 104-191 and referred to as HIPAA). HIPAA includes: 1) privacy standards for the use and disclosure of individually identifiable private health information; 2) transaction standards for the electronic exchange of health information; and 3) security standards to protect the creation and maintenance of private health information. The HIPAA regulations apply to protected health information (PHI), whether transmitted orally, in writing, or electronically, that is generated by an employer, a health plan, a health clearinghouse, or a health care provider, or in connection with financial or administrative activities related to health care (Fisher, 2003). Failure to implement the standards can lead to civil and criminal penalties (USDHHS, n.d.). The two techniques that are used to protect the privacy of program participants are anonymity and confidentiality. **Anonymity** exists when no one, including those conducting the program, can relate a participant's identity to any information pertaining to the program. In applying this concept, health education specialists would need to ensure that collected information had no identifying marks attached to it such as the participant's name, social security number, or any other less common information. In practice, because of the nature (the need to know about the participants) of most health education/promotion programs, anonymity is not often used. Its most common application in health education/promotion is in conducting research projects.

On the other hand, the concept of confidentiality is common in health education/promotion programs. **Confidentiality** exists when only those responsible for conducting a program can link information about a participant with the individual and do not reveal such information to others. Thus, health education specialists need to take every precaution to protect participants' information. Often this means keeping the information "under lock and key" while the program is being conducted, then destroying (e.g., shredding) the information when it is no longer needed.

Having identified problems that may cut across all professions, let us examine those that are more specific to health education/promotion. First, Penland and Beyrer (1981) state that ethical issues are defined by two criteria. "First they must be 'issues'; that is, there must be controversy related to the problem or topic. There must be 'two sides,' supported by people with two different viewpoints" (p. 6). Issues, by definition, are controversial. For example, the need for youth to know sexual information is not an issue; however, from whom and when such information should be provided may be an issue.

"The second criterion for an ethical issue in health education is that it must involve a question of right and wrong" (Penland & Beyrer, 1981, p. 6). "Can health education/

promotion programs in the worksite change health behavior?" may be a controversial issue, but it does not deal with rightness and wrongness. Thus, it is not an ethical issue, but "does an employer have the right to make all employees attend the health education/ promotion program?" is an ethical issue.

Now that we know what comprises an ethical issue, let us look at some of the ethical issues health education specialists are likely to face. The literature is abundant with examples of ethical issues in health education/promotion. Issues cited include abstinence-only and abstinence-plus sexuality education (Wiley, 2002), community organization and community participation (Minkler & Pies, 2005), ethics instruction (Modell & Citrin, 2002), health education research (Bastida, Tseng, McKeever, & Jack, 2010; Buchanan et al., 2002; Minkler et al., 2002; Minkler, Vasquez, Tajik, & Petersen, 2008), health literacy (Marks, 2009), health promotion evaluation (Thurston, Vollman, & Burgess, 2003), health risk appraisals (SPM, 1999), practice of health education (Shive & Marks, 2006), research/scientific inquiry/publishing (Margolis, 2000; McKenzie, Seabert, Hayden, & Cottrell, 2009; Pigg, 1994 & 2006; Price & Dake 2002; Price, Dake, & Islam 2001), service by health education specialists (Price, Dake, & Telljohann, 2001; Young & Valois, 2010), social marketing (Rothschild, 2000; Siegel & Lotenberg, 2007), the teaching of health (Telljohann, Price, & Dake, 2001), topical areas (Eve, Marty, McDermott, Klasko, & Sanberg, 2008), and the teaching of ethics (Goldsmith, 2006). McLeroy, Bibeau, and McConnell (1993) have identified other areas of ethical concern, which reflect the inclusion of health education as a component of health promotion. The major categories of issues raised by McLeroy and colleagues (1993) include:

1. "Assigning individual responsibility to the victim for becoming ill due to personal failures" (p. 314)—for example, becoming ill because one does not exercise, or continues to use tobacco products.

2. "Attempting to change individuals and their subsequent behaviors rather than the social environment that supports and maintains unhealthy lifestyles" (p. 314)—for example, telling employees to manage their stress when it is environmental stressors causing the stress.

3. Using "system interventions to promote health behaviors" (p. 315)—for example, public policy strategies or coercive strategies to modify unhealthy actions.

4. Overemphasizing behavior change as a program outcome instead of focusing more on changes in the social and physical environment.

5. Overemphasizing the importance of health, forgetting that health is a means to an end, not an end in itself.

6. Educating the public on the concept of risk and how to properly use risk factor information.

7. Underemphasizing professional behavior, regardless of the health education/ promotion setting—for example, keeping up-to-date, serving as a role model, and providing ethics education for the next generation of health education specialists.

As you can see, there are a number of ethical issues that can arise in the process of carrying out the work of a health education specialist. Rabinowitz (2010) has provided several issues that need to be considered when planning, implementing, and evaluating community interventions. They are presented in **Box 5.3**.

**Box 5.3**    ETHICAL ISSUES THAT NEED TO BE CONSIDERED WITH COMMUNITY INTERVENTIONS

1. **Confidentiality.** Probably the most familiar of ethical issues—perhaps because it's the one most often violated—is the expectation that communications and information from participants in the course of a community intervention or program (including conversations, written or taped records, notes, test results, etc.) will be kept confidential.

2. **Consent.** There are really three faces of consent: program participants giving program staff consent to share their records or information with others for purposes of service provision; participants giving informed consent to submit to particular medical or other services, treatment, research, or program conditions; and community members consenting to the location or operation of an intervention in their neighborhood.

3. **Disclosure.** Like consent, disclosure in this context has more than one meaning: disclosure to participants of the conditions of the program they're in; disclosure of participant information to other individuals, agencies, etc.; and disclosure—by the program and by the affected individuals—of any conflict of interest that the program represents to any staff or board members.

4. **Competence.** By offering services of any kind, an organization is essentially making a contract with participants to do the job it says it will do. Implied in that contract is that those actually doing the work, and the organization as a whole, are competent to accomplish their goals under reasonable circumstances.

5. **Conflict of interest.** A conflict of interest is a situation in which someone's personal (financial, political, professional, social, sexual, family, etc.) interests could influence his judgment or actions in a financial or other decision, in carrying out his job, or in his relationships with participants. In community interventions, conflicts of interest may change—to the community's disadvantage—how a program is run or how its money is spent.

6. **Grossly unethical behavior.** This is behavior far beyond the bounds of the normally accepted ethical standards of society. In some cases, grossly unethical behavior may stem from taking advantage of a conflict of interest situation. In others, it may be a simple case of dishonesty or lack of moral scruples. Both individuals and organizations can be guilty of some instances of it, and in both cases it is often a result of someone managing to justify the unjustifiable. Community programs need to be clear about their own ethical standards, and to hold individuals to them and to any other standards their professions demand. In most cases, staff members guilty of grossly unethical behavior should be dismissed as quickly as possible, and prosecuted where that is appropriate.

7. **General ethical responsibilities.** Ethical behavior for a community intervention is more than simply following particular professional codes and keeping your nose clean. It means actively striving to do what is right for participants and for the community, and treating everyone—participants, staff members, funders, the community at large—in an ethical way.

*Source:* From Rabinowitz, P., edited by Berkowitz and Brownlee. (2010). "Ethical Issues in Community Interventions," *The Community Tool Box: Ethical Issues in Common Interventions.* Reproduced by permission of the Work Group for Community Health and Development, The Community Tool Box: http://ctb.ku.edu.

## Ensuring Ethical Behavior

The majority of this chapter has been used to identify and deal with ethical issues and discuss why it is important to act ethically. What we have yet to discuss is how the profession can ensure that professionals will behave ethically. It cannot. Professionals who act unethically usually do so (1) for personal financial gain and reputation and (2) for the benefit of clients or employers without considering the effects on others (Bayles, 1989). However, a profession can put procedures into place to work toward ethical behavior by all.

Some procedures put in place by professions are limited, in some form, to those who are in professional preparation programs and those who have already been admitted to the profession. Traditional ways of doing this have been through (1) selective admissions into academic programs, (2) retention standards to remain in academic programs, (3) graduation from academic programs, (4) completion of internships, (5) the process of becoming credentialed (i.e., certified or licensed to practice), and (6) continual updating to retain the credential. While proceeding through these steps, individuals may have to provide evidence of good moral character.

Once in the profession, professionals are expected to behave according to a system of norms. As noted earlier in this chapter, this system of norms (or professional moral consensus, as some refer to it) is often placed in writing and referred to as a code of ethics. More specifically, a **code of ethics** is a "document that maps the dimensions of the profession's collective social responsibility and acknowledges the obligations individual practitioners share in meeting the profession's responsibilities" (Feeney & Freeman, 1999, p. 6). Such a document is usually useful not only for the professional but also for those who use the services of the professional. An ethical code's principal function is to "organize in a systematic way basic ethical standards, rules, and principles of professional conduct" (Pritchard, 2006, p. 85). In other words, "codes serve to *constrain* and set limits by identifying behaviors that should be avoided. They *guide* or instruct by identifying obligations and desirable qualities" (Svara, 2007, p. 75). And, "they can *inspire* and set forth the board goals that the adherents are supposed to promote" (Svara, 2007, p. 76). They also provide the consumers of health education/promotion services with an understanding of what they should expect from the provider.

Svara (2007) has noted that most codes of ethics have four different types of statements in them. They include (1) "don't" statements (which cover prohibited activities or behaviors), (2) obligations and responsibilities (which set forth the things one must or should do), (3) virtues, personal qualities, and/or values (which state how one should be rather than what one should do), and (4) aspirations (which state desirable conditions that one seeks to promote as opposed to actions or personal qualities). **Box 5.4** lists these four different types of statements and references to where they may be found in the *Code of Ethics for the Health Education Profession* (CNHEO, 1999).

In addition to a code of ethics, a profession should also have a means by which to deal with (discipline) professionals who violate the code of ethics. "A wide range of enforcement mechanisms are possible" (Taub, Kreuter, Parcel, & Vitello, 1987, p. 82). Such mechanisms may range from self-monitoring (also referred to as self-regulating) to a more formal process in which ethics cases are reviewed by a committee of peers. When self-monitoring is used, charges of the ethical violation "might be conveyed directly to

| **Box 5.4** | TYPES OF ETHICAL STATEMENTS AND EXAMPLES FOUND IN THE *CODE OF ETHICS FOR THE HEALTH EDUCATION PROFESSION* |

### "Don't" statements

Ex. There are no "Don't" statements in the *Code of Ethics for the Health Education Profession* (CNHEO, 1999), but they are assumed. All statements are made in the positive of what health education specialists will do, not what they shouldn't do. For example, instead of saying that health education specialists should never violate one's right to privacy, Article I, Section 6 states "Health Educators protect the privacy and dignity of individuals" (CNHEO, 1999, p. 1).

### Obligations and Responsibilities

Ex. Article IV, Section 5—"Health Educators communicate the potential outcomes of proposed services, strategies, and pending decisions to all individuals who will be affected" (CNHEO, 1999, p. 3).

### Virtues, Personal Qualities, and/or Values

Ex. Article I, Section 9—"Health Educators provide services equitably to all people" (CNHEO, 1999, p. 2).

### Aspirations

Ex. Article VI, Section 2—"Health Educators strive to make the educational environment and culture conducive to the health of all involved, and free from sexual harassment and all forms of discrimination" (CNHEO, 1999, p. 3).

the professional charged with the violation. That person would then be responsible for resolving the situation. This procedure works well when there is peer pressure for professionals to behave consistent with a clearly identifiable set of standards and rules of professional conduct" (Gold & Greenberg, 1992, p. 143). When ethical violations are reviewed by an ethics committee of the profession or as part of a professional organization, the "committees usually have the authority to recommend sanctions against members who are judged to behave unethically" (Gold & Greenberg, 1992, p. 143). First and/or minor violations of ethical behavior often carry disciplinary measures of "warnings." Repeated and/or major violations can lead to more serious penalties like limitations on the ability to practice and "even outright expulsion from the profession (that is, decertification or rescinding the member's license to practice)" (Gold & Greenberg, 1992, p. 145). In determining the sanctions, review committees may base their decision on a variety of factors including but not limited to (1) the type of violation (e.g., violation of privacy vs. sexual misconduct), (2) number of prior violations by the professional, (3) the willfulness of the violation, and (4) the level of responsibility of the professional (Svara, 2007).

## Ensuring Ethical Behavior in the Health Education/Promotion Profession

In the previous section, we identified a number of steps that a profession can take to try to ensure ethical behavior from its professionals. Let's look at how the health education profession has dealt with this, starting with admission into a health education professional preparation program at a college or university.

Currently, the admission procedure into the profession of health education/promotion is not clear. Some colleges and universities preparing health education specialists have selective admission standards, but most have open admissions, meaning that students can enter the health education/promotion program if admitted to the institution. Once in the program, all academic institutions have retention standards and graduation requirements, however minimal they may be—minimum grades in certain courses or a grade point average of 2.0 on a 4-point scale. Other institutions may have a minimum overall grade point average or minimum grade point average in certain professional courses in order to be admitted into student teaching an and/or an internship. With regard to the amount of education required in the profession, a bachelor's degree is required to sit for the certified health education specialist (CHES) examination (see Chapter 6); however, there is no consensus in the profession that a bachelor's degree should be the standard. Many feel a master's degree is more appropriate. Regardless of whether a bachelor's or master's degree is required to take the credentialing examination, the earned credentials (CHES or MCHES) are not universally accepted, either in or out of the profession, as necessary to practice health education/promotion.

The profession of health education/promotion has had a code of ethics for a number of years. The first was created in 1976 by the Society for Public Health Education (SOPHE). That code was later revised in 1983 and abridged in 1993. Though that code was developed more than twenty years ago, it was not universally adopted by the profession. In 1984, SOPHE and the Association for the Advancement of Health Education (AAHE; now known as the American Association for Health Education) appointed a joint committee to develop a profession-wide code of ethics. That committee was not able to create a profession-wide code of ethics. Further, in April 1994, AAHE developed another code, the "Code of Ethics for Health Educators." However, in 1995, the National Commission for Health Education Credentialing, Inc. (NCHEC) (see Chapter 6 for more on NCHEC) and Coalition of National Health Education Organizations (CNHEO) (see Chapter 8 for more on CNHEO) co-sponsored a conference, "The Health Education Profession in the Twenty-First Century: Setting the Stage," at which it was recommended that efforts be expanded to develop a profession-wide code of ethics. Soon after that conference the CNHEO began work on such a code. After several years of work, in 1999 the *Code of Ethics for the Health Education Profession* was created and approved by all members of CNHEO, thus replacing the earlier codes developed by SOPHE and AAHE (see Appendix A for a copy of the code and more information on its development). However, like the codes before it, this code does not include a formal procedure for enforcement. So currently, the profession has informal enforcement via "the subtle influences colleagues exert on one another" (Iammarino et al., 1989, p. 104). "One of the true weaknesses of our present code of ethics is no accountability to its standards" (Goldsmith, 2006, p. 36). [Note: At the time this book was being written, the *Code of Ethics for the Health Education Profession* was being revised by the Coalition of National Health Education Organizations (CNHEO). Readers should check the CNHEO Web site for the revised copy.]

As can be seen from this analysis, the health education/promotion profession is moving in the right direction but still has much opportunity to refine its ethical foundations.

## SUMMARY

Ethical questions impact all aspects of life. Individuals on both a personal and professional level are constantly being confronted with ethical dilemmas. To deal with these situations, people must have a basic understanding of how to make an ethical decision. To prepare readers for this task, this chapter presented key terms, such as philosophy, ethics, and morals; the philosophical, practical, and professional viewpoints of why people and professionals should work from an ethical base; the two major categories of theories (deontology and teleology) used to create ethical "yardsticks" for making ethical decisions; a set of principles and a guide for ethical decision making; a sampling of the ethical issues facing health education specialists today; and a discussion about how a profession can ensure that its professionals will act ethically.

## REVIEW QUESTIONS

1. What are the three major areas of philosophy? What does each of them mean?
2. In your own words, how do you define *ethics?*
3. What do the definitions of *ethics* and *morals* share? How are they different?
4. Why is it important to act ethically?
5. What is meant by the term *professional ethics?* What is *research ethics?*
6. How would you summarize the difference between the two major categories of ethical theories (deontology and teleology)?
7. What are Thiroux's five principles that create a common ground for all ethical theories?
8. What should be included in a process for making ethical decisions?
9. What is meant by the term *moral sensitivity?*
10. Name five ethical issues currently facing the profession of health education/promotion.
11. What can a profession do to ensure that its professionals will act ethically?
12. Define *code of ethics.*

## CASE STUDY

Sue accepted a position as a patient educator with the Franklin County Hospital after graduating with her bachelor's degree last spring. She is one of five health education specialists employed by the patient education department. About three months after Sue was hired, she observed Tom, the most experienced patient educator in the department, engage in what she believed was unethical behavior. Sue observed Tom accepting a really nice windbreaker (worth about $80) from a pharmaceutical company representative. In return, the pharmaceutical rep asked Tom to recommend the pharmaceutical company's glucometer during the diabetes education sessions he ran. Tom said that

"that would be no problem." Do you agree with Sue—do you think this is unethical behavior? On what ethical principles do you base your response? Is there something in the *Code of Ethics for the Health Education Profession* (Appendix A) that supports your position? Say you agree with Sue; what would be your course of action? Do you think Tom's supervisor should be involved? Why or why not? Do you think Tom should be sanctioned by the profession? If so, how could it be enforced?

## CRITICAL THINKING QUESTIONS

1. If you were asked by one of your professors to help design a professional ethics course for health education/promotion majors/minors at your college/university, what would you suggest be included in the course? Why?

2. Several professions (e.g., medicine and law) have procedures for dealing with members' unethical behavior. In fact, if the offense is extreme enough a lawyer can be disbarred and a physician could lose his or her license to practice medicine. Do you think the profession of health education/promotion should create a similar process to review unethical behavior and if necessary take away the certification of certified health education specialists (CHES)? Defend your response.

3. Do you think that all health education/promotion majors/minors should be required to take an ethics course while in college? Why or why not? If you responded yes to the question, do you think that a general ethics course open to all university students would be sufficient, or do you think the course should be specific to the profession? Why?

## ACTIVITIES

*Directions for activities* 1–4. You will find four scenarios that include an ethical dilemma. Using the ten-step decision-making process put forth in this chapter, write a response to one of the scenarios. Include in your response a paragraph for each of the ten components. Your ten paragraphs should state your course of action.

1. You have been hired to work for the city health department to complete a project that was begun by your predecessor and funded with money from a local foundation. The grant requires the health department to develop X number of programs on the topic of hepatitis and then to present these programs to X number of people representing very specific priority groups in the community. After being hired, you discover that the administrator of the grant, your supervisor, has not adhered to the grant guidelines. Only half the number of programs have been developed as the grant required. Further, the number of presentations is less than required, and presentations have been given to people not in the identified priority groups. In addition, your supervisor has taken some of the travel funds allocated to pay for your travel to and from presentations and has diverted them into his personal travel fund to attend a national conference in Las Vegas. It is now time for you to develop your year-end report, which will be sent directly to the local foundation

office. Your supervisor has provided you with a copy of the original grant proposal and says to make sure your figures agree with those in the proposal. In other words, he expects you to "fudge" the data. What will you do?

2. As the health and fitness director of a large corporate wellness program, you have been asked to provide data to your supervisor that supports the effectiveness of your program. The trend in the company has been to cut programs that do not "carry their weight." The "bottom line" is important. In your review of the data related to your program, it is obvious that the data are not very strong. However, in fairness to you, the program has been in operation for only two years, and it is too early to see the type of results management is looking for. You are the only one who has access to the data, and no one will know if the data you submit are accurate. How will you handle this situation?

3. You are a high school health teacher. The board of education has just adopted a policy that prohibits the teaching or discussing of information related to contraceptives or abortion in the district. The only approach that can be mentioned in the classroom is abstinence. You have read that the abstinence approach is ineffective. After class one day, one of your students approaches you and informs you that she is pregnant. She requests your help and asks for the name and location of an abortion clinic. She also asks that you not tell anyone else about this. What will you do?

4. You are the health education specialist for a large city hospital. Your supervisor has asked you to develop a program on "safer sex" practices for the gay and lesbian population. The program is to be provided to each HIV-positive person who enters the hospital, and it is to be made available to lesbian and gay groups in the community. Because of your strong religious convictions, your personal values and beliefs are opposed to the gay/lesbian lifestyle and the "safer sex" approach. In addition, you feel very uncomfortable dealing with homosexuals in general and especially with anyone who is HIV-positive. How will you handle this situation?

5. Read thoroughly the *Code of Ethics for the Health Education Profession* presented in Appendix A, then provide written answers to the following questions.
   - What is your overall opinion of the code? Does it include everything you thought it would? Were there any surprises?
   - Do you think it should include any "Don't" statements? (Refer back to Box 5.4.) If yes, which ones? If no, why not?
   - Is there anything in the code you feel should not be there? If so, what and why?
   - If you could add something else to the code, what would it be?
   - Do you think the profession should incorporate a means of enforcement in the code? Why or why not?

6. Select one of the ethical theories presented in Table 5.1 to study further. Find and read from other sources explaining the theory. Then write a three-page paper on the theory's application to the practice of health education/promotion.

7. Make an appointment to meet with one of your professors or with a practicing health education specialist. Inform him/her that you would like to spend about fifteen to twenty minutes discussing professional ethics. At the meeting ask him/her if

he/she has ever observed a professional situation that involved an ethical dilemma. If so, ask him/her to describe the situation without revealing the parties who were involved. Then ask how the dilemma was resolved. After your meeting, summarize in writing the discussion and compare the steps taken in the situation to the components of the ten-step process presented in this chapter. Do you think the dilemma was handled properly? Why or why not?

## WEBLINKS

1. http://www.cnheo.org

   Coalition of National Health Education Organizations (CNHEO)

   This is the home page for the CNHEO. The Coalition has as its primary mission the mobilization of the resources of the health education/promotion profession in order to expand and improve health education/promotion, regardless of the setting. At this site you can print out a copy of the *Code of Ethics for the Health Education Profession*.

2. http://www.ethics.org/

   Ethics Resource Center (ERC)

   The ERC is a nonprofit, nonpartisan educational organization dedicated to independent research that advances high ethical standards and practices in public and private institutions.

3. http://www.usoge.gov/index.html

   U.S. Office of Government Ethics (OGE)

   The OGE, a small agency within the executive branch, exercises leadership in the executive branch to prevent conflicts of interest on the part of government employees, and to resolve conflicts of interest that do occur. This site provides a view of what an employer—the federal government in this case—expects in terms of ethical behavior.

4. http://www.professionalethics.ca/

   Professional Ethics

   This is a Canadian Web site that provides a wide variety of resources on various topics related to professional ethics. One special feature of this Web site is the presentation of a number of up-to-date articles on professional ethics. It also has links to several other ethics-related Web sites.

5. http://www.hhs.gov/ocr/privacy/

   United States Department of Health and Human Services (USDHHS)

   This is a page at the USDHHS Web site where you can get more information about the National Standards to Protect the Privacy of Personal Health Information.

6. http://ohsr.od.nih.gov/info/sheet6.html

   Office of Human Subjects Research

   This is a page at the National Institutes for Health (NIH) Web site where you can get more information about informed consent.

# REFERENCES

Balog, J. E., Shirreffs, J. H., Gutierrez, R. D., & Balog, L. F. (1985). Ethics and the field of health education. *The Eta Sigma Gamma Monograph Series, 4* (1), 65–110.

Bastida, E. M., Tseng, T-S., McKeever, C., & Jack, Jr., J. (2010). Ethics and community-based participatory research: Perspectives from the field. *Health Promotion Practice, 11* (1), 16–20.

Bayles, M. D. (1989). *Professional ethics* (2nd ed.). Belmont, CA: Wadsworth.

Buchanan, D., Khoshnood, K., Stopka, T., Shaw, S., Santelices, C., & Singer, M. (2002). Ethical dilemmas created by the criminalization of status behaviors: Case examples from ethnographic field research with injection drug users. *Health Education & Behavior, 29* (1), 30–42.

Coalition of National Health Education Organizations (CNHEO). (1999). *Code of ethics for the health education profession.* Retrieved August 11, 2010, from http://www.cnheo.org/index.html

Cottrell, R. R., & McKenzie, J. F. (2011). *Health promotion and education research methods: Using the five-chapter thesis/dissertation model* (2nd ed.). Sudbury, MA: Jones & Bartlett.

Dorman, S. M. (1994). The imperative for ethical conduct in scientific inquiry. In R. M. Pigg (Ed.), Ethical issues of scientific inquiry in health science education. *The Eta Sigma Gamma Monograph Series, 12* (2), 1–5.

Eve, D. J., Marty, P. J., McDermott, R. J., Klasko, S. K., & Sanberg, P. R. (2008). Stem cell research and health education. *American Journal of Health Education, 39* (3), 167–179.

Feeney, S., & Freeman, N. K., (1999). *Ethics and the early childhood educator.* Washington, DC: National Association for the Education of Young Children.

Fisher, C. B. (2003). *Decoding the ethics code: A practical guide for psychologists.* Thousand Oaks, CA: Sage Publications.

Fox, R. C., & Swazey, J. P. (1997). Medical morality is not bioethics: Medical ethics in China and the United States. In N. S. Jecker, A. R. Jonsen, & R. A. Pearlman (Eds.), *Bioethics: An introduction to history, methods and practice* (pp. 237–251). Sudbury, MA: Jones and Bartlett.

Gold, R. S., & Greenberg, J. S. (1992). *The health education ethics book.* Dubuque, IA: Wm. C. Brown Publishers.

Goldsmith, M. (2006). Ethics in health education: Issues, concerns, and future directions. *The Health Education Monograph Series: Foundations of Health Education, 23* (1), 33–37.

Greenberg, J. S. (2001). *The code of ethics for the health education profession: A case study book.* Boston: Jones and Bartlett Publishers.

Hiller, M. D. (1987). Ethics and health education: Issues in theory and practice. In P. M. Lazes, L. Kaplan, & G. A. Gordon (Eds.), *The handbook of health education* (pp. 87–108). Rockville, MD: Aspen.

Iammarino, N. K., O'Rourke, T. W., Pigg, R. M., & Weinberg, A. D. (1989). Ethical issues in research and publication. *Journal of School Health, 59* (3), 101–104.

Kimmel, A. J. (2007). *Ethical issues in behavioral research: Basic and applied perspectives* (2nd ed.). Malden, MA: Blackwell Publishing.

Margolis, L. (2000). Commentary: Ethical principles for analyzing dilemmas in sex research. *Health Education & Behavior, 27* (1), 24–27.

Marks, R. (2009). Ethics and patient education: Health literacy and cultural dilemmas. *Health Promotion Practice, 10* (3), 328–332.

McGrath, E. Z. (1994). *The art of ethics: A psychology of ethical beliefs.* Chicago: Loyola University Press.

McKenzie, J. F., Neiger, B. L., & Thackeray, R. (2009). *Planning, implementing, and evaluating health promotion programs: A primer* (5th ed.). San Francisco: Benjamin Cummings.

McKenzie, J. F., Seabert, D. M., Hayden, J., & Cottrell, R. R. (2009). Textbook writing: A form of professional development. *Health Promotion Practice, 10* (1), 10–14.

McLeroy, K. R., Bibeau, D. L., & McConnell, T. C. (1993). Ethical issues in health education and health promotion: Challenges for the profession. *Journal of Health Education, 24* (5), 313–318.

Mellert, R. B. (1995). *Seven ethical theories.* Dubuque, IA: Kendall/Hunt.

Minkler, M., Fadem, P., Perry, M., Blum, K., Moore, L., & Rogers, J. (2002). Ethical dilemmas in participatory action research: A case study from the disability community. *Health Education & Behavior, 29* (1), 14–29.

Minkler, M., & Pies, C. (2005). Ethical issues and practical dilemmas in community organization and community participation. In M. Minkler (Ed.). *Community organizing and community building for health* (2nd ed.), pp. 116–133. New Brunswick, NJ: Rutgers University Press.

Minkler, M., Vasquez, V. B., Tajik, M., & Petersen, D. (2008). Promoting environmental justice through community-based participatory research: The role of community and partnership capacity. *Health Education & Behavior, 35* (1), 119–137.

Modell, S. M., & Citrin, T. (2002). Ethics instruction in an issues-oriented course on public health genetics. *Health Education & Behavior, 29* (1), 43–60.

Morrison, E. E. (2006). *Ethics in health administration: A practical approach for decision makers.* Sudbury, MA: Jones & Bartlett.

Morrison, E. E. (2009). *Health care ethics: Critical issues for the 21st century* (2nd ed.). Sudbury, MA: Jones & Bartlett.

National Commission for Health Education Credentialing, Inc. (2010). *Health educator job analysis—2010: Executive summary and recommendations.* Retrieved August 10, 2010, from http://www.nchec.org/news/docs/nch-mr-tab2-169.htm

Office of Human Subject Research (OHSR). (2006). *Guidelines for writing informed consent documents.* Retrieved August 11, 2010, from http://ohsr.od.nih.gov/info/sheet6.html

Patterson, S. M., & Vitello, E. M. (1993). Ethics in health education. The need to include a model course in professional preparation programs. *Journal of Health Education, 24* (4), 239–244.

Penland, L. R., & Beyrer, M. K. (1981). Ethics and health education: Issues and implications. *Health Education, 12* (4), 6–7.

Pigg, R. M. (Ed.). (1994). Ethical issues of scientific inquiry in health science education. *The Eta Sigma Gamma Monograph Series, 12* (2).

Pigg, R. M. (2006). Conflict and consensus on ethics in publishing. *The Health Education Monograph Series: Foundations of Health Education, 23* (1), 38–41.

Pigg, Jr., R. M. (2010). Three essential questions in defining a personal philosophy. In J. M. Black, S. Furney, H. M. Graf, & A. E. Nolte (Eds.), *Philosophical foundations of health education* (pp. 11–15). San Francisco, CA: Jossey-Bass.

Price, J. H., & Dake, J. A. (2002). Ethical guidelines for manuscript reviewers and journal editors. *American Journal of Health Education, 33* (4), 194–196.

Price, J. H., Dake, J. A., & Islam, R. (2001). Ethical issues in research and publication: Perceptions of health education faculty. *Health Education & Behavior, 28*, 51.

Price, J. H., Dake, J. A., & Telljohann, S. K. (2001). Ethical issues regarding service: Perceptions of health education faculty. *American Journal of Health Education, 32* (4), 208–215.

Pritchard, M. S. (2006). *Professional integrity: Thinking ethically.* Lawrence: University Press of Kansas.

Rabinowitz, P. (2010). *The community health toolbox: Ethical issues in community interventions.* Retrieved August 10, 2010, from http://ctb.ku.edu/en/tablecontents/sub_main_1165.aspx

Reamer, F. G. (2006). *Social work values and ethics* (3rd ed.). New York: Columbia University Press.

Remley, T. P., & Herlihy, B. (2007). *Ethical, legal, and professional issues in counseling* (2nd ed.). Upper Saddle River, NJ: Merrill, Prentice Hall.

Rest, J., Narvaes, D., Bebeau, M. J., & Thoma, S. J. (1999). *Postconventional moral thinking: A neo-kohlbergian approach.* Mahwah, NJ: L. Erlbaum Associates.

Rothschild, M. L. (2000). Ethical considerations in support of marketing of public health issues. *American Journal of Health Behavior, 24* (1), 26–35.

Shive, S. E., & Marks, R. (2006). The influence of ethical theories in the practice of health education. *Health Promotion Practice, 7* (3) 287–288.

Siegel, M., & Lotenberg, L. D. (2007). *Marketing public health: Strategies to promote social change,* (2nd ed.). Sudbury, MA: Jones & Bartlett.

Sperry, L. (2007). *Dictionary of ethical and legal terms and issues: The essential guide for mental health professionals.* New York: Routledge.

Summers, J. (2009). Principles of healthcare ethics. In E. E. Morrison, *Health care ethics: Critical issues for the 21st century* (2nd ed.) (pp. 41–58). Sudbury, MA: Jones & Bartlett.

Svara, J. (2007). *The ethics primer for public administrators in government and nonprofit organizations.* Sudbury, MA: Jones & Bartlett.

Taub, A., Kreuter, M., Parcel, G., & Vitello, E. (1987). Report of the SOPHE/AAHE joint committee on ethics. *Health Education Quarterly, 14* (1), 79–90.

Telljohann, S. K., Price, J. H., & Dake, J. A. (2001). Selected ethical issues in the teaching: Perceptions of health education faculty. *American Journal of Health Education, 32* (2), 66–74.

The Society of Prospective Medicine Board of Directors (SPM). (1999). Ethics guidelines for the development and use of health assessments. In G. C. Hyner, K. W. Peterson, J. W. Travis, J. E. Dewey, J. J. Foerster, & E. M. Framer (Eds.), *SPM handbook of health assessment tools* (pp. xxii–xxvi). Pittsburgh, PA: The Society of Prospective Medicine.

Thiroux, J. P. (1995). *Ethics: Theory and practice* (5th ed.). Englewood Cliffs, NJ: Prentice-Hall.

Thompson, I., Melia, K., & Boyd, K. (2000). *Nursing ethics* (4th ed.). Edinburgh, Scotland: Churchill Livingstone.

Thurston, W. E., Vollman, A. R., & Burgess, M. M. (2003). Ethical review of health promotion program evaluation proposals. *Health Promotion Practice, 4* (1), 45–50.

Tschudin, V. (2003) *Ethics in nursing: The caring relationship* (3rd. ed.). Edinburgh, Scotland: Butterworth Heinemann.

United States Department of Health and Human Services (USDHHS). (n.d.). *Health information privacy.* Retrieved August 12, 2010, from http://www.hhs.gov/ocr/privacy

Westin, A. F. (1968). *Privacy and freedom.* New York: Atheneum.

White, T. I. (1988). *Right and wrong: A brief guide to understanding ethics.* Englewood Cliffs, NJ: Prentice-Hall.

Wiley, D. C. (2002). The ethics of abstinence-only and abstinence-plus sexuality education. *Journal of School Health, 72* (4), 164–167.

Young, M., & Valois, R. F. (2010). Magic, morals, and health: Plus 40 years. *American Journal of Health Education, 41* (1), 18–19.

# 6

# The Health Education Specialist: Roles, Responsibilities, Certifications, Advanced Study

## CHAPTER OBJECTIVES

After reading this chapter and answering the questions at the end, you should be able to:

- Define *credentialing*.
- Discuss the history of role delineation and certification.
- Explain the differences among *certification*, *licensure*, and *accreditation*.
- List and describe the seven major responsibilities of a health education specialist.
- Discuss the need for advanced study in health education/promotion.
- Outline factors to consider in applying for master's degree programs.

Although education about health has been around since the beginning of human intelligence, health education/promotion as a profession is, relatively speaking, an infant. When any infant begins to mature, it takes on its own identity. This chapter chronicles major historical events that have helped shape the identity of health education/promotion since the 1970s. The current identity of health education/promotion is also presented in terms of roles, responsibilities, certification, and accreditation. The importance of advanced study and continuing education in the health education/promotion profession is also discussed.

## Quality Assurance and Credentialing

Quality assurance and credentialing often go hand-in-hand. It is important to be familiar with these terms as they apply to health education/promotion. In the business world, the term **quality assurance** means, "the planned and systematic activities necessary to provide adequate confidence that the product or service will meet given requirements" (Quality Assurance Solutions, 2010). **Credentialing** is the means by which professions such as health education/promotion demonstrate quality assurance. In other words, credentialing would be the "planned and systematic activities" used to increase confidence that the product or service—in this case, health education specialists—is meeting the requirements of the profession. Credentialing is a process whereby an individual, such as a health education specialist, or a professional preparation program demonstrates that established standards are met. When people or programs meet specific standards established by a credentialing body, they are recognized for having done so. We say, "They earned their credentials," which indicates they are meeting their profession's requirements. Credentialing can take the form of accreditation, licensure, or certification.

**Accreditation** "is the process by which a recognized professional body evaluates an entire college or university professional preparation program" (Cleary, 1995, p. 39). Thus, the health education/promotion program at any particular institution may be accredited by one of several outside agencies discussed later in this chapter. For example, the health education/promotion program at Alpha University could be accredited by Beta Accrediting Group. Such a process takes place after the program at Alpha University creates a self-study document that shows how it meets the Beta Accrediting Group's standards. Accrediting procedures also include an on-campus visit by representatives from Beta. Throughout the process, factors such as student–teacher ratio, curriculum, and faculty qualifications are closely examined.

**Licensure** is "the process by which an agency or government [usually a state] grants permission to individuals to practice a given profession by certifying that those licensed have attained specific standards of competence" (Cleary, 1995, p. 39). Licensure applies to most medical professionals, such as doctors, nurses, dentists, and physical therapists. The only health education specialists who are licensed in the United States at the present time are school health education specialists.

**Certification** "is a process by which a professional organization grants recognition to an individual who, upon completion of a competency-based curriculum, can demonstrate a predetermined standard of performance" (Cleary, 1995, p. 39). Note that certification is granted to an individual, not a program, and it is given by the profession, not by a governmental body. Certification is available for all health education specialists, regardless of specialty area. One who is certified is recognized as a **Certified Health Education Specialist** and may use the initials **CHES** after one's name and academic degree. In fall 2010, an advanced certification became available. Those who obtain this advanced certification are **Master Certified Health Education Specialists** and may use the initials **MCHES** after their names.

## History of Role Delineation and Certification

Certification in health education got its formal start around 1978. At that time, individual certification for health education specialists was not available, except for school health education specialists, who had to be licensed or certified in the state where they taught. Program accreditation was available only for school health and public health professional preparation programs. Many public health programs outside schools of public health, and all community health programs, were not accredited, nor was accreditation available for these programs. This gave rise to a situation in which there were great discrepancies in professional preparation. One program might look very different from another program. To say that an individual was a health educator had little meaning. In

**Figure 6.1** Helen P. Cleary—the person most responsible for establishing certification for health education specialists

(Dr. Helen P. Cleary)

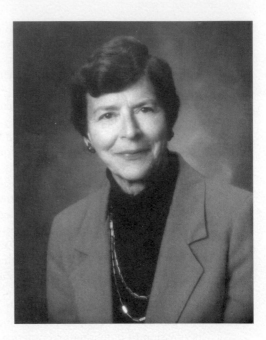

describing the situation, Helen Cleary (see **Figure 6.1**), who was president of the Society for Public Health Education (SOPHE) in 1974, wrote the following:

> What I found in my travels [as SOPHE president] was a profession in disarray. Many, many health educators could neither define themselves nor their role. It was clear that the preparation of most was so varied that there was no common core. There was no professional identity, no sense of a profession. Numbers of competent, bright, young professionals were leaving health education for greener pastures. (Cleary, 1995, p. 2)

As a result of this situation, Cleary began to pursue the idea of credentialing health educators and/or health education programs. To undertake such a project, outside expertise and funding were needed. Thomas Hatch, director of the Division of Associated Health Professions in the Bureau of Health Manpower of the Department of Health, Education and Welfare, expressed an interest in the project. Prior to funding the project, however, he needed assurances that members of the profession would work together to create a credentialing system. Hatch wanted to be certain that those who practiced health education in different settings would have enough in common to develop one set of standards.

In response to Hatch's concern, a conference, known today as the Bethesda Conference on Commonalities and Differences, was held in February 1978 in Bethesda, Maryland. The conference's planning committee was made up of representatives from the eight organizations comprising the Coalition of Health Education Organizations. This planning committee formulated two questions to be answered at the conference: (1) What are the commonalities and differences in the function of health educators practicing in different settings? and (2) What are the commonalities and differences in the preparation of health educators? (Cleary, 1995, p. 3).

After much discussion, conference attendees concluded that health education was one profession and that a credentialing system was necessary. "It was the consensus of the participants that standards were essential if they were to provide quality service to the public and if they were to survive as a viable profession" (Cleary, 1986, p. 130).

**Table 6.1**   Organizations represented on the national task force on the preparation and practice of health educators, 1978

American College Health Association

American Public Health Association, Public Health Education Section

American Public Health Association, School Health Education and Services Section

American School Health Association

Association for the Advancement of Health Education (AAHE)

Conference of State and Territorial Directors of Public Health Education

Society for Public Health Education, Inc.

Society of State Directors of Health, Physical Education and Recreation

Further, the conference planning committee members were asked to continue as a task force to develop the credentialing system. Thus, the **National Task Force on the Preparation and Practice of Health Educators** was born (see **Table 6.1**).

In January 1979, funding became available to embark on the project, and **role delineation** for health educators got under way. Alan Henderson was hired as the project director. Under his leadership, a working committee of the task force began the difficult job of defining the health education specialist's role. In describing this process, Cleary (1995) notes, "For the first time in the profession's history, specialists in school health education and in community health education faced each other across the table and learned that each was dealing with similar concepts, but using different terminology and, as well, applying them in different settings" (p. 5).

Once the initial phase of role delineation was completed, the next step was to verify and refine the role of a health educator. Funding for this became available in March 1980. Health education specialists working in all areas of health education were surveyed to verify the role of a health educator. Survey results were very positive; there were no significant differences among practitioners in different settings.

In addition to the survey, a conference for college and university health education faculty members was held in Birmingham, Alabama, in February 1981. The conference provided the opportunity for academics to review the initial role delineation work and discuss its potential impact on the field. The planning committee chairman was Warren E. Schaller from Ball State University, and 238 academics from 125 institutions attended.

Many conference participants were happy with the work and direction of the task force, but others were not. Differences of opinion surrounding the health educator as a content expert versus a process expert emerged and probably reflected the different types of professional preparation programs the faculty represented. Although these differences were very real, they were not divisive enough to alter the work of the task force.

The third step in the role delineation process involved creating a curriculum framework based on the verified role of a health educator. Initially, the task force decided to develop a curriculum guide, which is a fairly specific set of rules used to develop a curriculum. Little room is left for interpretation, as the curriculum must meet the standards established in the guide. Betty Mathews from the University of Washington and Herb L. Jones from Ball State University were recruited to do the actual writing.

After a draft copy of the curriculum guide was developed, it had to be pretested. Eleven regional workshops were held around the country to obtain feedback on the guide. Again, differences surfaced regarding whether health educators were specialists in content or process. Further, some felt entry-level preparation should be at the bachelor's degree level, while others believed it should be at the master's degree level. Feedback was also obtained from professional associations and practitioners in the field.

To deal with some of the criticisms and to make the curriculum guide less rigid, it was ultimately transformed into a curriculum framework. A framework merely provides a frame of reference around which a curriculum can be developed. As Cleary (1995) notes, "It does not tell a faculty what to teach or how to teach it. It simply tells them what the students should know when they have completed the program of studies" (p. 9). Marion Pollock was the individual responsible for transforming the curriculum guide into a curriculum framework.

At this juncture, it was important to check with those in the profession to determine if they wanted to continue with the development of a credentialing system and, if so, what kind of system they wanted. The Second Bethesda Conference was held in February 1986, with 99 attendees. Participants were divided into five groups and asked to answer several predetermined questions. When reports from the groups were analyzed, four of the five were in favor of a certification system for individuals and some form of credentialing for professional preparation programs. They recommended that the task force continue to develop the credentialing system.

Over the next two years, the task force continued to work toward the development of a certification system for individual health education specialists. The Professional Examination Service (PES), which developed certification and licensure exams for many other professions, was contracted to assist with this process. Not only was its experience in test development vital to the process, but it was also willing to provide start-up funds to get the process off the ground.

By June 1988, the National Task Force on the Preparation and Practice of Health Education had functioned for ten years. With the certification of individual health education specialists about to become a reality, it was time to establish a more permanent structure to manage the certification process. As a result, the **National Commission for Health Education Credentialing, Inc. (NCHEC)** was formed to replace the national task force. Today, NCHEC still oversees and administers the health education certification process. NCHEC's mission "is to enhance the professional practice of Health Education by promoting and sustaining a credentialed body of Health Education Specialists. To meet this mission, NCHEC certifies health education specialists, promotes professional development, and strengthens professional preparation and practice" (National Commission for Health Education Credentialing, 2010a).

## Individual Certification

When a new certification program is initiated, charter certification is usually available for a limited time. Charter certification allows qualified individuals to get certified on the basis of their academic training, work experience, and references, without taking an exam. After the charter period expires, anyone seeking certification must meet all criteria for certification and pass the examination. The CHES charter certification period began in October 1988 and ended in 1990. When the first exam was held in 1990, 644 candidates passed it to become Certified Health Education Specialists.

The CHES voluntary professional certification program established for the first time a national standard for health education practice. All health education/promotion students are strongly urged to obtain national certification upon graduation (see **Box 6.1**).

## Box 6.1 Practitioner's Perspective    CHES

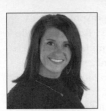

(Reprinted by permission of Lauren A. Clark)

NAME: Lauren A. Clark, B.S., CHES, CPST

CURRENT POSITION/TITLE: Injury Prevention Coordinator

EMPLOYER: Riley Hospital for Children

DEGREE/INSTITUTION: B.S., Ball State University, 2010

MAJOR: Health Science

MINORS: Psychology of Human Development, Marketing

**Job Responsibilities:** I coordinate and implement injury prevention programs within the local school systems and throughout the community. My primary focus is on low-income areas that do not have many resources. However, children everywhere can benefit from the variety of services we have to offer. I teach CPR and first aid courses for a variety of children's organizations, churches, daycares, and schools in the area. I also oversee and teach Safe Sitter® classes to children ages 11 to 13. During this 12½ hour course, the students learn the basics of babysitting, how to work with children of different ages and developmental stages, and how to handle emergency situations. These not only are skills they can use now but also are life-long skills that they can use when raising their own children in the future.

With my position, I also have the opportunity to plan and implement programs that teach children about different safety topics such as pedestrian safety, bicycle safety, water safety, sports injuries, and more! Child Passenger Safety is another one of my job responsibilities and is also a passion of mine. Data show that 80 percent of children nationwide are not correctly restrained in vehicles. Without proper restraint, children are put at serious risk should a crash occur. I am certified (CPST) as a technician to perform car seat checks and clinics for parents/guardians who have children in car seats. Beyond all of the programming, one of my most important roles is serving as a resource person for the community. I am regularly contacted by community members with questions regarding injury prevention. By serving as a resource person, I can answer their

questions or help find them additional resources. I am also frequently asked to give presentations at conferences, forums, and community events. At these events, I have the opportunity to impact a large number of individuals who also have a child's best interest at heart.

**How I obtained my job:** I was finishing up my internship in Indianapolis, IN, and knew that I wanted to stay in the area. I was ecstatic when my internship coordinator contacted my graduating class about a job opportunity available at Riley Hospital for Children. It seemed like a great fit because my career goal was to become a health education specialist and I have always loved working with children and families. I applied for the position online and received a phone call a few weeks later to set up an interview. During the first round of interviews, I was interviewed by two individuals in the department that I work directly with on a day-to-day basis. For my second interview, I was asked to give a presentation on bicycle safety to the entire department, which consisted of eight individuals at the time. Following my presentation, the department members had a chance to interview me. Now, here I am!

**What I like most about my job:** One thing I considered while applying for jobs was "will I make a difference?". With this position, I have an opportunity to make a difference in the lives of others. I also enjoy the variety that comes with my position. I am constantly implementing different programs within the school systems and community. By doing this, I also have the opportunity to work with

**Box 6.1 Practitioner's Perspective**   Continued

different groups and organizations every day. For example, one day I might be teaching CPR and first aid skills to daycare workers in a high-risk area of Indianapolis, and the next day I might be fitting and distributing bicycle helmets to a group of kids at a children's museum. No matter what I am doing day-to-day, I know that I am making a difference in the lives of children.

I am also blessed to work for a company that encourages life-long learning. My department has paid for all of my trainings and certifications. For example, they have sent me to trainings to become a CPR and First Aid Instructor, Safe Sitter® Instructor, Child Passenger Safety Technician, and Playground Safety Inspector. They also encourage me to attend conferences where I can network with other professionals and broaden my expertise.

**What I like least about my job:** My position is a part of the Trauma Services Department at Riley Hospital for Children. I receive notice every time a child comes into the Emergency Department for a trauma-related injury or incident. It is sad and hard to constantly see children being hurt, disabled, and even killed from situations that could have easily been prevented.

**How the Certified Health Education Specialist (CHES) credential has helped me:** I believe my CHES certification helped me get the position I have now. Out of the 30+ individuals they interviewed, I was the only one scheduled to take the CHES examination. Others were open to it, but I was the only one that had taken the initiative to sign up and start studying. Not only has my initiative to take the exam helped me, but I also feel like it has made me more qualified for my position. Everything I do at work, I use one or more of the CHES responsibilities and competencies. Without the background knowledge I have gained from my CHES credential, I would not be as confident or successful at what I do.

**How my work relates to the responsibilities and competencies of a CHES:** Everything I do at work can relate to one or more of the CHES responsibilities and competencies. Based on data and other related information we receive through our trauma registrar, it makes it easy to assess the individual, organizational, and community health needs. I can easily see what types of programs are needed to help reduce injury among our local children. Based on those needs and the interests of the community, I plan and implement injury prevention programs for the children, parents/guardians, and caregivers. For example, if we see a dramatic increase in the number of children injured by bicycle crashes, I know there is a need for education and I can start planning and implementing these types of programs. Evaluation is also the key component of any program I implement. Not only do we want to see how effective our efforts are, we want to improve programs for the future. I am constantly changing programs based on process and impact evaluation methods. Through my programs and on a day-to-day basis, I consistently act as a health education resource person advocating for health and health education. Whether I answer questions, find answers, or find additional resources for individuals in the community, people view me as a reliable resource.

**Recommendations for those preparing to become health education specialists:** I strongly suggest studying for and taking the CHES exam prior to graduating. Not only are you still in the "studying mode," but it will help you become more prepared for your future career. I would also suggest forming strong relationships with the professors you have now in school. Not only are they a wealth of knowledge, they can serve as a great resource and mentor to you in the future. I still keep in contact with several of my professors. The same goes for your classmates. Once they start their careers as health education specialists, they can all be a great resource to you. This is also a great way to network within the field!

Certification includes the following benefits listed (National Commission for Health Education Credentialing, 2010d):

- Establishes a national standard of practice for all health education specialists.

- Attests to the individual health education specialist's knowledge and skills.

- Assists employers in identifying qualified health education practitioners.

- Develops a sense of pride and accomplishment among certified health education specialists.

- Promotes continued professional development for health education specialists.

Currently, eligibility to sit for the CHES exam is based exclusively on academic qualifications. You must "possess a bachelor's, master's or doctoral degree from an accredited institution of higher education; *AND* (1) an official transcript (including course titles) that clearly shows a major in health education, e.g., Health Education/Promotion, Community Health Education, Public Health Education, School Health Education, etc. Degree/major must explicitly be in a discipline of Health Education/Promotion; *OR* (2) an official transcript that reflects at least 25 semester hours or 37 quarter hours of course work (with a grade 'C' or better) with specific preparation addressing the Seven Areas of Responsibility and Competency for Health Educators" (National Commission for Health Education Credentialing, 2010b).

## Graduate Health Education Standards

The roles and responsibilities document, *A Competency-Based Framework for Professional Development of Certified Health Education Specialists* (National Commission for Health Education Credentialing, 1996), defined the skills needed for the entry-level health education/promotion professional. This document provided guidance for professional preparation programs at the bachelor's degree level, but not at the graduate degree level. Although many health education specialists with advanced degrees had obtained certification, it attested only to the fact that they had entry-level skills.

In June 1992, the Joint Committee for Graduate Standards was established by the Association for the Advancement of Health Education (now called the American Association for Health Education [AAHE]) Board of Directors. Committee membership was initially composed of Society of Public Health Education (SOPHE) and AAHE members serving on their respective accreditation bodies. To obtain a broader perspective, committee membership was expanded to include members from the Council on Education for Public Health (CEPH) and the National Commission for Health Education Credentialing, Inc. (NCHEC). After much work, discussion, and review, the Joint Committee for Graduate Standards developed a draft document that contained additional responsibilities, competencies, and sub-competencies specific to graduate-level preparation (Joint Committee for Graduate Standards, 1996).

In February 1996, 134 health education specialists from over 100 colleges and universities gathered at the National Congress for Institutions Preparing Graduate Health Educators. At this meeting in Dallas, Texas, the draft document of graduate-level competencies was presented to attendees. After thoroughly discussing and debating these competencies, recommendations for improvement were presented to the planning committee. Despite some dissension, the general mood was in favor of the competencies, and the planning committee was urged to move on with the approval process. After revisions were made, the final version was presented to the AAHE and SOPHE boards of directors, who granted approval in March 1997.

## Competencies Update Project

Since the initial Role Delineation Project began over thirty years ago, health education/promotion has evolved and matured. Changes in the profession created a need to reverify the competencies and sub-competencies of a health education specialist. The **Competencies Update Project (CUP)** began in 1998 and was completed in 2005. The majority of the CUP work was conducted by a three-person steering committee comprised of Gary Gilmore, chair, Allison Taub, and Larry Olsen (see **Figure 6.2**). The profession owes a deep debt of gratitude to these individuals for the time and effort they invested in this project.

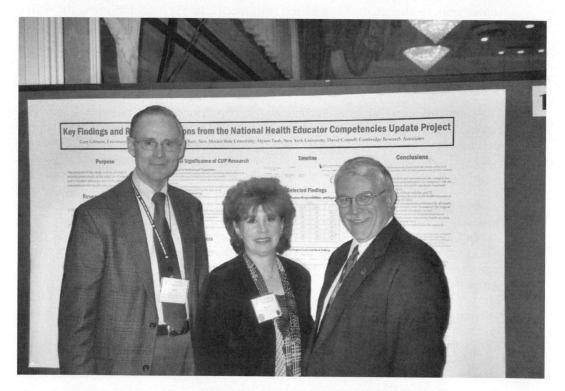

**Figure 6.2** CUP Steering Committee. From left, Gary Gilmore; Chair: Allison Taub; and Larry Olsen

(Gary D. Gilmore, MPH, Ph.D, CHES Professor and Director Graduate Community Health Programs University of Wisconsin-La Crosse)

The final CUP report, released in November, 2005, was based on the largest national dataset ever created of practicing health education specialists. Over 4,000 health education specialists from every state in the United States, and from all major employment settings, completed the 19-page questionnaire. The survey response rate was 70 percent and the total database contained more than 1.6 million data points (Gilmore, Olsen, Taub, & Connell, 2005). The results of this study helped direct the curriculum of U.S. health education/promotion professional preparation programs and served as the basis for the CHES exam from 2005 to 2010.

## Health Education Job Analysis 2010

The National Commission for Certifying Agencies (NCCA) accredits accrediting agencies. To obtain a "gold standard" endorsement from NCCA, an accrediting agency must follow recognized best practices. One of these best practices is updating the job analysis for the agency's field every five years.

In August, 2008, the National Commission for Health Education Credentialing (NCHEC) received a "gold standard" endorsement from NCCA (NCHEC 2010c). To meet the five-year update requirement, NCHEC along with AAHE and SOPHE commissioned the 2010 job analysis study (AAHE, NCHEC, & SOPHE, 2010). This study was needed in order to update the health education competencies, last revised in 2005 by the CUP project. Results of the study were released in 2010, called the Health Education Job Analysis 2010 model (*HEJA 2010* model). The areas of responsibility remained essentially the same as in the initial entry-level framework and the CUP project with only minor wording changes. This can be seen in **Table 6.2**. The fact that the responsibilities have remained fairly consistent with only minor wording changes confirms the earlier work of the role delineation project and the CUP project.

The important point here is that the health education/promotion profession has carefully and systematically reviewed and validated the competencies of a health education specialist. The CHES exam is based on these standards, and the health education/promotion curricula of professional preparation programs should be grounded on them.

## International Efforts in Quality Assurance

Outside the United States, efforts to ensure quality in health education/promotion have also occurred. According to Allegrante, Barry, Auld, Lamarre, and Taub (2009), Canada, Australia, New Zealand, member states of the European Union and Council of Europe, Spain, Japan, Israel, the People's Republic of China, India, and Taiwan have all endeavored to improve health education or health promotion practice.

In an effort to promote international exchange and understanding related to the core competencies of health education/promotion and various credentialing mechanisms, a working group of 26 health education/promotion scholars and leaders from around the world met at the National University of Ireland in the summer of 2008.

**Table 6.2**   Comparison of areas of responsibility (1985–2010)

| Entry-Level Framework (1985) | Graduate-Level Framework (1999) | CUP Model (2006) | HEJA Model (2010) |
|---|---|---|---|
| I. Assessing individual and community needs for health education | I. Assessing individual and community needs for health education | I. Assessing individual and community needs for health education | I. Assess needs, assets, and capacity for health education |
| II. Planning effective health education programs | II. Planning effective health education programs | II. Plan health education strategies, interventions, and programs | II. Plan health education |
| III. Implementing health education programs | III. Implementing health education programs | III. Implement health education strategies, interventions, and programs | III. Implement health education |
| IV. Evaluating effectiveness of health education programs | IV. Evaluating effectiveness of health education programs | IV. Conduct evaluation and research related to health education | IV. Conduct evaluation and research related to health education |
| V. Coordinating provision of health education services | V. Coordinating provision of health education services | V. Administer health education strategies, interventions, and programs | V. Administer and manage health education |
| VI. Acting as a resource person in health education | VI. Acting as a resource person in health education | VI. Serve as a health education resource person | VI. Serve as a health education resource person |
| VII. Communicating health and health education needs, concerns, and resources | VII. Communicating health and health education needs, concerns, and resources | VII. Communicate and advocate for health and health education | VII. Communicate and advocate for health and health education |
|  | VIII. Applying appropriate research principles and techniques in health education |  |  |
|  | IX. Administering health education programs |  |  |
|  | X. Advancing the profession of health education |  |  |

NOTE: CUP = Competences Update Project.
From National Commission for Health Education Credentialing, Inc. (NCHEC), Society for Public Health Education (SOPHE), American Association for Health Education (AAHE). (2010a). A COMPETENCY-BASED FRAMEWORK FOR HEALTH EDUCATION SPECIALISTS-2010. Whitehall, PA: Author. By permission.

This meeting, now known as the Galway Consensus Conference, was a first effort to identify and codify agreement around quality assurance and credentialing on an international basis.

At this conference, the Domains of Core Competencies were developed (Allegrante, Barry, Airhihenbuwa et al., 2009). The domains are broader than competencies, but using these broad domains, competencies and credentialing systems can be developed by nations around the world. Review **Box 6.2** to see how the responsibilities of a health education specialist in the United States align with the Domains of Core Competency.

| Box 6.2 | Domains of Core Competency from the Galway Consensus Conference |

1. **Catalyzing Change**—Enabling change and empowering individuals and communities to improve their health.

2. **Leadership**—Providing strategic direction and opportunities for participation in developing healthy public policy, mobilizing and managing resources for health promotion, and building capacity.

3. **Assessment**—Conducting assessment of needs and assets in communities and systems that leads to the identification and analysis of the behavioral, cultural, social, environmental, and organizational determinants that promote or compromise health.

4. **Planning**—Developing measurable goals and objectives in response to assessment of needs and assets and identifying strategies that are based on knowledge, derived from theory, evidence, and practice.

5. **Implementation**—Carrying out effective and efficient, culturally sensitive, and ethical strategies to ensure the greatest possible improvements in health, including management of human and material resources.

6. **Evaluation**—Determining the reach, effectiveness, and impact of health promotion programs and policies. This includes utilizing appropriate evaluation and research methods to support program improvements, sustainability, and dissemination.

7. **Advocacy**—Advocating with and on behalf of individuals and communities to improve their health and well-being and building their capacity for undertaking actions that can both improve health and strengthen community assets.

8. **Partnerships**—Working collaboratively across disciplines, sectors, and partners to enhance the impact and sustainability of health promotion programs and policies.

*Source:* John P. Allegrante et al. (2009). "Domains of Core Competency, Standards, and Quality Assurance for Building Global Capacity in Health Promotion: The Galway Consensus Conference Statement." *Health Education & Behavior 36* (3): 476–482. Copyright © 2009 Society for Public Health Education. Reprinted by permission of Sage Publications.

## Program Accreditation

"Accreditation is a process by which a recognized professional body evaluates an entire program against predetermined criteria or standards" (Cleary, 1995). In most cases, colleges and universities that train students to enter a given profession are accredited by a recognized professional body that operates independently of the school. If a program does not meet the standards of the recognized professional body, it can lose its accreditation. A nonaccredited program might have difficulty recruiting new students and may be restricted in its participation in the profession. Therefore, accreditation helps ensure that all students entering the profession have similar training and preparation.

In health education/promotion, accreditation is available through four accrediting bodies. Health education/promotion programs that are affiliated with a college of education and train students for positions in school health may be accredited through the

National Commission for the Accreditation of Teacher Education (NCATE) or the Teacher Education Accreditation Council (TEAC). When this text was written, TEAC and NCATE were in negotiations to combine efforts to develop a unified accreditation system for schools and colleges of education.

The Council on Education for Public Health (CEPH) accredits schools of public health and graduate public health programs. Undergraduate public health programs in the same unit as a Master of Public Health (MPH) degree program may be accredited along with the MPH program. Undergraduate programs in school health or public/community health that are not affiliated with an MPH program may elect to obtain approval through the Society for Public Health Education/American Association for Health Education (SOPHE/AAHE). This is done through the SOPHE/AAHE Baccalaureate Program Approval Committee (SABPAC) process. As of August, 2010, 20 institutions had chosen to obtain SABPAC approval, with an additional two programs in the process of obtaining approval.

Having four accreditation-approvals available is considered by many a weakness in the profession. As Cleary (1995) noted, "There were (and are) huge gaps and great discrepancies in the accreditation/approval process" (p. 16). Professional preparation is not at all uniform in the profession (Cleary, 1986). Some programs focus more on content, such as drugs, sexuality, stress, and physical fitness, while other programs emphasize process courses, such as planning, implementing, and evaluating. Some programs stress individual behavior change, while others stress population-based approaches to change. In 1987, the National Task Force on the Preparation and Practice of Health Educators attempted to develop a registry of health education programs. This effort, however, had to be abandoned. There was too much variety in faculty, administrative arrangements, courses, and philosophies of the various professional preparation programs to agree on criteria for inclusion in the registry (Cleary, 1995). Currently, there are 273 programs listed in the 2009 edition of the AAHE *Directory of Institutions Offering Undergraduate and Graduate Degree Programs in Health Education* (M. Goldsmith, personal communication, August 3, 2010). Most of these programs are neither approved nor accredited, and there is no professional body monitoring their efforts. This clearly indicates a lack of consistency and quality control in the profession.

## Accreditation Task Forces

Accreditation has been a major focus for the health education/promotion profession since 2000. In January 2000, the Society for Public Health Education and the American Association for Health Education co-sponsored a meeting in Dulles, Virginia, to explore the issue of accreditation. Twenty-four professionals who were broadly representative of health education/promotion professional preparation programs or other stakeholders were invited to attend. Meeting participants reached consensus that a "coordinated accreditation system" was needed.

As a result of this meeting, the SOPHE/AAHE National Task Force on Accreditation in Health Education was established and charged to (1) "gather background information and refine plans for a comprehensive, coordinated quality assurance system that meets commonly accepted standards of accreditation, and (2) develop processes for ensuring profession-wide involvement in the discussion and design of such a system to foster its adoption and utilization" (Society for Public Health Education, 2000, p. 5).

After a comprehensive study of the issue, the task force completed its work in the spring of 2004 and submitted its final report to the AAHE and SOPHE boards of directors (Allegrante et al., 2004). In this report, four principles (see list below) were given to guide the profession. On the basis of these four principles, the task force included seven important recommendations with the study's final results (see **Box 6.3**).

1. Health education is a single profession, with common roles and responsibilities.

2. Professional preparation in health education provides the health education specialist with knowledge and skills that form a foundation of common and setting-specific competencies.

3. Accreditation is the primary quality assurance mechanism in higher education.

4. The health education profession is responsible for assuring quality in professional preparation and practice (Allegrante et al., 2004, p. 676).

Both boards accepted the final report and then instituted a second committee to transition from the National Task Force recommendations to an implementation phase of the process. Dr. David Birch, Southern Illinois University, and Dr. Kathleen Roe, San Jose State University, co-chaired this committee called the National Transition Task Force on Accreditation in Health Education

The work of this task force culminated in a three-day meeting of health education/promotion professional preparation programs in Dallas, February 23–25, 2006 (Taub, Birch, Auld, Lysoby, & King, 2009). At this "Third National Congress on Institutions Preparing Health Educators," accreditation issues were presented, discussed, and debated. Some attendees felt accreditation should move forward as quickly as possible. Others seemed reluctant to move in the direction of accreditation and wanted more discussion and debate. Several small programs expressed concern that they would not be able to meet accreditation requirements. Some present were concerned that the Council on Education in Public Health (CEPH) was being considered as the accreditation body and that using CEPH would push all health education/promotion programs to become public health programs. Others felt that if the roles and responsibilities identified by the CUP were used as the basis of accreditation, CEPH would be a suitable accrediting body. At the end of the conference, most participants supported the initiation of a coordinated accreditation system (Taub et al., 2009).

To follow up the work of the National Transition Task Force and the Third National Congress, a third task force was initiated late in 2006. This task force, co-chaired by Dr. David Birch and Dr. Randy Cottrell, was named the National Implementation Task Force for Accreditation in Health Education. It is still functioning today with the charge to continue preparing the health education/promotion profession for accreditation (Cottrell et al., 2009).

Much progress has been made in meeting the recommendation of the first National Task Force on Accreditation in Health Education. Advanced certification for health education specialists began in fall 2010 with initial testing in 2011. At the time this text was written, CEPH had agreed to initiate a new accreditation process for free-standing undergraduate public/community health programs, but a definite timeline was still unknown. Also, NCHEC agreed, in principle, that it will only certify health education

| Box 6.3 | RESULTS AND RECOMMENDATIONS FROM THE NATIONAL TASK FORCE ON ACCREDITATION IN HEALTH EDUCATION |

1. That accreditation be the quality assurance mechanism for health education professional preparation institutions, and should replace existing approval processes in orderly transition.

2. That there be a unified accreditation system, comprising two parallel, coordinated accreditation mechanisms for community and school health education preparation institutions, which are responsive to the needs of the health education profession. These mechanisms must assure that common and specific competencies in health education are addressed at the undergraduate and graduate levels.

   a. That the National Council for the Accreditation of Teacher Education (NCATE) is the preferred accrediting entity to provide a single coordinated accreditation mechanism for school health education programs at the undergraduate and graduate levels. If a dual teacher certification program is in place, health education is to be reviewed as a separate program.

   b. That the Council on Education for Public Health (CEPH) is the preferred accrediting entity to provide a single coordinated accreditation mechanism for community/public health education programs at the undergraduate and graduate levels.

3. That the coordinated accreditation system should build upon the best practices of existing community and school health accreditation mechanisms.

4. That graduate professional preparation programs must assure that students perform all health education competencies, and that their performance reflect graduate-level proficiency.

5. That new designations should be created to distinguish the practice level of health educators at the undergraduate and graduate levels, parallel with other professional disciplines such as nursing and social work. We recommend that these designations be:

   a. Health Education Specialist (HES) for undergraduate-level practitioners from an accredited program.

   b. Master Health Education Specialist (MHES) for the graduate-level practitioners from an accredited program.

6. That the National Commission for Health Education Credentialing (NCHEC) is an appropriate entity to oversee the process of individual certification at both the undergraduate and graduate levels. We further recommend that:

   a. Persons who successfully complete the certification processes should be designated as a Certified Health Specialist (CHES) (undergraduate level) or Master's-level Certified Health Education Specialist (MCHES) (both master's and doctorate graduate level). Only students from accredited programs/schools should be eligible for CHES and MCHES certification; however, those individuals who held the CHES certification prior to the implementation of this process would remain certified.

   b. Appropriate deeming of those undergraduate-level practitioners holding CHES should be considered, with students currently from nonaccredited undergraduate programs/schools permitted to sit for CHES for a reasonable, multiyear period of time. After such time, only students from accredited undergraduate programs/schools should be eligible to sit for CHES. A multiyear window of time should allow the new accreditation system to be fully functioning, while offering a transition period for programs/schools to prepare and qualify for accreditation.

c. Appropriate deeming of those master's- or doctorate-level practitioners holding CHES be considered, with a window of time of up to 24 months to earn MCHES designation.

**7.** That the results of the work of the Task Force be articulated to the American Public Health Association, Association of Schools of Public Health, Association of Teachers of Preventive Medicine, Coalition of National Health Education Organizations, National Commission for Health Education Credentialing, and other relevant groups.

The implementation of the Task Force recommendations will require a profession-wide effort and the commitment of new resources over several years from a broad range of stakeholders beyond SOPHE and AAHE.

*Source:* John P. Allegrante et al and the National Task Force on Accreditation in Health. 2004. "Toward a Unified System of Accreditation for Professional Preparation in Health Education: Final Report on the National Task Force on Accreditation in Health Education." *Health Education & Behavior* 31 (6): 668–683 (December 2004). Copyright © 2004 Society for Public Health Education. Reprinted by permission of Sage Publications.

specialists who graduate from accredited programs. The implementation of this recommendation will, however, have to wait until there are a sufficient number of accredited undergraduate public/community programs and a sufficient number of graduates from these programs to support the continued operations of NCHEC.

## Responsibilities and Competencies of Health Education Specialists

The skills needed to practice health education/promotion are clearly delineated as responsibilities, competencies, and sub-competencies. **Responsibilities** essentially specify the overall scope of practice for health education specialists. They provide a general idea of what health education specialists do, but do not provide the detail necessary to practice health education/promotion.

Under each responsibility there are four to seven **competencies**. A competency "reflects the ability of the student to understand, know, etc." (National Commission for Health Education Credentialing, 1996, p. 12). Each competency is further divided into one to five **sub-competencies**. A sub-competency "reflects the ability of the student to list, describe, etc." (National Commission for Health Education Credentialing, 1996, p. 12). All health education specialists should be able to demonstrate at least minimal skills to meet all of the competencies and sub-competencies of a health education specialist.

The responsibilities, competencies, and sub-competencies of health education specialists were first described in the *Framework for the Development of Competency-Based Curricula for Entry Level Health Educators* (National Task Force on the Preparation and Practice of Health Educators, 1985). This document was later modified and reformatted based on the results of the CUP project, previously discussed in this chapter. The *Competency-Based Framework for Health Educators—2006* (NCHEC, SOPHE, &

**Table 6.3** HEJA 2010 model hierarchical approach

| Level of Practice | Sub-Competencies |
|---|---|
| **Entry-Level** (less than 5 years of experience; baccalaureate or master's degree) | 162 entry-level sub-competencies |
| **Advanced 1** (5 or more years of experience; baccalaureate or master's degree) | 162 entry-level sub-competencies<br>**PLUS**<br>Advanced 1 sub-competencies |
| **Advanced 2** (doctorate and 5 or more years of experience) | 162 entry-level sub-competencies<br>**PLUS**<br>Advanced 1 sub-competencies<br>**PLUS**<br>Advanced 2 sub-competencies |

Note: Information regarding the Advanced 1 and Advanced 2 sub-competencies had not been released at the time of this writing but should be released in future NCHEC reports to the profession.

From National Commission for Health Education Credentialing, Inc. (NCHEC), Society for Public Health Education (SOPHE), American Association for Health Education (AAHE). (2010a). A COMPETENCY-BASED FRAMEWORK FOR HEALTH EDUCATION SPECIALISTS-2010. Whitehall, PA: Author. By permission.

AAHE, 2006) combined the 1985 Entry-Level Framework responsibilities and the 1999 Graduate-Level Framework responsibilities into one set of seven responsibilities. These responsibilities were applicable to all health education specialists regardless of degree held, years of experience, or work setting.

The Health Education Job Analysis 2010 model (*HEJA 2010* model) is the most recent update of health education roles, responsibilities, competencies, and sub-competencies. It has 39 competencies within seven major areas of responsibility. The areas of responsibility remain essentially the same as those in the initial entry-level framework and the CUP project, with only minor wording changes (see **Table 6.3**). However, the total number of sub-competencies in the HEJA 2010 model is now 223, compared to 163 in the CUP framework. Additional sub-competencies are identified in areas related to ethics, partnership development, training, consultative relationships, influencing policy, and promoting the health education/promotion profession. Of the 223 sub-competencies, 162 are designated as entry-level competencies, while 61 are designated as advanced-level competencies (AAHE, NCHEC, & SOPHE, 2010).

The *HEJA 2010* document should be used by health education/promotion students on a regular basis during their professional preparation program (see Appendix B). The National Commission for Health Education Credentialing (1996) suggested that the competencies be used "as a personal inventory to assess progress toward becoming a health educator; that is to determine which competencies and sub-competencies have been mastered. It is suggested that the student assess his or her progress at intervals during the student's course of study and do a final review at the completion of the health education program" (p. 7). Students who are diligent in monitoring their progress and who can perform the competencies and sub-competencies have a much greater chance of passing the credentialing exam to become a Certified Health Education Specialist.

Because the seven major responsibilities identified in the *HEJA 2010 model* are the core of what a health education specialist does, it is important to have a basic understanding of them. The following sections briefly describe each responsibility.

## Responsibility I: Assess Needs, Assets, and Capacity for Health Education

The first major area of responsibility listed for health education specialists involves assessing needs, assets, and the capacity for health education/promotion. This responsibility provides the foundation for program planning (Bensley & Brookins-Fisher, 2003). In fact, "Assessing the needs of the priority population may be the most critical step in the planning process . . ." (McKenzie, Neiger, & Thackeray, 2009, p. 80). A **needs assessment** is a process that helps program planners determine what health problems might exist in any given group of people, what assets are available in the community to address the health problems, and the overall capacity of the community to address the health issues. Other terms used to describe this process include community analysis, community diagnosis, and community assessment (McKenzie et al., 2009).

In a needs assessment, "**Capacity** refers to both individual and collective resources that can be brought to bear for health enhancement" (Gilmore & Campbell, 2005, p. 7). More specifically, assessing capacity identifies the assets—skills, resources, agencies, groups, and individuals—that can be brought together in a community to solve problems and empower a community. "**Community Empowerment** is about helping people help themselves in a way that encourages them to take ownership of their health problems and use their abilities and resources to develop solutions" (Doyle & Ward, 2001, p. 125). For that reason, it is critical to include members of the community on any planning team.

All health education specialists, regardless of the setting in which they are employed, must have the skills to assess the needs and capacity of those groups or individuals to whom their programs are directed. For example, a school health education specialist needs to base curriculum on the needs of the students, a health education specialist in the corporate setting needs to plan programs based on the needs of the company's employees, and public health education specialists should base their health education/promotion efforts on the needs of the community they serve.

Health education/promotion programs should not be based on the whim of the health education specialist or any small group of decision makers. Resources are too valuable to waste on programs that do not address the needs of the population being served. As McKenzie et al. (2009) notes, ". . . failure to perform a needs assessment may lead to a program focus that prevents or delays adequate attention directed to a more important health problem" (p. 80). Conversely, "We know our health education programs are on target when we base them on accurate needs assessment data and a careful interpretation of their meaning" (Doyle & Ward, 2001, p. 124). Ultimately, a well-conceived and well-conducted needs assessment determines if a health education/promotion program is justified. It also defines the nature and scope of a program (Gilmore & Campbell, 2005).

To conduct a needs assessment, health education specialists should know how to locate and obtain valid sources of information related to their specific population(s) with similar characteristics. For example, this may entail a literature review or accessing information from local, county, or state health departments. In addition to examining pre-existing information, called **secondary data**, it may be necessary for health education specialists to gather data of their own, known as **primary data**. They may have to conduct mail, electronic, and/or telephone surveys; hold focus group meetings (see **Figure 6.3**); and use a nominal group process. After all this information is collected, the health education specialist must be able to analyze the data and determine priority areas for health education/promotion programming.

The following example demonstrates the importance of a needs assessment. A health education internship student was placed with the Shriners Hospital for Burned

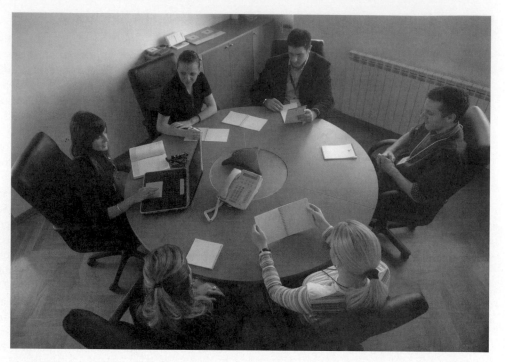

**Figure 6.3** A group of health education specialists meeting to discuss information gathered during the assessment phase that will be used to guide the planning phase. (Lucky winner/Alamy)

Children in Cincinnati, Ohio. The hospital identified a problem with children being burned around campfires during the summer months and asked the student to develop a fire safety program for young campers. Fortunately, the site supervisor required the student to conduct a needs assessment before planning the program. After conducting focus groups, interviewing camp counselors, and reviewing the literature, it was concluded that campers were the wrong group to target with the program. Instead, a program for the camp leaders and counselors was needed. If the needs assessment had not been done, valuable time and resources would have been spent developing a program for the wrong audience.

## Responsibility II: Plan Health Education

Planning involves more than just determining a location and time for a health education/promotion program. Planning begins by reviewing the health needs, problems, and concerns of the priority population obtained through the needs assessment. Early in the planning process, it is important to recruit interested stakeholders, such as community leaders, representatives from community organizations, resource providers, and representatives of the population, to support and help develop the program. Without the help of these stakeholders, it may be impossible to develop effective programs. To be effective in the planning process, the health education specialist should have strong written and oral communication skills, leadership ability, and the expertise to help diverse groups of people to reach consensus on issues of interest.

As part of the planning process, health education specialists must be competent to develop goals and objectives specific to the proposed health education/promotion program. These goals and objectives are the foundation on which the program is established. Writing specific and measurable objectives is critical. No health education/promotion program should be initiated without objectives, or considered complete until an evaluation of the objectives is conducted. Writing good objectives is a skill you can only obtain through guided practice and experience. After program goals and objectives are written, the next step is to develop appropriate interventions that will meet these goals and objectives.

Consider the following example of the planning process. A health education specialist, who is working in the university health service wellness center, analyzes the results of a recently conducted needs assessment. Next, the health education specialist recruits a variety of individuals to develop a plan for the university. This group includes representatives of the Greek system, student life organization, resident life (dorms), athletics, health education/promotion program, provost's office, campus security, and local chamber of commerce. Together, they review the needs assessment data and agree that alcohol-related incidents are a problem on campus that needs to be addressed.

First, the planning group utilizes existing baseline data on alcohol-related incidents to establish written objectives for the overall program. Next, they plan a variety of strategies to increase awareness of alcohol-related problems, modify alcohol-drinking behaviors, and reduce the number of reported alcohol incidents on campus. They organize a campus-wide alcohol awareness day, and they devise strategies with local bar owners to reduce excessive drinking. They also establish an agreement with campus security and the provost to refer any student involved in an alcohol-related incident to a mandatory alcohol education program. In addition, they develop posters and flyers promoting responsible drinking, train a bevy of peer student leaders to speak to dorm and Greek groups, and plan a variety of nonalcohol alternative events for campus. For each and every strategy, they write specific objectives, establish implementation timelines, assign tasks to committee members, and establish a budget. If the planned strategies are successful, the program objectives will be met.

An important aspect of planning includes observing the **Rule of Sufficiency**. This rule states that any strategies chosen must be sufficiently robust, or effective enough, to ensure the stated objectives have a reasonable chance of being met. For example, in the above scenario, do you think the primary objective (e.g., reduce the number of alcohol-related incidents on campus by 20 percent) has a reasonable chance of being reached if all the listed program strategies are implemented? On the other hand, if the only strategy utilized was to hand out a pamphlet on alcohol abuse to students, the intervention will not be robust enough to achieve the stated objective. In that case, the Rule of Sufficiency would not be met. Either the intervention strategies need modification, or the program should not be implemented. Time and resources are wasted if interventions are not effective enough to create the desired change. Further, if interventions fail to meet their objectives, then both the reputation of the health education specialist and the health education/promotion profession suffer.

## Responsibility III: Implement Health Education

After a needs assessment is conducted and analyzed, objectives are written, and intervention strategies are developed, it is time to implement the program. For many health education specialists, implementation is the most enjoyable of the responsibilities because it involves putting the program into action.

To successfully implement a program, the health education specialist must have a thorough understanding of the people in the priority population. What is their current level of understanding regarding the issue at hand? What will it take to get the people to participate? Do they need financial assistance or childcare? What time of the day should the program be offered? What location(s) would be most convenient? While some of these questions can be answered from the initial needs assessment, it may also be necessary to obtain additional information about the priority population before proceeding with implementation.

When conducting various health promotion and education programs, it is important for the health education specialist to be comfortable using a wide range of educational methods or techniques. In school health, for example, it is not enough to simply lecture to students about "proper" health behaviors. A successful health education specialist uses many teaching strategies such as brainstorming, debate, daily logs, position papers, guest speakers, problem solving, decision making, demonstrations, role playing, drama, music, and current events. In community health, most programs require going beyond developing and distributing a simple pamphlet on a given health topic. Again, a wide variety of strategies should be used, including television, radio, newspapers, billboards, celebrity spokespersons, behavioral contracting, community events, contests, incentives, support groups, and many more. As a general rule, health education specialists should always use multiple intervention activities when planning and implementing programs.

Health education specialists should also include population-based approaches to create health-improvement changes. Instead of focusing on individuals, population-based approaches focus on policies, rules, regulations, and laws to modify behaviors of a priority group or population. For example, instead of working one-on-one with individuals to enhance exercise levels, it might be more effective to work toward funding new walking and biking trails, having bike racks available at bus stations, initiating a city-wide walk/bike-to-work day, advocating for improved pedestrian safety laws, and so forth.

After a program is in place and operating, the responsibility of the health education specialist is not over. The health education specialist should continue to monitor the program to make certain everything is going as planned. If problems are noted, it may be necessary, even while the program is in progress, to revise the objectives or the intervention activities.

When implementing program strategies or interventions, health education specialists may need to apply a variety of sub-competencies such as presentation skills, group facilitation skills, pretest/posttest administration, data collection, and technology utilization, all of which must be demographically and culturally sensitive. During the intervention phase, a health education specialist typically has the most contact with the public. The Code of Ethics for health education specialists (see Appendix A) should be strictly followed, and one should always dress and act in an appropriate professional manner.

## Responsibility IV: Conduct Evaluation and Research Related to Health Education

Accurate evaluations must be conducted to measure the success of health education/promotion programs. These evaluations help reveal whether or not implemented programs are meeting their specified objectives. Programs not properly evaluated may be wasting valuable time, money, and other resources. Further, an unevaluated program cannot "prove its worth." So, it may risk being cut back or even eliminated when resources are short and downsizing occurs.

To conduct an effective evaluation, the health education specialist must first establish realistic, measurable objectives. As previously mentioned, this is an important part of the planning process. After objectives are in place, the health education specialist must develop a plan that will accurately assess if the program objectives have been met. Depending on the setting, this process may involve developing and administering tests, conducting surveys, observing behavior, tracking epidemiological data, or other methods of data collection. Evaluation plans can be very simple or extremely sophisticated, depending on the program being evaluated, the expectations of the program planners, and the requirements of the funding agents.

After data is collected, it must be analyzed and interpreted. Reports are then developed and distributed to the appropriate parties. Ultimately, the evaluation results should be used to modify and improve current or future program efforts. In some cases, evaluation results may indicate that a program needs to be discontinued and funding redirected to other, more productive efforts. Health education specialists must have the fortitude to make these difficult decisions when needed.

In addition to evaluation, research is a vital activity for any profession, including health education/promotion. A profession moves forward and improves in large part due to the quality of its research and the new information it generates. **Health education research** can be defined as "a systematic investigation involving the analysis of collected information or data that ultimately is used to enhance health education knowledge or practice, and answers one or more questions about a health-related theory, behavior or phenomenon" (Cottrell & McKenzie, 2011, p. 2). While more complex research skills are required at advanced levels, entry-level health education specialists should be able to read, synthesize, and utilize research results to improve their practice.

## Responsibility V: Administer and Manage Health Education

A great deal of administration, management, and coordination is needed to bring a health education/promotion program to fruition. Even though some administrative tasks may be performed by entry-level health education specialists, administration and management responsibilities are generally handled by professionals at more advanced levels of practice. For example, experienced health education specialists often become program managers or staff supervisors. "Good management and supervisory skills require training in a variety of organizational, psychological and business environments. Good management incorporates effective 'people skills' and knowledge of budgeting, task assignments and performance evaluation" (NCHEC, SOPHE, & AAHE, 2006, p. 33).

Health education specialists must facilitate cooperation among personnel, both within programs and between programs. Many public school systems, for example, have initiated coordinated school health programs. This involves coordinating the activities and services of school nurses, counselors, psychologists, food service personnel, physical educators, health education specialists, teachers, administrators, support staff, parents, and public health agencies. The ultimate goal is to develop both curricular and extracurricular programs to improve the health status of students, faculty, staff, and the community as a whole. Further, health education specialists in school settings may serve as curriculum coordinators or project directors and can be responsible for managing grants and program budgets.

Similar examples can be seen in the community setting. For example, a health department decides to apply for grant funds to reduce the incidence of tobacco use in its community. The health education specialist may form a coalition by bringing together individuals and/or groups with a vested interest in reducing tobacco use. Coalition members might include representatives from the American Cancer Society, American Lung Association, American Heart Association, local medical society, local dental association, public health department, public school system, and YMCA/YWCA. Coordination and integration of the services offered by these various groups would be critical to the successful development of a grant proposal and ultimately to the success of the funded program. It may even be necessary for the health education specialist to conduct or coordinate in-service training programs to ensure that all coalition members have similar knowledge related to tobacco prevention programs. Obviously, administrative and management skills are needed throughout this entire process.

### Responsibility VI: Serve as a Health Education Resource Person

Health education specialists are often called to serve as resource persons. It is not unusual for a student to seek out the health teacher for assistance when having a health-related problem. In the corporate setting, health education specialists get questions about a wide range of topics, including nutritional supplements, cancer signs and symptoms, the best type of shoe to wear for jogging, and many more.

Because it is impossible for health education specialists to know all the information that could be needed in a given position, they must have the skill to access resources they need. It may be necessary to visit the library; use computerized health retrieval systems; access health databases; find information on specific diseases; obtain local, regional, state, and national epidemiological data; and so on. As part of this process, it may also be necessary for health education specialists to select or develop effective educational resources for distributing information to their priority populations.

Consider, for example, the entry-level health education specialist who was hired by a large metropolitan hospital. Her duties included developing health education/promotion programs for the community and resource materials for patients. Her first assignment was to develop educational materials on the problem of incontinence in older adults. This subject had not been covered in her professional preparation program. However, because of the skills she had previously learned, she was able to locate a variety of resources on the topic, evaluate their validity, select relevant information, and then develop an educational video and pamphlet on the topic.

Being able to simply retrieve information is not enough. Health education specialists must be able to establish effective consultative relationships with people who seek assistance, whether they are students, clients, employees, or other health education specialists. They must instill confidence and communicate effectively in a nonthreatening manner. In some situations, health education specialists may decide to market their skills to individuals or groups, as resource consultants. They may even decide to focus their career entirely as a resource person.

### Responsibility VII: Communicate and Advocate for Health and Health Education

Health education specialists must interact with various groups of people, including other health professionals, consumers, students, employers, employees, and fellow health education specialists. They must be skilled in written communication, oral communication, and mass media use. Health education specialists need to feel comfortable working with individuals, small groups, and large groups, as the situation warrants. In essence, communication is the primary tool of the health education specialist.

It is often necessary for health education specialists to serve as communication filters between medical doctors/researchers and students or clients. Health education specialists must be able to "translate" difficult scientific concepts so that constituents can understand the information necessary to improve and protect their health. For example, a physician may tell a patient to start an exercise program, reduce fat in the diet, or manage stress better. Although many patients have a general idea of what these recommendations mean, they may not have the knowledge or skills to implement them. Most physicians cannot take the time to teach patients how to incorporate these changes into their lifestyles. Health education specialists can communicate detailed information on exercising safely, teach the client to recognize high-fat foods by reading food labels, and instruct the patient in progressive neuromotor relaxation. This may involve conducting one-on-one instruction, developing a videotape for patients to watch, developing brochures for distribution to patients, teaching classes, or coordinating support groups.

Beyond communicating health information, Responsibility VII requires health education specialists to "advocate" for health and health education/promotion. This means they should initiate and support legislation, rules, policies, and procedures that will enhance the health of the populations with which they work. Health education specialists should be involved in supporting nonsmoking laws, mandatory helmet laws, seatbelt laws, antidrug policies, rules to prevent selling "junk foods" in school cafeterias, initiatives to develop walking/biking trails, gun safety laws, and so forth.

Further, health education specialists should "advocate" for their profession. They should educate potential employers about the value of hiring professionally trained and degreed health education specialists with CHES status. When health education specialists hold positions with hiring authority, they should advertise for and hire qualified health education specialists. It is important that health education specialists talk to legislators, policy makers, personnel directors, allied health workers, co-workers, family, and friends about the value of health education/promotion. They should join health education professional associations and support the national initiatives designed to move the profession forward. These include the development of National Health Education Standards and the current initiative for program accreditation. While advocating for the profession may seem awkward and somewhat akin to "blowing one's own horn," if health education specialists do not promote their profession, who will?

## Summary of Responsibilities and Competencies

The responsibilities, competencies, and sub-competencies required for health education specialists do not function independently; they are highly interrelated. All of the responsibilities demand excellent communication skills. Conducting an accurate needs assessment requires research skills to identify and gather appropriate resources. Planning should be based on a valid and reliable needs assessment. When implementing programs, be prepared to serve as a resource person when asked. Evaluation relies on goals and objectives established during the planning process. Coordinating people and administering programs are necessary in planning, implementing, and evaluating programs.

It is not enough to be proficient in one, two, or even six of the responsibility areas. All seven responsibilities are critical for effective health education/promotion to take place. It is beyond the scope of this book to teach the reader how to do these tasks. Rather, it is the intent of this text to familiarize readers with the responsibilities, competencies, and skills they will be taught in later classes and ultimately practice in their employment settings.

## Multitasking

It is often necessary for health education specialists to use several competency-related skills simultaneously. This requires **multitasking**: the skill of coordinating and completing multiple projects at the same time. In college, health education/promotion students are often given a project at the beginning of a term. There is a specific amount of time to complete the project, and when the term ends the project is completed. In the work world, things do not function this way. Health education specialists work on multiple projects at the same time, and each project is usually in a different stage of completion.

Organization is the key to successful multitasking. For example, one health education/promotion internship student used a visual concept to help her stay organized while working on multiple projects. Using a bulletin board, unfinished projects and tasks were represented by floating balloon images. Once completed, these "balloons" were placed at the bottom of the bulletin board in the hand of a stick figure that represented the health education specialist. Other effective tools for multitasking include spreadsheets, timelines, and "to do" lists.

## Technology

As in most professions, health education specialists must be familiar with and comfortable using computers and other forms of technology. Since computer software and hardware are constantly changing, it is important to keep up-to-date on the latest technological aids. Entry-level health education specialists are expected to have required technology skills by the time they enter their internships and certainly by the time they accept their first position. See **Box 6.4** for a list of entry-level computer skills.

**Social networking** is another aspect of technology that needs to be fully explored and utilized by health education specialists. According to Wikipedia (2010), a social network is, "a social structure made up of individuals (or organizations) called 'nodes,' which are tied (connected) by one or more specific types of interdependency, such as friendship, kinship, common interest, financial exchange, . . . beliefs, knowledge or prestige." Facebook, Myspace, Cyworld, Bebo, Twitter, and podcasts are just a few examples of how people are communicating. These social networking services can be used by health education specialists to connect people with similar health interests, such as losing weight or reducing stress. They can also be used to link people who have a common cause, such as passing nonsmoking legislation. In addition, they are helpful for sending information or updates about programs sponsored by a given health agency. The list of uses is limited only by one's creativity.

| **Box 6.4** | ENTRY-LEVEL TECHNOLOGY SKILLS (NOT PRIORITIZED) |

- Basic word processing/text editing skills including use of writing tools like spell checkers, electronic thesaurus, etc.
- Basic to advanced electronic spreadsheet use, beginning with elementary worksheets and progressing to more sophisticated "what-if" analyses
- Introductory statistical analysis software and data entry (assuming that statistics applications are also learned)
- Preparing effective PowerPoint presentations
- Critiquing components of computer-assisted health education software (health assessments to computer-assisted instruction)
- Electronic retrieval of quality health information—search engines, databases, and indexes of health literature
- Electronic health information media literacy, including evaluating the quality of health Web sites
- Utilizing a Web page editor to design and develop effective health-based Web pages. This would include skills needed to upload pages to a server and then marketing the site to specific Internet audiences.
- Professional electronic mail and discussion list etiquette
- Use of common technological innovations in health education/promotion such as digital video/photography, scanners, personal digital assistants, and computer-assisted interviews and surveys

*Source:* List provided by Dr. Ernesto Randolfi, Montana State University–Billings. Posted to HEDIR Listserve, 2002.

## Role Modeling

Being a healthy role model is not listed anywhere in the roles and responsibilities of a health education specialist, but it has been discussed and debated as much as any other aspect of the profession (Davis, 1999; Bruess, 2003). Some people feel that health education specialists should not be expected to be healthy role models. This expectation may discriminate against professionals who suffer from disease conditions that cause obesity or preclude a regular exercise regimen. Others think that being a healthy role model puts too much pressure on health education specialists, especially since there is no accepted definition for what "healthy" means. On the other hand, many in the profession believe that being a healthy role model is important to effectively carry out the responsibilities of the profession. Some even argue that ethically, health education specialists must be role models.

The authors of this text tend to believe that role modeling is an important aspect of being a health education specialist. The purpose of presenting this issue is to stimulate health education/promotion students to enter the debate. Do you feel health education specialists should be role models? Do you think health education specialists who are not role models will be less effective in their work? What does it mean to be a role model? Are you a role model now? Do you want to be a role model in the future?

## Advanced Study in Health Education

After receiving a bachelor's degree in health education/promotion, students should not stop the educational process. At the very least, health education specialists should continue to learn on their own. One way of doing so is to participate in one or more professional associations (see Chapter 8). Such memberships allow the opportunity to read professional publications and attend state, regional, and national meetings of the associations.

If you are a Certified Health Education Specialist, an average of 15 continuing education contact hours are required each year (75 over five years) to maintain certification. These may be obtained by reading professional journals and submitting responses to questions on selected articles, by attending various professional meetings and workshops, by taking additional coursework, or by participating in other professional development activities.

At some point, health education specialists with a bachelor's degree should consider getting a master's degree. In some areas of the country and in some health education/promotion settings, such as medical care and worksite health education/promotion, the master's degree is often considered the entry-level degree. In other words, to be considered for employment in these settings, the health education specialist must hold an appropriate master's degree (see **Box 6.5**).

In school settings, the master's degree brings additional financial rewards and, in some states, progress toward more permanent teaching certificates. It is usually advised, however, not to complete a master's degree in teaching prior to obtaining your first teaching position. Hiring a new teacher with a master's degree, versus one with a bachelor's degree, is more expensive for a school district. This factor may put a person with a master's degree at a disadvantage in the hiring process.

In community or public health settings, the master's degree may bring additional financial rewards, as well as promotions within the agency. It may also open the door to higher-level positions with other public health agencies or public health departments.

## Master's Degree Options

There are multiple types of master's degrees. Typical choices include a Master's of Education (**M.Ed.**), Master's of Science (**M.S.**), Master's of Arts (**M.A.**), Master's of Public Health (**M.P.H.**), and Master's of Science in Public Health (**M.S.P.H.**) (Bensley & Pope, 1994). Some colleges and universities may offer only one degree option, while others may offer more than one.

The M.Ed. degree is typically found in institutions where the health education/promotion program is located in a College of Education or Teacher's College. Although many students in these programs focus on school health, this does not mean that everyone who obtains this degree must pursue a career in public schools. Some colleges and universities offer M.Ed. degrees, which emphasize areas such as community health and corporate health promotion.

The M.S. and M.A. degrees are usually found in universities where the health education/promotion program is located in colleges other than education. Because there is no accepted accreditation for these programs, schools have much flexibility to develop programs that meet the needs of the local job market. These degrees offer a variety of emphasis areas, including public health, community health education/promotion, and corporate health promotion.

## Box 6.5 Practitioner's Perspective    Graduate Level Study

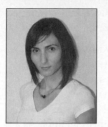

(Reprinted by permission of Lavinia S. Streza)

NAME: Lavinia S. Streza, M.S. Health Education

CURRENT POSITION/TITLE: Wellness/Fitness Specialist

EMPLOYER: TriHealth Corporate Services

DEGREE/INSTITUTIONS: B.A., Classics and Greek Studies, Hellenic College, Boston, MA; M.S. Health Promotion and Education, University of Cincinnati

UNDERGRADUATE MAJOR: Classics and Greek Studies

MINOR/EMPHASIS: Elementary Education with concentration on Inner City schools

**Background:** I was born in Romania, where there are few Health Promotion Programs. The notions of wellness and disease prevention have not yet penetrated the culture. Growing up, I had no idea I wanted to be a health educator. In 2003, I was offered a scholarship to attend Hellenic College to pursue my bachelor's degree in Classics Studies. Full of energy and enthusiasm for this new opportunity, I moved to Boston to begin my college degree. Being an international student in a challenging, new environment, I developed a strict personal discipline and lifestyle that focused almost solely on my studies. Gradually, I realized that such discipline was detrimental to my overall health. Therefore, in parallel with my classics studies, I developed a genuine interest for health-related topics. As my knowledge improved, so did my health behaviors and general wellness. Just like someone who discovers something precious and wants to share it with the world, I found I wanted to share my healthy lifestyle with others. In order to achieve this, I added to my curriculum a minor in education, hoping that it would equip me with essential teaching skills. After graduation from Hellenic College, I knew I wanted to learn more about health and how to help others improve their health. In 2009, I was offered a graduate assistantship and admission to the Health Promotion and Education MS degree program at the University of Cincinnati. Serving as a graduate assistant really enriched my overall graduate experience and provided me with much needed experience.

**Overall impressions of graduate school:** Considering my graduate degree, I can think of three distinct learnings that impacted me. First, as an international student, it provided an understanding of health issues at the individual, community, and society levels. I can now see how health issues are treated in my home country of Romania and can compare that to what I see in the United States. The cultural environment conditions behaviors, and studying them taught me much about the values, lifestyle, and standards of Americans. Second, graduate school made me a better parent. I am the mother of a beautiful two-year old daughter. Having a child was a continuous motivation to learn more not only for her now, but to be able to teach her and others the importance of a healthy family lifestyle. Third and above all, I believe that grad school made me a competent health educator. When I graduated from my undergraduate degree program, I completely changed my area of studies. While I was excited to finally be studying health, I was also nervous, as the notions of health promotion and education were still vague in my mind. The curriculum, faculty, and personal research gradually shaped and outlined various areas of expertise (i.e., personal coaching, community education, corporate wellness), and with every class that I took, I was more certain that this was what I loved doing. In other words, when I started the program, I knew that I wanted to change the world as a health educator. During the program, I feel that I was given the tools and the confidence that I could practice health

**Box 6.5 Practitioner's Perspective** Continued

education and make an impact in many different ways and different levels.

**Motherhood and Health Promotion:** In 2008 before beginning graduate school, I became the mother of a wonderful little girl. The entire pregnancy, the experience of birth and care for a newborn, was not only a life-changing experience, but also drew me even closer to health information and health research. Health Promotion truly covers all stages of life; it deals with wellness "from womb to tomb." Prenatal health promotion is a fast growing field and I hope in the future I will be able to share with many expectant women the importance of diet, exercise, and overall health during the nine months of pregnancy. While attending grad school, I was also caring for my newborn. Even if, at times, it added to my stress, parenting kept me grounded and focused during my studies. I, as any responsible parent, needed to tend to her wellbeing and health. I want to be the health education specialist who educates and advocates for healthy habits, active lifestyle, and disease prevention for the sake of our generation and for the generations to come. Children should not inherit destructive and unhealthy behaviors from their parents.

**What I liked most about graduate school:** A graduate degree program opens countless opportunities for further study or employment. From personal exercise management to community-wide education programs, from grant proposals to policy making, from immediate employment to further academic research at the doctoral level, the Health Promotion and Education Graduate Program helps students identify their skills and talents and to further shape their professional or academic career. I felt that the courses provided me with the needed skills and competencies, while the internship program provided a safe environment to apply and advance my skills. Throughout the study period, the faculty did an outstanding job mentoring

and offering me personal direction according to my individual areas of interest.

**What I liked least about graduate school:** During my graduate studies, I was expected to fulfill various roles and sometimes I found it difficult to find a balance between them. As a mother, my instinct was to spend as much time as possible with my daughter. As a wife, I felt that the academic workload took away some of our family time. As a graduate assistant I was expected to teach, assist in research, and invest energy and time. I fulfilled all these responsibilities while maintaining my high academic standards, but it was not easy. Overall, what I liked least about the program was the constant need to prioritize among responsibilities that were all important. I was never able to fully enjoy or immerse myself in any of my varied roles; nevertheless, I truly believe it was worth the sacrifice and effort. It is possible to be a full-time international graduate student, graduate assistant, mother, and wife all at the same time.

**Recommendations for Health Education students considering graduate study:** If you are interested in graduate study, know that it is more than a job training program; it is a life-changing experience. It is a stage of a journey, which began when you first became interested in your health. It is the transitional point when you evolve from being self-serving in regards to your health to serving others, educating and promoting a way of life. No matter what direction your academic work will take, always keep in mind the people whose lives you will change (i.e., the pupils, the employees, the communities that benefit from your programs). This way, your career will be fulfilling, dynamic, and exciting. The program may be a year or two long, but it is the beginning of a life-long endeavor, especially in such a dynamic field as Health Education/Promotion. Dedicate yourself to your studies, focus on your goals, balance your life, and you will be successful in graduate school.

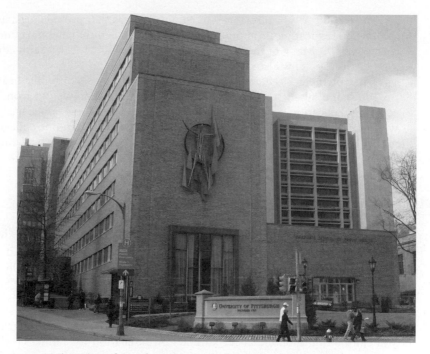

**Figure 6.4** University of Pittsburgh Graduate School of Public Health
(Wikipedia)

When considering differences between the M.S., M.A., and M.Ed. degrees, remember that the M.S. may be the more scientific or research-oriented degree, while the M.A. and M.Ed. may be more practitioner oriented. This distinction, however, is not always true. Prospective students need to carefully examine the stated mission and degree requirements for any graduate-level health education/promotion program.

As their names imply, the M.P.H. and M.S.P.H. are degree choices for those wishing to work in the field of public health. The M.S.P.H. degree is typically more research oriented than the M.P.H. degree; otherwise, the degrees are similar. The M.P.H. can be awarded in a variety of specialty areas such as nursing, dietetics, or epidemiology. The M.P.H. with an emphasis in health education/promotion is the degree of most interest to health education specialists.

Most M.P.H. degree-granting colleges and universities are accredited by the Council on Education for Public Health (CEPH). Thus, the requirements to obtain an M.P.H. are more standardized than the requirements to obtain the M.S., M.A., or M.Ed. degrees, which typically are not accredited by any professional body. Due in part to accreditation, the M.P.H. degree may enjoy a higher status and more credibility than other health education/promotion degree designations. To obtain M.P.H. accreditation, the curriculum must contain five specific areas of knowledge: biostatistics, epidemiology, health services administration, social and behavioral sciences, and environmental health.

The M.P.H. in health education/promotion has the reputation of being a more prestigious degree than the M.S., M.A., or M.Ed. There are, however, more health education specialists with M.S., M.A., or M.Ed. degrees than there are with the M.P.H.

degree. The 2009 AAHE directory lists 96 institutions that provide master's-level non-M.P.H. health education/promotion degrees (M. Goldsmith, personal communication, August 3, 2010). Many of the institutions that offer non-M.P.H. health education/promotion degrees are now also offering the M.P.H. degree.

As of September 2010, there were 44 accredited schools of public health (up from 38 in 2007) and 84 accredited graduate public health programs (up from 68 in 2007) (Council on Education for Public Health, 2010). Not all of these public health programs, however, provide a focus in health education/promotion. From one college to another, there are great variations in degree program requirements. Carefully examine program requirements and master's degree options within the context of your future career goals.

## Selecting a Graduate School

Determining which college or university to attend is a decision that goes hand-in-hand with deciding which degree to pursue. In terms of practicality, factors such as cost, location, and size must be considered (Cottrell & Hayden, 2007). For listings of graduate programs, see the American Association for Health Education's *Directory of Institutions Offering Undergraduate and Graduate Degree Programs in Health Education* (M. Goldsmith, personal communication, August 3, 2010). This resource lists institutions by state and type of degrees offered. The best listing of accredited programs in public health can be found online at the Council on Education for Public Health Web site, http://www.ceph.org.

College or university reputation is an important factor to consider when selecting a health education/promotion graduate program. There is a definite hierarchy among colleges and universities in the United States. Graduating from one of the more prestigious institutions may lend instant credibility to the graduate degree and enhance job opportunities.

Next, consider the reputation of the health education/promotion program at a given institution. To learn about various programs, bachelor's-level health education specialists can talk to other professionals in the field whom they admire and trust. A visit or call to former college professors may also be a good source of information.

After narrowing your list to several programs, contact the program administrator for each one. Ask for materials describing the program, application forms, admission requirements, a copy of the graduate catalog, and a list of recent graduates and where they are employed. Much of this information may be obtained online. Contacting recent graduates is also a good way to learn about a particular program (Cottrell & Hayden, 2007).

Finally, most colleges and universities now have home pages on the World Wide Web that provide extensive information about graduate programs. These sites often allow students to complete the entire application process electronically.

## Admission Requirements

As an undergraduate health education/promotion student, it is not too early to be concerned about admission requirements to graduate school. Although admission requirements vary greatly from one university to another, the undergraduate grade point average (GPA) has traditionally been important. In general, a student should strive to achieve an overall undergraduate GPA of at least a 3.0 on a 4.0 scale in order to be considered by most graduate programs. Some institutions do not specify a minimum GPA (Bensley & Pope, 1994). Instead, they tend to use more individual and subjective criteria in their admission process. In either case, it is important for new health education/promotion students to attempt from the first term of their freshman year to achieve the best grades possible. Too often, low grades in the first two years of college prevent otherwise good students from being accepted into the master's degree program of their choice.

In addition to GPA requirements, most graduate programs require a completed application form, a letter of application, and several letters of reference. To be considered for admission, some programs also require students to submit scores from a standardized performance test such as the Graduate Record Exam or Miller Analogy Test. These scores may be a major component in the decision-making process, or they may simply be used in conjunction with other applicant information to provide a more well-rounded view of the prospective student.

## Financing Graduate Study

Funding a graduate degree may not be as burdensome as funding undergraduate education. Many colleges and universities award assistantships or fellowships to graduate students on a competitive basis. Typically, these graduate awards pay all or part of the graduate tuition and provide students with a monthly stipend to cover living expenses during their graduate studies. In return, students agree to work for the health education/promotion program.

If the award is a **graduate teaching assistantship** (or fellowship), the student teaches a specified number of undergraduate courses each term. These are usually introductory health education/promotion courses that meet general university requirements, or they are the first courses for health education/promotion majors. If the award is a **graduate research assistantship** (or fellowship), the student usually works closely with one or more faculty members on a particular research project. Students might be assigned to do literature reviews, assist with data collection, enter data into the computer, or a host of other research-related activities (Cottrell & Hayden, 2007).

Graduate assistantships and fellowships not only provide an excellent alternative for funding graduate education but also provide valuable health education/promotion work experience for the student. Further, a graduate assistantship may provide an advantage in the job market after the degree program is completed.

### SUMMARY

Since the late 1970s, many people have dedicated much time and hard work to defining and developing the roles and responsibilities of a health education specialist. The initial stages of this work were known as the Role Delineation Project. Eventually, a set of responsibilities, competencies, and sub-competencies were agreed on for health education specialists, regardless of whether they ultimately wished to work in schools, communities, clinics, or corporate settings. These responsibilities, competencies, and sub-competencies encouraged college and university professional preparation programs to develop their curricula based on a standardized set of skills for teaching all health education/promotion students. These standards were also the basis for establishing individual certification within the profession.

In 1997, three additional responsibilities with accompanying competencies and sub-competencies were identified for graduate preparation in health education/promotion. With the completion of the Competencies Update Project (CUP) in 2005, the initial seven responsibilities and the three graduate responsibilities were united into seven revised responsibility areas that are now common to all health education specialists regardless of setting, degree, or experience. In 2010, the results of the Health Education Job Analysis study were released, which increased the number of competencies to 39 and sub-competencies to 223. All health education/promotion professional preparation programs should now be training students based on the HEJA 2010 standards.

Continued study in health education/promotion is necessary to stay current with health information and new techniques for conducting health education/promotion programs. All health education specialists should read professional journals, join one or more professional associations, and take an active role in their functioning. Certified Health Education Specialists (CHESs) must obtain continuing education credits to maintain their certification. Most bachelor's-level health education specialists should consider a master's degree at some point in their career. Decisions concerning graduate study should not be taken lightly. Undergraduate health education/promotion students need to be aware of the admission requirements for graduate school, and work toward meeting those requirements. Graduate assistantships or fellowships provide an excellent alternative to fund graduate education.

## REVIEW QUESTIONS

1. Define *credentialing* and explain the differences among certification, licensure, and accreditation.

2. Outline the major events of the Role Delineation Project. How does the Competencies Update Project (CUP) relate to role delineation? What is the significance of the CUP? How does the HEJA 2010 relate to role delineation and what is its significance?

3. Review the "Responsibilities and Competencies for Entry-Level Health Educators" (Appendix B). Do you think they are more focused on health content or the process skills needed to be a health education specialist? Defend your position and explain why you believe the health education/promotion profession has moved in this direction.

4. Identify two ways health education specialists can stay up-to-date in the field.

5. What are the differences among the following academic degrees: M.A., M.Ed., M.S., M.P.H., M.S.P.H.?

6. What technology skills are important for current and future health education specialists?

7. Briefly describe the process for applying to graduate school and discuss the potential benefits of serving as a graduate assistant.

## CASE STUDY

Anita considers herself a school health education specialist. She graduated from college with a major in health education/promotion and an emphasis in school health. She is licensed by the state in which she lives to teach health education in the schools. She is also a Certified Health Education Specialist (CHES) and has been very vocal in advocating that all school health education specialists should be CHESs. Anita has been asked to provide a thirty-minute presentation at the state AAHPERD convention on the importance of CHES. This audience will be mostly school health education specialists. Your task is to help Anita develop the main points of her presentation. Why should school health education specialists become CHESs? Also, be the devil's advocate. What arguments will she likely hear from those who are not certified and do not feel certification is important? How can she respond to these arguments? (Note: This same case study can be replicated with Anita being a community health education/promotion specialist, worksite health education/promotion specialist, or clinic/hospital health education/promotion specialist.)

## CRITICAL THINKING QUESTIONS

1. If Helen Cleary and her contemporaries had not begun the Role Delineation Project, and if there were no certification (CHES) available to health education specialists, how do you think the profession would be different today? Think in terms of professional preparation, recognition, employment opportunities, and so on.

2. Suppose that an accreditation system were developed and implemented that required all health education/promotion professional preparation programs to meet the same guidelines and standards. How do you think such a system would impact the profession? What do you see as the potential positive outcomes and the potential negative outcomes of such accreditation? Do you feel that only students graduating from accredited programs should be allowed to sit for the certification exam?

3. Review the National Health Education Competencies that resulted from the HEJA 2010 model (see Appendix B). Do you feel they accurately represent professional practice? Why or why not? What changes do you think should be made in terms of eliminating competencies, adding competencies, and/or moving sub-competencies from one level to the other?

## ACTIVITIES

1. Read each competency and entry-level sub-competency of a health education specialist (see Appendix B). Score each competency and sub-competency using the following scale:
   a. I currently have the skill to meet this competency/sub-competency.
   b. I am uncertain if I have the skill to meet this competency/sub-competency.
   c. I do not have the skill to meet this competency/sub-competency.

After rating each competency and sub-competency, make a list of things you can do to enhance your skills. Keep this table, and periodically reevaluate your skills throughout your program of study.

2. Write to one or more universities you may wish to attend and request information on their graduate health education/promotion programs or go online to find this information. Try to learn about their admission requirements, degree options, and financial aid opportunities.

3. Make an appointment with a professor at your school to talk about graduate school. Ask about schools the professor attended and the degrees earned. Finally, ask for advice on what degree to earn and what school to attend.

## WEBLINKS

1. http://www.nchec.org/

   National Commission for Health Education Credentialing (NCHEC)

   Use this Web site to learn more about becoming a Certified Health Education Specialist (CHES). The site provides helpful information about health education certification including application procedures.

2. http://www.ceph.org/

   Council on Education for Public Health

   The Council is responsible for accrediting programs in public health. A complete list of accredited schools and programs of public health can be found at this site.

3. http://www.csuchico.edu/cjhp/2/1/index.htm

   *California Journal of Health Promotion*

   Read the article titled, "Improving the Quality of Professional Life: Benefits of Health Education and Promotion Association Membership" by Kathleen Young and Whitney Boling. This article clearly explains the benefits of professional association membership for keeping up-to-date with the profession. It also provides a list of health education professional associations to consider joining. While at this site, also read the article titled, "Graduate School in Health Education: A Challenge to Consider" by Michele Pettit. It provides insight and helpful points to ponder when considering graduate school.

## REFERENCES

Allegrante, J. P., Airhihenbuwa, C. O., Auld, M. E., Birch, D. A., Roe, K. M., & Smith, B. J. (2004). Toward a unified system of accreditation for professional preparation in health education: Final report of the National Task force on Accreditation in Health Education. *Health Education & Behavior, 31* (6), 668–683.

Allegrante, J. P., Barry, M. M., Airhihenbuwa, C. O., Auld, M. E., Collins, J. L., Lamarre, M., & Mittelmark, M. B. (2009). Domains of core competency, standards, and quality assurance for building global capacity in health promotion: The Galway Consensus Conference Statement. *Health Education & Behavior, 36* (3), 476–482.

Allegrante, J. P., Barry, M. M., Auld, M. E., Lamarre, M., & Taub, A. (2009). Toward international collaboration on credentialing in health promotion and health education: The Galway Consensus Conference. *Health Education & Behavior, 36* (3), 427–438.

American Association for Health Education, National Commission for Health Education Credentialing, & Society for Public Health Education. (2010). Health Educator Job Analysis—2010: Executive Summary and Recommendations. Available at: http://www.nchec.org/_files/_items/nch-mr-tab2-169/docs/health%20educator%20job%20analysis%20ex%20summary-final-2-19-10.pdf.

Bensley, L. B., Jr., & Pope, A. J. (1994). A study of graduate bulletins to determine general information and graduation requirements for master's degree programs in health education. *Journal of Health Education, 25* (3), 165–171.

Bensley, R. J., & Brookins-Fisher, J. (2003). *Community health education methods: A practical guide* (2nd ed.). Boston: Jones and Bartlett Publishers.

Bruess, C. (2003). The importance of health educators as role models. *American Journal of Health Education, 34* (4), 237–239.

Cleary, H. P. (1986). Issues in the credentialing of health education specialists: A review of the state of the art. In William B. Ward (Ed.), *Advances in health education and promotion,* Greenwich, CT: Jai Press, Inc. (pp. 129–154).

Cleary, H. P. (1995). *The credentialing of health educators: An historical account 1970–1990.* New York: The National Commission for Health Education Credentialing, Inc.

Cottrell, R. R., & Hayden, J. (2007). The why, when, what, where and how of graduate school. *Health Promotion Practice 8* (1), 16–21.

Cottrell, R. R., Lysoby, L., Rasar King,, L., Airhihenbuwa, C. O., Roe, K. M., & Allegrante, J. P. (2009). Current developments in accreditation and certification for health promotion and education: A perspective on systems of quality assurance in the United States. *Health Education & Behavior, 36* (3), 451–463.

Cottrell, R. R., & McKenzie, J. F. (2011). *Health promotion and education research methods.* Boston: Jones and Bartlett Publishers.

Council on Education for Public Health. (2010). *U. S. Schools of Public Health and Graduate Public Health Programs Accredited by the Council on Education for Public Health.* Available at: http://www.ceph.org/

Davis, T. M. (1999). Health educators as positive health role models. *Journal of Health Education, 30* (1).

Doyle, E., & Ward, S. (2001). *The process of community health education and promotion.* Mountain View, CA: Mayfield Publishing.

Gilmore, G. D., & Campbell, M. D. (2005). *Needs and capacity assessment strategies for health education and health promotion.* Boston: Jones and Bartlett.

Gilmore, G. D., Olsen, L. T., Taub, A., & Connell, D. (2005). Overview of the National Health Educator Competencies Update Project, 1998–2004. *American Journal of Health Education, 36* (6), 363–370.

Joint Committee for Graduate Standards. (1996). *National Congress for Institutions Preparing Graduate Health Educators.* Program Booklet, 1.

McKenzie, J. F., Neiger, B. L., & Thackeray, R. (2009). *Planning, implementing & evaluating health promotion programs* (5th ed.). San Francisco: Pearson, Benjamin Cummings.

National Commission for Health Education Credentialing. (1996). *A competency-based framework for professional development of certified health education specialists.* New York: National Commission for Health Education Credentialing.

National Commission for Health Education Credentialing. (2010a). *Mission statement.* Available at: http://www.nchec.org/aboutnchec/mission/

National Commission for Health Education Credentialing. (2010b). *Eligibility for the CHES exam.* Available at: http://www.nchec.org/exam/eligible/ches/

National Commission for Health Education Credentialing. (2010c). *What's new at NCHEC.* Available at: http://www.nchec.org/news/what/

National Commission for Health Education Credentialing. (2010d). *Why certify? Credentialing and benefits of certification.* Available at: http://www.nchec.org/credentialing/credential/

National Commission for Health Education Credentialing, Society for Public Health Education, & American Association for Health Education. (2006). *A competency–based framework for health educators—2006.* NCHEC: Whitehall, PA.

National Task Force on the Preparation and Practice of Health Educators. (1985). *Framework for the development of competency-based curricula for entry level health educators.* New York: National Commission for Health Education Credentialing, Inc.

Quality Assurance Solutions. (2010). *Quality assurance definition.* Available at: http://www.quality-assurance-solutions.com/Quality-Assurance-Definition.html

Society for Public Health Education. (2000). Future directions for quality assurance of professional preparation in health education. *News & Views, 27* (3).

Taub, A., Birch, D. A., Auld, M. E., Lysoby, L., & King, L. R. (2009). Strengthening quality assurance in health education: Recent milestones and future directions. *Health Promotion Practice, 10* (2), 192–200.

Wikipedia. (2010). Social Network. Available at: http://en.wikipedia.org/wiki/Social_network

# The Settings for Health Education/Promotion

After reading this chapter and answering the questions at the end, you should be able to:

- Identify the four major settings in which health education specialists are employed.
- Describe the major responsibilities for health education specialists in the four major settings.
- Discuss the advantages and disadvantages of the four major settings.
- Explain the qualifications and major responsibilities of health education specialists working in colleges and universities.
- Identify a variety of "nontraditional" settings in which health education specialists may be employed.
- State several action steps that can be taken to help procure one's first job in health education/promotion.

Today, most Americans live a healthier and longer life than ever before. Despite this fact, however, it is clear that many, if not most, Americans are not living at their optimal level of health. Hereditary, environmental, societal, and behavioral factors predispose too many U.S. citizens to disease, suffering, disability, and premature death. Health education specialists are professionally trained to help individuals and communities reduce their health risks. According to the U.S. Department of Labor Bureau of Labor Statistics (2010b), in 2009 there were 63,320 health education specialists employed in the United States earning a mean annual wage of $49,060 or a mean hourly wage of $23.59. The challenge for health education specialists is to help people reduce their risk and increase the probability of a long, happy, and productive life.

To meet this challenge, health education specialists conduct programs in a variety of settings (National Commission for Health Education Credentialing [NCHEC], 2010). The use of multiple settings is important, as it allows health education specialists to reach the greatest number of people in the most convenient, efficient, and effective ways possible. Although the goals of health education/promotion and the skills needed to carry out the responsibilities are nearly the same in all settings (English & Videto, 1997), the actual duties of a job may differ greatly from setting to setting.

Professional preparation programs in health education/promotion should prepare students to meet the various competencies and sub-competencies of a health education specialist and thus prepare students for employment in one or more of four major settings. These settings are schools, hospitals/clinics, public/community health agencies, and business/industry. On obtaining advanced degrees, students from any of these settings may seek employment as college or university health education faculty. In addition, health education specialists can work in a variety of nontraditional employment areas.

This chapter discusses each of the four major settings for health education/promotion. After a short introduction to the setting, a description of one day in the career of a health education specialist from that particular setting is presented. This is designed to give the reader a general idea of what a workday is like. Because of the great diversity in duties from one health education specialist to another even within the same setting, it is impossible to say that this is a typical day. For most health education specialists, there is no such thing as a typical day. Following this is a section that describes additional responsibilities that might be assigned to health education specialists in the setting. Again, this is not intended to be an exhaustive list but rather to further the reader's understanding of job responsibilities in that setting. Finally, each section ends with a listing of some advantages and disadvantages for that setting. As students become interested in one or more settings they are encouraged to contact, interview, and job shadow health education specialists working in those settings.

## School Health Education/Promotion

School health involves "all the strategies, activities, and services offered by, in, or in association with schools that are designed to promote students' physical, emotional, and social development" (American School Health Association, 2010). **School health education/promotion,** as the name implies, primarily involves instructing school-age children about health and health-related behaviors. The initial impetus for school health stemmed from the terrible epidemics of the 1800s and the efforts of the Women's Christian Temperance Movement to promote abstinence from alcohol in the early 1900s. Many states mandated school health education/promotion to inform students about these health hazards. Unfortunately, these mandates have seldom been strictly enforced. Further, teachers often have been underqualified, with only an academic minor or a few elective courses to prepare them for the health classroom. Frequently they hold a dual certification in health education/promotion and physical education with the majority of their professional preparation being in physical education. As a result, the quality of school health programs often has been compromised (Breckon, Harvey, & Lancaster, 1998; Naidoo & Wills, 2000).

Despite these limitations, the potential for school districts and health instruction programs in particular to impact students is tremendous. Jalloh (2007) noted that "school-based health education is an opportunity waiting to be taken advantage of; an opportunity for you to discover the best way to influence positive health-related change in the lives of youth and to maximize the use of some education dollars to achieve synergistic health and education goals" (p. 18). It is easier and more effective to establish healthy behaviors in childhood than it is to change unhealthy behaviors in adulthood.

The goal of health education/promotion in schools is to help students adopt and maintain healthy behaviors (Joint Committee on National Health Education Standards, 2007). Each school day provides the opportunity to reach 56 million students. The 132,000 schools in the United States should provide a laboratory where students can eat healthy foods, participate in physical activity, and learn how to take care of their health and well-being (CDC, 2010b). School health programs have demonstrated effectiveness when they are well planned, sequential, provided significant time in the curriculum, and taught by a trained health education specialist (Fisher et al., 2003).

The sophistication of school health education/promotion programs has increased dramatically over the years. Today's school health education specialist needs to be well trained and prepared to deliver a comprehensive and demanding curriculum. Comparing the 1922 "Rules of Good Health" with the 2007 National Health Education Standards (Joint Committee on National Health Education Standards, 2007) clearly illustrates this point (see **Tables 7.1** and **7.2**).

**Table 7.1**     Rules of good health—1922

1. Take a full bath more than once a week.
2. Brush teeth at least once a day.
3. Sleep long hours with window open.
4. Drink as much milk as possible, but no coffee or tea.
5. Eat some vegetables or fruit every day.
6. Drink at least four glasses of water a day.
7. Play part of every day outdoors.
8. Have a bowel movement every morning.

*Source:* "Rules of the Health Game" in *Milk and Our School Children,* U.S. Dept. of the Interior, Bureau of Education, Health Education, No. 11 (1922).

**Table 7.2**     National health education standards

1. Students will comprehend concepts related to health promotion and disease prevention to enhance health.
2. Students will analyze the influence of family, peers, culture, media, technology, and other factors on health behaviors.
3. Students will demonstrate the ability to access valid information and products and services to enhance health.
4. Students will demonstrate the ability to use interpersonal communication skills to enhance health and avoid or reduce health risks.
5. Students will demonstrate the ability to use decision-making skills to enhance health.
6. Students will demonstrate the ability to use goal-setting skills to enhance health.
7. Students will demonstrate the ability to practice health-enhancing behaviors and avoid or reduce health risks.
8. Students will demonstrate the ability to advocate for personal, family, and community health.

*Source:* Reprinted with permission from the American Cancer Society. *National Health Education Standards: Achieving Excellence, Second Edition.* Atlanta, GA: American Cancer Society, 2007. http://www.cancer.org/bookstore.

When the school health education/promotion component is made a part of a broader, district-wide approach known as a **coordinated school health program,** the potential to impact students in a positive way is even greater. Allensworth and Kolbe (1987) were the first to envision a comprehensive and coordinated school health program. They defined it as

> an integrated set of planned, sequential, school-affiliated strategies, activities, and services designed to promote the optimal physical, emotional, social, and educational development of students. The program involves and is supportive of families and is determined by the local community based on community needs, resources, standards and requirements. It is coordinated by a multidisciplinary team and accountable to the community for program quality and effectiveness. (p. 60)

In other words, a coordinated school health program coordinates and integrates various aspects of a school district to best impact the health of the students, faculty, staff, administration, and community as a whole. This includes food services, nursing services, school counseling and psychology, health instruction, physical education, administration, school environment, community involvement, and faculty/staff wellness (CDC, 2010a).

A health education specialist choosing to work in the school setting will find a challenging and rewarding career. Given the number of school districts in the United States, it is obvious that a large number of people teach health education/promotion in the schools. Unfortunately, many of these people are not health education specialists. Some school districts have used biology, physical education, home economics or family life, and consumer science teachers to teach health. Even when certified health education teachers are employed, they may have only a minor in health education/promotion and are not fully prepared. A further problem confounding the employment situation in the schools is that the requirement for health education/promotion is usually less than for other academic subjects. Students typically need only one or two semesters of health education/promotion to graduate from high school, while they probably are required to complete four years of English. With such a minimal requirement, the number of health teachers needed and the resulting demand for health teachers are low. The bottom line is that, in many parts of the country, it is difficult to obtain a job in school health.

Those students who are really committed to being outstanding health teachers, however, should not be deterred from this career path. With time, dedication, networking, and perseverance, those who really want to teach health in the schools can usually find employment. Substitute teaching, coaching, and volunteering are good ways to make oneself known in a school district and increase the likelihood of eventual employment. Students are encouraged to talk to their own professors to determine the job market for school health education/promotion in their area.

Beyond teaching in the classroom, the school health education specialist should also take a leadership role in advocating for and the development of school health policy. Policies are written statements that guide the school district related to many health issues (McKenzie, Pinger, & Kotecki, 2008). For example, a school district may have policies related to tobacco use on school property, the food and snack items available in the cafeteria (see **Figure 7.1**), safety measures, violence, suicide, staff wellness programs, community advisory committees, and many more issues. Further, once policy is developed, it needs to be carefully implemented and then monitored.

**Figure 7.1** Food service is one component of a coordinated school health program.
(David Buffington, Getty Images)

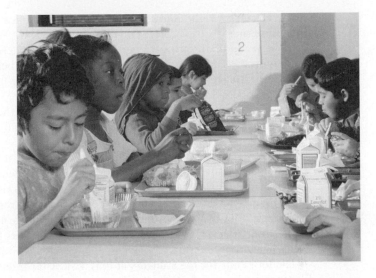

Policy work is not easy, but it is extremely important for a school district (McKenzie et al., 2008).

## A Day in the Career of a School Health Education Specialist

At 5:45 A.M. the alarm goes off, and Ms. Bell's day starts. Ms. Bell teaches seventh- and eighth-grade health at a junior high school in a suburban school district. After going through the normal morning routine, she arrives at the school building around 7:00 A.M. There is a half hour before homeroom, so she picks up her mail and duplicates a test that she prepared the night before for her eighth-grade health class. Essentially, homeroom involves administrative responsibilities and a considerable amount of paperwork.

In homeroom she takes attendance, gets a lunch count, listens to announcements over the loudspeaker, and collects money from a fruit sale fund-raiser. The fruit sale is being conducted by the PTA to raise money for new computers in the school. The PTA used to sell candy, but because of a new district policy that Ms. Bell and the Coordinated School Health team advocated for, candy sales are no longer allowed as fund raisers.

At 7:45 A.M. the first period starts. This school has eight fifty-minute periods, with only four minutes between periods. In the first three periods, Ms. Bell teaches seventh-grade health. Today's lesson is on refusal skills related to alcohol and drug use. Ms. Bell has written three scenarios that students could find themselves in. The scenarios are open ended, so after each one Ms. Bell leads a discussion on how to use refusal skills to get out of a bad situation. She then asks students to role-play the situations to gain further practice in using refusal skills. Unfortunately, only two of her three classes will get this lesson today. The second-period class is one day behind due to an assembly that was held a week ago. Ms. Bell has to find a way to catch this group up with the rest of the classes.

Ms. Bell's fourth period is divided in half. The first half, she has lunch room duty. It is her responsibility to monitor the lunch room while students are eating. This is a very noisy and somewhat stressful duty. In today's lunch room, two boys become unruly and nearly get into a fight. She sends them to the office for discipline, but the situation is quite upsetting.

The second half of fourth period is Ms. Bell's lunch time. She usually has twenty-five minutes to eat lunch and relax before fifth period begins. Today, however, she must use part of that time to drop by the office for a follow-up discussion with the assistant principal concerning the incident in the lunch room.

In fifth period, Ms. Bell teaches eighth-grade health. Today is a test day. While the students are taking their test, Ms. Bell works at her computer to update the online Web page that lists student assignments for the week.

Sixth period is Ms. Bell's planning period. Today she tries to make a phone call to the parents of one of her students who is having problems in health class, but no one is home. She then grades the test papers from her previous class and records the grades. She averages the grades and starts to develop interim reports for the fifth-period class, but she runs out of time. Seventh and eighth periods are also eighth-grade health classes. While students take their tests, Ms. Bell grades papers from the previous classes and writes her interim reports.

School ends for the students at 2:57 P.M. After monitoring the hall while students leave the building, Ms. Bell hurries to the cafeteria for the monthly teachers' meeting. General information and announcements are presented by the principal. The meeting ends at 4:00 P.M.

In addition to her teaching responsibilities, Ms. Bell coaches the junior high girls' volleyball team. Practice usually goes from 3:15 P.M. to 5:00 P.M. Today's practice will go from 4:00 P.M. to 5:00 P.M. due to the teachers' meeting. After practice, Ms. Bell waits until the last girl leaves the locker room, then returns to her classroom to prepare for the next day's classes. She leaves the school at around 5:30 P.M.

After dinner and her family responsibilities, Ms. Bell spends twenty minutes on the phone with the student's parents who were not at home earlier in the day. She then finishes grading the tests she gave in class and continues working on interim reports. It will take her at least one more evening to finish the interims. At 11:00 P.M. she turns off the light and goes to bed.

## Additional Responsibilities

In addition to the lesson planning, grading, parent meetings, disciplining, coaching, and the various administrative duties, teachers may have still more responsibilities. They may be involved in curriculum development, the review of materials for classroom use, the chaperoning of dances or other after-school activities, fund-raising, and the advising of student groups such as yearbook, debate, or student council. Many teachers now keep active Web pages that can be accessed by students and parents. These Web pages may contain announcements, assignments, and grades or progress reports. Teachers need to be responsive to their e-mail accounts as parent, student, and school district communication is often conducted in this manner. School health education specialists should also be active members of their professional organizations. This allows them to network with other health education specialists and to stay up-to-date in the field. Finally, school health education specialists should be strong advocates for health and health education/promotion (see **Box 7.1**). They must make certain that fellow faculty, administrators, school boards, and the community as a whole are aware of the unique contributions of a school health program. (See **Table 7.3**.)

**Box 7.1 Practitioner's Perspective** | School Health Education/Promotion

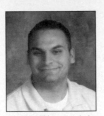

NAME: Brian Jones
CURRENT POSITION: Health Education Specialist
EMPLOYER: Lake Central School Corporation, Indiana
DEGREE/INSTITUTION: Bachelor of Science, Ball State University, 2008
MAJORS: Physical Education, Health Education
EMPHASIS: Standards Based Learning

(Reprinted by permission of Brian Jones)

**Responsibilities:** As the only health education specialist at my school, I am responsible for teaching age-appropriate material that aligns with the state standards for grades 6, 7, and 8. This includes creating a health curriculum for the middle school that meets the state standards. My responsibilities, however, do not stop there.

There is a lot more that goes into teaching than creating a curriculum and lesson plans. I am responsible for maintaining communication with staff, other faculty members, the school staff, parents, and other community members. Maintaining a constant line of communication is very important for the students and me as a professional. Communication takes time and effort and is facilitated through phone calls, newsletters, meetings, and an up-to-date Web site.

I have made it a priority of mine to make my school and town known for its health and wellness program. I have collaborated with other faculty and staff members, created a wellness team at my middle school, implemented wellness activities throughout the school year, and became a member of my school corporation's coordinated school health program (CSHP) committee. I am also very active in writing grant proposals to seek additional external funds for my school programs. I also have the responsibility of coaching and being a role model for my students. In both my role as a teacher and coach, I try to "practice what I preach" while making all of the content meaningful for each and every student.

**Obtaining my position:** The moment I saw the posting on the Lake Central School Corpora-

tion Web site for a Physical Education/ Health Education teacher, I knew it was mine. I knew in my mind that I have done everything I can to be better than any candidate that applied for this job. The day after the posting I entered the school with the full intention of grabbing the principal's attention. I explained to the principal my desire for the job and how I was the right fit for this school. That same day I received a call for an interview.

I was extremely nervous waiting for the interview. When the principal called my name I entered the office and was greeted by an interview committee of eight individuals whose job was to weed out candidates. As soon as I was asked the first question, all of the anxiety went away. I was told that I would find out if I had the job within 5–7 days. I knew that my interview went well, but having to wait 5–7 days seemed awful. That next day I performed my normal routine and went to work. Around 9:00 A.M. I received a call asking, "So, do you want to be a Coyote?" Those eight words took the weight of the world off of me. I now had a job that I knew would make me happy.

**What I enjoy most:** It sounds like a cliché, but I enjoy absolutely everything about being a teacher and coach. I sometimes think to myself, "I can't believe I get paid to do this!" However, the thing I can say that I enjoy most is the day-to-day interaction with my students. Every class, every student, and every lesson is so diverse that it keeps things fresh, fun, exciting, and sometimes challenging. This challenge is what pushes me to make myself, my lessons, my projects, and my discussions better each and

**Box 7.1 Practitioner's Perspective** Continued

every class. By eliminating the monotony and complacency that some teachers have, I have been able to evolve and reflect daily on ways to improve myself as an educator.

**What I enjoy least:** The most difficult/ least enjoyable aspect I had to change when I started teaching was the attitude and perception that some others had about health education/ promotion. Some students, parents, and even a few teachers had the preconceived notion that little learning goes on inside the health classroom. I knew I had to target these individuals and prove that health education/promotion was not only an important subject, but necessary for the growth of these teenagers.

Some of the things I have had to deal with have been parent phone calls asking "how can you give me son a D in HEALTH . . . it's health!" I also had to deal with fellow teachers popping their head into my room and pulling kids out for retesting, late homework, etc., during my instructional periods. Cognitively, thinking that what I was teaching was considered unimportant to some motivated me once again to go above and beyond my daily work to change the culture of the health curriculum.

As time has gone on I have started to win over the students and parents. Creating a meaningful learning environment and keeping a consistent line of communication with parents was the key. I have made sure that the students were receiving "real world" applications during each and every unit that I taught.

The last group I needed to "pull in" were the few teachers. Throughout my employment, I have volunteered, joined committees, written grant proposals, and created staff wellness activities. I believe I was able to win over the other faculty members at my school when they saw the time and dedication I put into everything I did.

The reason why I "enjoyed" this aspect the least is because of the feeling I had many days after school after all the hard work and time I put in. Throughout my employment things definitely changed; success has carried over into the new school year, and it is evident through the students' behavior and attitude within the classroom. It took a lot of hard work, but it surely paid off.

**Recommendations:** I recommend a variety of things at all levels when preparing for your future profession. Start building connections, resources, and references that you can take with you throughout your career. Take advantage of the additional courses and certifications that your school offers. Everything extra you do now will pay off with dividends in the future. You never want to say "what if . . ."

During the job application process you need to stay optimistic and portray the best "you." This is where you are trying to show your future employers the sculptured educator you have become. Remember to stay professional throughout the interview process and be confident and honest to every question.

Once you have earned your job you will be placed in an environment that is unlike school and your student teaching environment. It is advantageous to make many positive relationships with your co-workers. Once again, be positive and show everyone around that you love what you are doing. That positive attitude will transcend and change the atmosphere of the school and your students' attitudes in your class.

Lastly, never be content with the minimum. We have entered this field because we care. Do everything you can in and out of school to make a positive change in your school, community, and students' lives. You truly never know how one lecture or conversation could change someone's life forever.

**Table 7.3**    Advantages and disadvantages of working in school health education/promotion

**Advantages**

- Health education specialists have the ability to work with young people during their developmental years.
- Health education specialists have the potential to prevent harmful health behaviors from forming instead of working with older people after such behaviors have been formed.
- Health education specialists have the opportunity to impact all students, because health education/promotion is usually a required course.
- A graduate degree is not needed for entry-level employment.
- There is good job security.
- Summer months are free and there are nice vacation periods in December and in spring.
- Benefits are good.
- There is a multifaceted career ladder.
- There are good retirement programs.

**Disadvantages**

- Good health education specialists usually spend many long hours at their job, including weekends and evenings that may compensate for the long vacation periods.
- Health education specialists may have relatively low status in a school district when compared with teachers of more traditional subjects such as math, science, and English.
- Pay is low when compared with professionals in other fields, but comparable with that of other health education specialists.
- Student discipline problems are often seen as a major disadvantage.
- Summer "free time" may be consumed with summer employment and/or returning to college for additional required coursework.
- It is difficult dealing with conservative school boards, parents, and community groups when teaching controversial issues such as sex education and drug education.
- Resources may be limited to support the program.

# Public/Community Health Education/Promotion

Within the health education/promotion profession, there has been much discussion concerning the terms community health education/promotion and public health education/promotion. Some believe these two terms are synonymous while others feel there are unique differences between them. It is the opinion of the authors that the terms are more alike than different and that the field is gradually evolving to accept the term public health education/promotion. Both community health education/promotion and public health education/promotion students have similar skill sets, meet the competencies of the National Commission for Health Education Credentialing, and compete for similar jobs in departments of public health and community health agencies. A survey of professional preparation programs (Miller, Birch, & Cottrell, 2010) found that 72.3 percent of respondents reported making modifications to their existing undergraduate health education/promotion program or concentration within the past three years to take on a more public health focus. Sixty-three percent of the programs surveyed indicated they would seek accreditation as a public health education/promotion program when available while only 19 percent indicated they would not seek accreditation as a public health education/promotion program. For that reason the authors use the term public health education/promotion to include both community health education/promotion and public health education/promotion programs.

According to the Association of Schools of Public Health (2010),

> [t]he work of public health educators (PHEs) is to change policies and environments as well as attitudes and behavior that affect health, and to operate in close association with community groups. PHEs plan and direct programs, design workshops and forums, work with community groups, and serve a broad public health agenda. They may conduct studies of public health education needs, evaluate the materials and methods used in programs, determine program effectiveness, and try to improve the general health in communities. They might do this by working with people and organizations addressing health-related issues such as pollution, drug abuse, nutrition, safety and stress management. These professionals also write health education materials such as fact sheets, pamphlets and brochures—a special and critical skill, as materials must often match the needs, preferences, and skills of underserved populations. (p. 82)

Public health programs target individuals, local communities, states, and the nation. There is a reciprocal relationship between these various targets. Over the years, it has become clear that the health of a community is closely linked to the individual health of community members. Likewise, the collective behaviors, attitudes, and beliefs of everyone who lives in the community profoundly affect the community's health. Indeed, the underlying premise of *Healthy People 2010* was that the health of the individual is almost inseparable from the health of the larger community, and that the health of every community in every state and territory determines the overall health status of the nation. This explains why the vision for *Healthy People 2010* was "Healthy People in Healthy Communities" (U.S. Department of Health and Human Services, 2000a).

The most likely sources of employment for community health education specialists are voluntary health agencies and public health agencies. **Voluntary health agencies** are created by concerned citizens to deal with health needs not met by governmental agencies (McKenzie, Pinger, & Kotecki, 2008). "Their missions can be public education, professional education, patient education, research, direct services and support to or for people directly affected by a specific health or medical problem. They may also serve families, friends, or loved ones of those affected" (Daitz, 2007, p. 4). As their name implies, they rely heavily on volunteer help and donations. There are usually paid staff members who are responsible for administration, volunteer recruitment and coordination, program development, and fund-raising. Health education specialists are hired to plan, implement, and evaluate the education component of the agency's programs (see **Box 7.2**). They often, however, are involved in other aspects of the agency as well. Voluntary health agencies are usually nonprofits and are funded by such means as private donations, grants, fund-raisers, and possibly United Way contributions. Examples of voluntary health agencies include the American Cancer Society (see **Figure 7.2**), American Heart Association, and American Lung Association. Most of these large, well-known voluntary agencies have national, state, and local divisions.

## Box 7.2 Practitioner's Perspective  Voluntary Health Agency

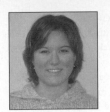

NAME: Laura Mackzum

CURRENT POSITION: Health Promotion Coordinator, Cancer Detection Programs

EMPLOYER: American Cancer Society, Ohio Division

DEGREE/INSTITUTION/MAJOR: B.S., University of Cincinnati, 2004, Health Education with Community Health Emphasis

(Reprinted by permission of Laura Mackzum)

**Job responsibilities in my current position:**
Under general supervision of the Regional Health Promotion Director, I build relationships with community-based organizations and health care providers to plan, organize, and develop effective breast and colorectal cancer prevention and early detection programs and activities. I collaborate with the Community Development Director to do targeted volunteer recruitment activities focused on advancing the Ohio Division's breast and colon cancer prevention and early detection strategic plan. Other activities include:

- Effectively represent the American Cancer Society and its mission in the community.

- Utilize the volunteer management model to work through volunteers. Volunteer management responsibilities include recruitment, training, and delegation to ensure successful implementation of the Breast and Colon Cancer Program of Work, and may include volunteer support of community mobilization; health care/plan, worksite and community-based systems initiatives; policy advocacy; as well as program delivery.

- Plan, organize, and implement community-level breast and colorectal cancer prevention and early detection initiatives, programs, and services.

- Establish and maintain relationships with health care organizations, health plans, and community organizations to increase the reach and impact of the Society's breast and colon cancer prevention and early detection strategic plan, particularly for uninsured or underinsured women.

- Identify opportunities to engage diverse populations and communities in breast and colon cancer prevention and early detection.

**How I obtained my current position:** I obtained my position through networking. I was involved in a group called the Greater Cincinnati Alliance for Health Promotions (GCAHP). A representative from the Southwest Region of ACS was also involved in the group and announced that the Hamilton County office was hiring a health education specialist. I followed up with her after the meeting and forwarded her my resume. Being involved in GCAHP and using the networking it promoted really paid off in moving my career forward.

**What I like most about my current position:** My position with the American Cancer Society is very different than most health education/promotion positions. The Southwest region of ACS covers 17 counties and we spend a lot of time traveling all over the region for meetings and appointments. Due to the large amount of travel and a schedule that can range from 7 A.M. to 9 P.M., the American Cancer Society, Ohio Division, recently made the decision to have all field workers operate from a home office. This arrangement allows tremendous flexibility in our positions. We have the flexibility to create our own schedules according to the hours our week demands.

The ACS has equipped my home office with a laptop, a phone, and an all-in-one printer/fax/copy/scanner. In the regional office each department has an administrative assistant to assist with mailings and other large projects that would normally be done in the office.

## Box 7.2 Practitioner's Perspective    Continued

Working from the regional office is an option if I need to spend a day in the office for any reason.

Our region staff meets bimonthly to update each other on what is happening in each department. The Health Promotion department meets monthly, and I meet monthly one-on-one with my supervisor to make certain we are both on the same page. Communication can be a challenge with the remote working situation. The technology ACS has provided really promotes the remote working environment and makes working from home a possibility. I have a follow-me-anywhere telephone and instant messaging software on my computer. It was a challenge to get used to working from home; however, the flexibility it allows really promotes a healthier work environment. In the past our staff had a lot of turnover due to burnout from working such long hours and odd schedules. This arrangement allows me to create a schedule that balances well with my personal and home life.

There are so many aspects of my position that I enjoy. Probably the thing I enjoy the most, however, is knowing that I am educating people on how to beat cancer. Meeting all the incredible cancer survivors and hearing their stories is really inspiring and keeps me motivated to continue educating people about cancer and the importance of screenings.

**What I like least about my current position:** The biggest downside to my position is educating people that need screenings but do not have access to screenings. This can be a very difficult part of my job. As a health education specialist it is my job to educate people about the importance of screenings and taking care of themselves. However, access to care for some uninsured people is impossible. I want to see everyone get screened for cancer, and it's very sad to see that for some people the free or reduced-cost screenings are not available, and if they are available the follow-up care for cancer is too costly for them to access.

**Recommendations for those preparing to be health education specialists:** My recommendations for students preparing to be health education specialists are to take advantage of any and every networking opportunity. Knowing people in the field makes life much easier when trying to get a job, and especially once you have a job in the field, the networks that you have can help you accomplish tasks much easier.

To network I would join professional organizations such as the Society for Public Health Education (SOPHE), the American Association for Health Education (AAHE), or local groups like the Greater Cincinnati Alliance for Health Promotions (GCAHP). The connections you make at these meetings are valuable for your career development.

**Public health agencies,** or official governmental health agencies, are usually financed through public tax monies. Government has long been responsible for doing for the people as a whole what individuals could not do for themselves. Thus, governments provide police protection, educational systems, clean air and water, and many other important services. Departments of public health, thus, are formed to coordinate and provide health services to a community. Health departments may be organized by the city, county, state, or federal government. They operate primarily with paid staff and typically provide health education/promotion services as part of their total program. They may also seek grants and hire health education specialists on grant funds. Public health agencies are known for their bureaucracies, protocols, policies, and procedures. It often takes considerable time to accomplish tasks, and work often needs to be reviewed and approved by higher-level administrators. On the positive side, public health agencies often work with the groups of people most in need of health services and offer good

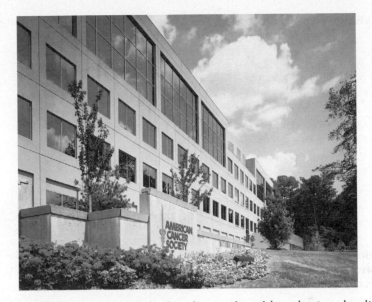

**Figure 7.2** The American Cancer Society is a nationwide voluntary health organization dedicated to eliminating cancer as a major health problem by preventing cancer, saving lives from cancer, and diminishing suffering from cancer through research, education, advocacy, and service. Health education specialists often work for voluntary agencies like the American Cancer Society.
(American Cancer Society/California Division)

benefit packages for employees (Hall, 2007). **Table 7.4** contains a list of agencies that have programs for which public health education specialists may be employed.

More diversity in terms of job responsibilities exists in the public/community health education/promotion setting than in the other major settings in which health education specialists are employed. This is due to the large number of community and public health agencies that exist and the vast differences in their missions, goals, and objectives. In some agencies, health education specialists serve administrative functions such as co-ordinating volunteers, budgeting, fund-raising, program planning, and serving as liaisons to other agencies and groups. They often use population-based strategies such as advocating for laws, policies, rules, and regulations that impact health. In other public/community agencies, the health education specialist may be more involved in direct program delivery to the clientele of that agency and/or the community at large. Most frequently, however, health education specialists are involved in a little bit of everything.

## A Day in the Career of a Community Health Education Specialist

Mr. Fischer is the health education specialist for a local division of the American Cancer Society (ACS). In that role, he has the responsibility of conducting health education/promotion programs in a four-county area of the state. Mr. Fischer usually arrives at the office between 8:30 and 9:00 A.M. Today, however, he had an 8:00 A.M. meeting with a local coalition that is trying to encourage school districts to implement comprehensive school health education/promotion into their curricula. This is an important

**Table 7.4**   Possible sources of employment in public/community health
education/promotion

State, local, city health departments
U.S. Public Health Service
U.S. Food & Drug Administration
U.S. or state departments of agriculture
U.S. or state departments of transportation
County extension services
U.S. Department of Health and Human Services
U.S. Centers for Disease Control and Prevention
National Institutes of Health
Environmental Protection Agency (EPA)
Health Resources and Services Administration (HRSA)
Substance Abuse and Mental Health Services Administration (SAMHSA)
Indian Health Service
U.S. or state penal institutions
Voluntary health agencies
Private foundations

issue, as the ACS has made comprehensive school health education/promotion one of its major priority areas at the national level. Mr. Fischer has been responsible for forming this coalition and was recently elected to serve as its chairperson. As such, he sets the agenda, runs the meetings, takes minutes, and always plans for juice and bagels to be served.

It is 9:30 A.M. when Mr. Fischer finally arrives at his office. He spends the next half hour opening his mail, responding to e-mail, and returning telephone calls. From 10:00 A.M. to 11:00 A.M. is the biweekly staff meeting, which is run by Mr. Fischer's supervisor, who is director of the local ACS unit. In these meetings, staff members provide updates on projects for which they are responsible. Issues and problems facing the local unit are discussed, with the intent of involving the group in identifying potential solutions. Information from the state and national levels is also provided.

From 11:00 A.M. to 12:00 P.M., Mr. Fischer has time to sit at his desk and work on the Great American Smokeout. This is a yearly campaign to help smokers quit smoking for at least one day and hopefully for the rest of their lives. Mr. Fischer is responsible for this event. He has to recruit local sponsors to donate money or prizes for the event, plan a variety of activities to promote the event, contact local media to cover the various events, distribute materials to numerous participating groups, coordinate volunteers to assist with or run various events, develop letters of understanding with each group assisting with the event, and provide letters of thanks to all groups and individual volunteers who assist with the event after it is over. Twice during this hour, Mr. Fischer is interrupted by phone calls from individuals needing information on various cancers. Mr. Fischer writes down their request on a referral slip, along with their name and address. Twice a week he has a volunteer who comes in and mails all of the information that has been requested. It is Mr. Fischer's responsibility to recruit, train, monitor, evaluate, and acknowledge all of the volunteers he uses in his program.

At 12:00 P.M. Mr. Fischer heads out for lunch. He usually eats lunch at his desk while working, but today he is speaking to the local Rotary Club about the Great American Smokeout. Although Mr. Fischer enjoys public speaking, he does not have enough time to handle all of the requests and frequently coordinates volunteers to speak on behalf of the ACS.

Mr. Fischer returns to his office shortly before 2:00 P.M. He takes another hour to answer phone calls and e-mails that have come in since the morning and writes some correspondence related to the Great American Smokeout and the Coordinated School Health Coalition. From 3:00 P.M. to 5:00 P.M., Mr. Fischer is on the phone, calling volunteers to participate in a fund-raiser called Relay for Life. At this event, teams of people camp out at a local high school, park, or fairground and take turns walking or running around a track or path. Each team is asked to have a representative on the track at all times during the 24-hour event. Donations are made to the teams by those wishing to support the event. This is a good fund-raiser and a lot of fun, but it takes considerable staff time to prepare for the event.

Mr. Fischer leaves the office at 5:00 P.M. to have dinner with his family. Tonight, however, he has to be back at the office at 7:30 P.M. for a meeting of the Youth Education Committee. As the name implies, this committee of volunteers is responsible for all local ACS programs dealing with youth. As the health education specialist, Mr. Fischer has to be present for all of their monthly meetings. In addition to the Youth Education Committee, there are also board meetings, volunteer recognition nights, Adult Education Committee meetings, and numerous other speaking engagements and responsibilities that require Mr. Fischer to work in the evenings. He usually spends one to three nights a week on the job. In addition, he occasionally has to work on weekends during special ACS events like Relay for Life.

### Additional Responsibilities

As can be seen from the Mr. Fischer example, public/community health education specialists are involved in numerous and varied activities (see **Box 7.3**). Planning, implementing, and evaluating programs and events are major tasks, but, in conducting these tasks, health education specialists get involved in fund-raising, coalition building, committee work, budgeting, general administration, public speaking, volunteer recruitment, grant writing, media relations, and advocacy. (See **Table 7.5**.)

## Worksite Health Education/Promotion

The Joint Committee on Health Education and Promotion Terminology (2001) defined **worksite health promotion** as "a combination of educational, organizational and environmental activities designed to improve the health and safety of employees and their families" (p. 103). Since the mid-1970s, business and industry in the United States have been offering worksite health promotion programs for their employees. Why are worksites interested in offering these programs and why are health education specialists interested in working in these settings? Chapman (2006) offers a very insightful and succinct response to these questions:

> Increasing employer-related health care costs continue to provide a serious threat to the economic life of virtually all American employers. Behavioral issues of employees and

## Box 7.3 Practitioner's Perspective — Community Health Education Specialist

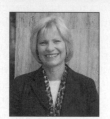

(Reprinted by permission of Patricia Stewart)

NAME: Patricia Stewart

CURRENT POSITION/TITLE: Director of Coordinated School Health Programs (CSHP)

EMPLOYER: Idaho State Department of Education (SDE)

DEGREE/INSTITUTION/YEAR: Bachelor's of Science, Dakota State University, Madison SD

MAJOR/MINOR: Physical Education and Health

**How I obtained my job:** My education and work experience prepared me well for my job. I have worked in the field of health education/promotion for over 30 years, starting my career teaching health and physical education at the secondary level. Teaching provided me with an opportunity to work with students from different cultural backgrounds, which broadened my perspective regarding health risks and protective factors influencing student behavior and educational outcomes. I worked as a consultant for a health education/promotion curriculum company training staff in school districts in several states, which increased my insight into the level of health education/promotion implementation occurring in the United States. My previous experience as director of CSHP in the South Dakota Department of Education is probably the best preparation for moving into my current position at the Idaho State Department of Education (SDE). Working in state government gave me the experience of writing grants, collecting data, informing policy, and evaluating the process and the outcomes of health-related projects/initiatives. Since CSHP is funded by the Centers for Disease Control and Prevention, Division of Adolescent School Health, I was exposed to the public health perspective. CDC bases funding and programming on data and research, so the importance of data collection and following research best practice to prioritize and focus programming became clearer to me. My involvement in professional organizations helped me build a broad network of health promotion partners across the country. This network has provided resources and funding support for various projects in programs and even opened doors for career opportunities. I am still a health educator, but now my opportunities to advocate for health education/promotion are expanded beyond the classroom to include community partners.

**How I utilize health education/promotion in my job:** As Director of CSHP, I collaborate with the Department of Health and Welfare and other organizations involved in health promotion to address health issues facing ID youth. Initially, I brought together lead health educators from pre-K to post-secondary, utilizing our partnership with the Idaho Association for Health, PE, Recreation and Dance to review and revise the ID Health Education Standards. I also worked closely with our physical education coordinator to follow the same process to revise the ID Physical Education Standards. I believe that these two content areas, although different, complement one another and are now closely aligned to the national standards. There has been a philosophical change in health education/promotion over the past ten years, resulting in a greater focus on skill building within each of the health education/promotion topics rather than focusing only on providing health information to students. Our program has provided significant professional development to health educators in schools focused on helping teachers align curriculum with standards and performance assessment to ensure that students have both the knowledge and the skills to practice healthy behavior for a lifetime. Our goal in

## Box 7.3 Practitioner's Perspective    Continued

providing this type of professional development is to help teachers change student health behaviors to reduce youth risk behaviors.

**What I like about my job:** My position provides a unique opportunity to work collaboratively with both government agencies and outside health-promoting organizations to gather data, garner resources, assist in policy change, and evaluate effectiveness of programs to promote the health of children and youth. Serving as a coordinated school health director allows me to work collaboratively with other areas to find the resources to address health needs. A CSHP Director has to look at the big picture and work collaboratively with health educators, physical educators, food service staff, school nurses, school counselors, the safe and drug-free school personnel, staff wellness, and parents and community partners. I enjoy providing professional development in health education/promotion and also helping school staff develop a coordinated approach to address health issues by utilizing their school and community partners.

**What I like least about my job:** Working in a state-level position in CSHP removes me from the direct contact I have with students, which is why I entered the education field initially. The CSHP staff are involved in so many initiatives and partnerships that sometimes one feels like it is difficult to follow a project from implementation to completion taking the time to fully evaluate both the process and the outcome. It is important to remain focused on key priority areas and recognize limitations in my time and resources. Funding from CDC for CSHP programs is highly competitive and very limited within states, so the need to continually write grants and seek funding to support programming through partnerships is an ongoing process. This challenge allowed me to grow in my skills to advocate for programs using data and collaborative partnerships to create an effective message of change.

**Recommendations for those preparing to be health educators:** To be effective you must remain committed to the hard work and passionate about what you do and why you do it. In order to remain dedicated to the profession, strive to be a lifelong learner with a commitment to seeking professional development. Join your professional organization(s) even before leaving your undergraduate program and stay connected by attending, presenting, and seeking leadership opportunities. Seek opportunities for internships to get experience and begin that networking process. Network and develop relationships with school, community, and state partners—you just never know how those partnerships may open doors of opportunity to benefit the people and programs you work within or provide you with a new and challenging career opportunity.

**The role of health educators/health promotion specialists in the future:** Primary prevention should be the most important priority of health care reform in this country. We cannot continue to react to chronic health issues and health care costs in this country, but must strive to be more proactive. Health educators will continue to have an ever-increasing role to play in schools and communities as part of a comprehensive health care system. Using the coordinated school health approach, health educators will work in partnership with public health and health care providers to plan, implement, and promote programs to reduce risk behaviors and increase the practice of health-enhancing behaviors significantly, reducing morbidity and mortality in the United States. Health educators should bring to these partnerships a passion for working with youth, knowledge of current best practices in health education/promotion, and teaching skills to effectively facilitate student learning. I believe these unique traits will impact positive health behavior change in youth and, ultimately, reduce the burden of health care costs in this country.

**Table 7.5** Advantages and disadvantages of working in public/community health education/promotion

| Advantages |
| --- |
| • Job responsibilities are highly varied and changing. |
| • There is a strong emphasis on prevention. |
| • There is usually a high community profile. |
| • Health education specialists work with multiple groups of people. |
| • There is a high degree of self-satisfaction. |
| • These positions typically offer good benefit packages. |
| • These positions typically allow flex time. |

| Disadvantages |
| --- |
| • Pay may be low, particularly in voluntary agencies. |
| • When hired directly by a community or public health agency, job security tends to be good. In such situations, the health education specialist is said to be employed on **hard money.** Sometimes, however, these agencies hire health education specialists on money secured through grants, which is known as **soft money.** In these situations, positions are terminated when grant funding is discontinued, so job security can be a concern. |
| • Relying heavily on volunteers can be frustrating. While most volunteers are great, some do not demonstrate the same level of commitment as might a paid employee. |
| • There never seems to be enough money to run all the programs that need to be offered in the way they should be offered. |
| • These positions often require irregular hours that may include evenings and weekends. |
| • There is a lot of bureaucracy in public health agencies. |

their family members continue to loom large as a major reason for increasing health costs. In addition more than 131 million individuals are in the U.S. work force and another 55–65 million are linked through family relationships or retirement relationships, putting employers in a key role related to health and wellness issues for approximately 80% of the U.S. population. This and several other characteristics of the worksite itself, such as the amount of time people spend at work each week and the economic role of employers in the health of employees, make it an excellent place to conduct wellness programs. (p. 6).

These worksite wellness programs offer an additional setting for health education specialists and allow them to reach segments of the population that are not easily reached through traditional community health programs.

In the United States health care expenditures surpassed 2.3 trillion dollars in 2008. This is more than three times the $714 billion spent in 1990, and over eight times the $253 billion spent in 1980. This averages to be $7,681 per resident and accounted for 16.2 percent of the gross domestic product (GDP) (Kaiser Family Foundation, 2010). Health care expenditures are projected to account for 17.7 percent of the GDP by 2012, which would be up from the 14.1 percent of the GDP in 2001 (U.S. Department of Health and Human Services, 2003). Many of these health care costs are picked up by business and industry in the form of health insurance premiums. Starbucks, for example, pays more for its U.S. employees' health insurance each year than it does for coffee

**Figure 7.3** Health education specialists are employed by business and industry to provide programs to improve the health of employees.

(iofoto/Shutterstock )

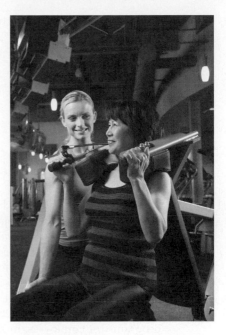

(Rubleski, 2007). Can worksite health promotion programs reduce these costs? According to the Wellness Councils of America (2006), the advantages of worksite health promotion are no longer a matter of speculation. In 2006 there were more than 600 articles that provided both circumstantial and direct evidence of the value of worksite health promotion programs. The tangible benefits include reduced sick leave absenteeism, reduced use of health benefits, reduced workers' compensation costs, reduced injuries, and reduced presenteeism losses (losses due to poor productivity in those employees that are present). Beyond the tangible benefits there are also intangible benefits including improved employee morale, increased employee loyalty, less organizational conflict, a more productive workforce, and improved employee decision-making ability.

Health promotion programs at worksites differ greatly from site to site (U.S. Department of Health and Human Services, 2003). Some are very extensive, include elaborate facilities, and are conducted by full-time staff members hired by the company (see **Figure 7.3**); others are minimal programs that may include only a brown bag lunch speaker's program or a discount at the local YMCA or health club (Chenoweth, 2007). For a list of worksite health promotion activities, see **Table 7.6**.

The proportion of employers who provide worksite health promotion programs has increased over the years. It is reported that health improvement programs of some kind are now being offered by over 80 percent of worksites with 50 or more employees and almost all large employers with more than 750 employees (U.S. Department of Health and Human Services, 2003). Despite these impressive numbers for large employers, more needs to be done. Many of these large employers have only minimal health promotion offerings. The majority of U.S. employees work in small and medium-sized companies that are much less likely to offer any health promotion opportunities. Certain types of employers, such as retailers, seldom offer health promotion programs, and any employer with a high rate of workforce turnover has no motivation to offer health promotion programs. Further, only

**Table 7.6** Worksite health promotion activities

| | | |
|---|---|---|
| Smoking cessation | Cancer risk awareness | Lending libraries |
| Stress management | Cardiovascular risk | Physical examinations |
| Weight loss | awareness | Smoke-free policies |
| Exercise/physical fitness | Skin cancer screenings | Counseling hot lines |
| Nutrition | Flu shots | Hypertension screenings |
| Safety | Health fairs | HIV/AIDS prevention |
| First aid & CPR | Bulletin boards | Paycheck stuffers |
| Mammography screenings | Newsletters | Website development |

28 percent of employees aged 18 years and over participate in employer-sponsored health promotion activities (U.S. Department of Health and Human Services, 2000b).

Worksite health promotion received a significant boost from the passage of the Patient Protection and Affordable Care Act. As a result of the wellness and prevention provisions in this act, a national worksite health policies and programs survey will be done to more thoroughly assess what employers are doing in relation to worksite health promotion. In 2011, five-year grants to small employers (< 100 employees) will be made available to provide technical assistance and other resources to establish wellness programs for employees. In 2014, employers will be permitted to provide employee rewards in the form of insurance premium discounts, waivers of cost sharing requirements, and so forth for employees participating in wellness programs and meeting certain health-related standards (Society for Public Health Education, 2010).

Though positions exist in the worksite health promotion setting that are strictly health education/promotion, more frequently expertise in exercise testing and prescription is also required. This is because many worksite health promotion programs are based in a fitness center. It is often the fitness center that is the most visible aspect of a worksite health promotion program and attracts many employees to health promotion activities. Therefore, skills related to exercise are important, and these skills are not part of the competencies required by a health education specialist. As a result, health education specialists preparing for employment in worksite health promotion should strongly consider a minor or second major in exercise science (see **Box 7.4**). Peabody and Linnan (2007) recommend that those wanting careers in the worksite setting consider getting two degrees: one a more generalist degree (health education, public health, health promotion), and the second a specialist degree (exercise physiology, nutrition science, nursing, athletic training). They indicate that it does not matter which degree is the undergraduate and which is the graduate, but that an individual with both a generalist and a specialist degree "will have many more options than someone with two degrees in either field" (Peabody & Linnan, 2007, p. 31). Beyond specialty expertise, a master's degree is also required for many entry-level health education/promotion positions in business and industry. In addition to the Certified Health Education Specialist (CHES) credential, certifications more specific to exercise are available from the American College of Sports Medicine and may be required at some worksite settings. Certifications for specific aspects of worksite health promotion, such as aerobic dance, first aid, and CPR, and for smoking cessation instructors are also available and encouraged. In general, the more degrees, certifications, and credentials one has, the better one will compete for worksite health promotion positions.

## Box 7.4 Practitioner's Perspective    Worksite Health Promotion

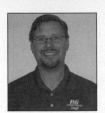

NAME: Robert Pabst

CURRENT POSITION: Fitness Coordinator II

EMPLOYER: TriHealth, Corporate Health

DEGREE/INSTITUTION: B.S. University of Cincinnati

MAJOR: Health Promotion, with an emphasis in Exercise Leadership

(Reprinted by permission of Robert Pabst)

**Job history:** I started in 1996 as an intern with TriHealth. I was located at Procter and Gamble Corporate Fitness Center in Cincinnati, which is operated by TriHealth. When I graduated, I obtained a job with TriHealth at their General Electric Fitness Center in Evendale, Ohio. I worked as a Fitness Technician (entry level position at the time) and later as a Fitness Specialist. In 2003 I moved back to the Procter and Gamble contract where I had started in 1996. Back at P&G I worked as a Specialist until the summer of 2006. I was then promoted to Coordinator (TriHealth's equivalent to a Fitness Center Manager). In the fall of 2008, I was again promoted to Fitness Coordinator level 2, giving me multisite management responsibilities.

**Current job responsibilities:** I currently manage Proctor and Gamble Fitness Centers at three locations. I rotate days that I am at each facility. I am responsible for making sure the Fitness Centers are staffed and classes are covered. To do this I hire several full- and part-time staff at various levels below me. I also manage the budget in relationship to my three sites. I control what new equipment and supplies we purchase on a yearly basis.

**What I like most about my position:** I must admit my favorite part of the position is still working with the members that we serve. I feel as if this will always be my favorite aspect of working in a Fitness Center, and it is the key to customer satisfaction. The design of individualized programs and follow-up exercise and fitness assessments to demonstrate results is the most enjoyable portion of my duties.

Another aspect of my job that has kept me engaged is hiring and retaining my own staff. I feel as if at my level I am building a team that should work together and strive for the same goal: to promote the well-being of our members. Being able to retain a staff over time is one indicator of a good manager. When there is a large turnover of staff it may mean that the management style or attitude is undesirable to staff.

Another aspect of my position that I enjoy is selecting and purchasing new equipment for the fitness center. Being a manager, I look to my frontline staff for opinions and recommendations, and then choose new equipment based upon their recommendations. It is exciting to work through all of the trends in the fitness industry and trying to predict our members' needs into the future.

**What I like least about my position:** As with most management positions, disciplining employees is very difficult. I try to avoid conflict by setting clear expectations. By being up front and direct, I am often able to avoid situations where I need to discipline an employee. At times there is still a need for interventions, but for the most part, unpleasant situations can be avoided by good direction and supervision.

Another unpleasant duty of a manager concerns dealing with employee relationships and conflict. When there is a large staff, all with strong personalities, it can be difficult at times to manage conflict between employees. Most large companies have management training programs, and I would encourage all new health education/promotion managers to attend every conflict resolution class that is offered.

**Recommendations for future students:** I cannot stress how important an internship is to

**Box 7.4 Practitioner's Perspective**   Continued

begin your career. I approach internships like a 10–15-week job interview. Managers are looking for enthusiasm, knowledge, and people skills. Entry-level positions in the fitness industry are extremely important. They are always on the front line and are the face of the Fitness Center. Managers will not even consider someone who does not show a high level of effort and really impress the manager during an internship. Over 85 percent of all of my staff were former interns with us. To be hired, these individuals had to demonstrate all of the traits that I would expect from a top employee. In a job interview, prospects can talk about how they are eager, outgoing, and knowledgeable, but in an internship I can observe and evaluate these traits for myself. If I had to choose between an outside candidate that looked great on

paper and interviewed very well and a former top intern, I would select the intern. Being able to observe the quality of an intern's work, the interactions with members, and the strengths they bring to the position is of tremendous importance to me.

Another recommendation for students is to work on practical skills. Practice your skills at general fitness assessments as much as you can. Learn to take blood pressures or measure body fat, and keep in mind that in health promotion there is a strong desire to hire someone that has knowledge of phlebotomy. With the growing diversity of the fitness and wellness industries, it is important to become diverse in your knowledge and competent in as many skills as possible. When you are in class, try to relate every subject to how it can be used in your future career.

## A Day in the Career of a Worksite Health Education Specialist

The day begins early for Alisa. The fitness center opens promptly at 5:00 A.M. so that employees who start work at 6:00 A.M. have time to work out prior to beginning their shift. Alisa has to be there at 4:45 A.M. to open the doors, turn on the lights, and greet the first members. The first two hours of her day are spent working the floor. This means she greets members as they enter the facility; walks around the machines, providing instruction where needed; chats with the members; answers health-related questions; and basically makes everyone feel important and welcome. By 7:00 A.M., all of the shift workers have left the fitness facility and, by 9:00 A.M., the managerial employees have cleared out.

From 9:00 A.M. to 11:00 A.M. is a slow time in the center. A few retired employees and their spouses use the machines, but this is basically the time for Alisa to get other tasks done. She begins by laundering the dirty towels and folding those that come out of the dryer. Next she provides the routine maintenance to the machines. This involves cleaning them with disinfectant and applying a lubricant to the moving parts. Once this is completed, Alisa has about an hour to work at her desk. Today she is writing an article on the different types of dietary fats, to be included in the Wellness Center newsletter she publishes each month. The newsletter is distributed to all active employees and retirees of the company. Alisa is always amazed at how important writing skills are to her position in worksite health promotion.

Between 11:00 A.M. and 12:15 P.M., Alisa teaches two aerobics classes for the employees. The first is a beginners' class for new members. The second is supposed to be a more advanced class. Unfortunately, many of the shift employees have no choice in their lunch time, so Alisa ends up with some very advanced members in the beginners' class and some beginners in the advanced class. This is frustrating and could be avoided if there were another fitness center employee. There are, however, only two employees in the center, and Rob, the other health education specialist, must work the floor with the lunch crowd while Alisa teaches. Alisa is going to pursue the possibility of hiring a part-time aerobics instructor just for the lunch hours. This would allow her to offer a beginning and an advanced class at each time slot.

From 12:15 P.M. to 1:00 P.M., Alisa runs an ongoing support group for employees trying to lose weight. All participants bring a brown bag lunch that is supposed to contain food appropriate for a weight-loss diet. They weigh in weekly, and Alisa provides each participant with a voluntary body composition (fat vs. lean) analysis every three months. At least twice a week, Alisa prepares a twenty-minute lecture on a weight-loss topic or invites a guest speaker from the community.

At 1:00 P.M. the employees are back at their work stations, and there is again a quiet time in the health promotion center. Alisa spends the next hour eating lunch at her desk and working on a new incentive program for employees to join the health promotion center that will be offered next month. She has to develop all of the brochures, promotional material, and registration forms and arrange for the purchase of incentive items.

At 2:00 P.M. she has a meeting with upper management of the company. She has been advocating for the company to establish a no-smoking policy for the past five years. Two years ago, the company did restrict smoking to specified smoking areas, which was a major accomplishment. Today she will present a proposal to phase out all smoking over a one-year period. Alisa would be responsible for offering several smoking cessation classes over the twelve-month period prior to the no-smoking policy taking effect. She has already decided that her next advocacy effort will be to have more healthy alternatives available in the vending machines, snack rooms, and cafeteria.

By 2:30 P.M. she is back in the health promotion center. The second shift employees are in the center now ahead of their shifts, so Alisa is again working the floor. Today she has to do initial fitness assessments on three new employees. This involves running the employees through a standardized series of tests. Based on the results of these tests and each employee's fitness objectives, she prescribes an individualized exercise program for each employee. She then takes the employees through the fitness center and teaches them how to use the equipment and maintain a record of their progress.

By 3:30 P.M. Alisa is finished with the assessments. Because she had the early shift, opening the facility, she is finished for the day. Rob, who came in later, will stay and close the facility at 8:00 P.M.

## Additional Responsibilities

The responsibilities involved in working in a corporate health promotion center are many and varied. In some facilities, maintaining records such as who is using the center, which programs are most popular, fitness assessment results, and health profiles is a major task. There are always many little things that need to be done, such as the creation and updating of bulletin boards, equipment maintenance, and towel distribution and laundering. Many times, annual health fairs, company-wide health screenings, and flu shot programs are the responsibility of the health promotion staff. In addition, advocating for population-based, corporate-wide policies, rules, and regulations to enhance the health of employees is important. These policies, rules, or regulations may relate to tobacco use, food service, safety, violence, stress, and so forth.

Being a health education specialist in a worksite setting is not easy. It is imperative that worksite health education professionals stay up-to-date with health information and the operational processes of running a worksite program. As noted by the American College of Sports Medicine (2003), "the worksite health promotion professional needs to have a good handle on where to find the information, knowledge, resources and expertise that are needed to access the underlying foundations on which programs are built, the operational processes that allow programs to flourish, and the motivation to continually keep a heads-up attitude toward new and innovative strategies that allow well-established programs to maintain their cutting edge" (p. xi). See **Table 7.7** for a listing of the advantages and disadvantages of employment in worksite health education/promotion.

Those who combine health education/promotion with a fitness background may find employment in settings beyond the business world. See **Table 7.8** for a partial listing of employment opportunities for those with both health education/promotion and exercise training.

**Table 7.7**　Advantages and disadvantages of working in worksite health promotion

| **Advantages** |
| --- |
| • It affords excellent opportunities for prevention. It provides access to individuals who may not participate in community programs. |
| • Health education specialists work with multiple and diverse groups of people, including everyone from upper management to shift workers. |
| • Most health education specialists in the corporate setting enjoy their positions and report a high degree of job satisfaction. |
| • Pay is usually higher than in other health education settings. Benefits are usually good, but they vary considerably from employer to employer. |
| • Health education specialists have access to fitness facilities for personal use. |

| **Disadvantages** |
| --- |
| • Hours are long and irregular. To cover employees on all shifts in a company may necessitate health education specialists' working hours very early in the morning or late in the evening. It is not unusual to work more than eight hours a day. |
| • Upward mobility may be a problem. Typically, there are only one or two managerial positions in health promotion at any given worksite. This makes it difficult for health education specialists to move up. In addition, those holding managerial positions as directors of health and fitness have nowhere to move up in a company unless they are willing to get out of the health promotion field. |
| • Health promotion programs and fitness centers often seem to be low on a company's priority list. Such programs are often the first to receive budget cuts in difficult times and often seem to be short of the staff necessary to run optimal programs. |
| • Some companies subcontract their health promotion and fitness programs to outside vendors. Some of these outside vendors hire part-time health education specialists, pay lower wages, and provide few or no benefits. |
| • Health education specialists have strong pressure to be extremely fit and be healthy role models for other employees. |

**Table 7.8**    Employment opportunities in health education/promotion with an emphasis in exercise and fitness

Corporations, business, and industry
Corporate/industrial parks
YMCAs/YWCAs
Private health and fitness clubs
Special-population clubs (women, elderly, etc.)
Community parks & recreation programs
Colleges/universities
Hospitals
Sports medicine centers
Insurance companies that offer health education/
    promotion programs to their corporate clients

Outside commercial vendors that provide programs
    to worksites
Entrepreneurial enterprises (aerobics studios,
    consulting, club owner, personal training)
Fitness product/service companies (sales and
    marketing)
Condos and apartment complexes
Hotels
Spas
Resorts and cruise lines

## Health Education/Promotion in Health Care Settings

Positions are available for health education specialists in a variety of **health care settings**, including clinics, hospitals, and managed care organizations (McKenzie, Neiger, & Thackeray, 2009). "Typically in the medical care field, health education specialists serve as administrators, directors, managers, and coordinators, supporting and consulting on health education programs and services" (Totzkay-Sitar & Cornett, 2007, p. 8). Health education specialists have also been used in health care settings to provide patient education (Byrd, Hoke, & Gottlieb, 2007). For example, a patient is diagnosed with heart disease. That patient is then referred to the health education specialist for information about exercise, nutrition, weight control, stress management, smoking cessation, and so on. This could involve one-on-one education or counseling sessions with the patient, or it might involve group programs in which multiple patients receive the same program at the same time.

In hospitals and other health care settings, health education specialists have also been hired to direct health and fitness programs for company employees, much the same as in other worksite settings (Breckon, Harvey, & Lancaster, 1998) (see **Figure 7.4**).

**Figure 7.4** Hospitals employ health education specialists to provide programs for employees, patients, or the community at large.
(Robert Clay/Alamy)

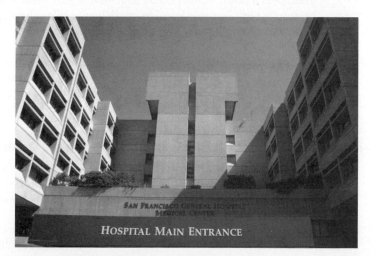

Sometimes these programs are also open as an outreach service to community members. Other times, health education specialists are responsible for developing and conducting health and fitness programs specifically designed for community members through fitness facilities that are affiliated with the hospital (see **Box 7.5**).

Unfortunately, patient education has not emerged as a major source of employment for health education specialists. Although it seems like an ideal activity for health education specialists, third-party reimbursement is not provided by health insurance companies to cover a health education specialist. Third-party reimbursement refers to the system whereby health care providers can submit their bills to the patient's insurance company for reimbursement (McKenzie et al., 2008). Thus, patient education does not happen or it may be done by nurses who can also serve other functions in the health care setting that are reimbursable. Although health insurance companies are certainly concerned about reducing health care costs, their strategies to date have been more short term. The impact of health promotion and education programs may not be seen for years, and cause-and-effect relationships are difficult to establish. Therefore, without the availability of third-party payment, there is a major disincentive for hospitals, clinics, and private practice physicians to offer health promotion and education services to their patients. In response to this problem, the Society for Public Health Education has made third-party reimbursement one of its major advocacy issues.

Of all health care settings, HMOs have been most receptive to hiring health education specialists. The first HMOs were established in the 1970s as a result of federal money that was made available to help with start-up costs and to study the effectiveness of this health care delivery mechanism. In essence, patients belonging to an HMO pay one set fee for all their medical services in a given year. It therefore benefits the HMO to provide preventive health services and health education/promotion programs to keep their patients healthy. The fewer services a patient uses, the greater the cost benefit to the HMO. In the initial HMO legislation, one of the criteria for establishing an HMO was providing health education/promotion. Unfortunately, there were no stipulations on the professional preparation of the health education/promotion provider. Often, nurses or other individuals with little or no health education/promotion preparation or experience were given the responsibility of providing health education/promotion programs. As a result, some HMOs have developed outstanding health education/promotion programs with health education specialists, while others do very little.

There is, however, reason to be optimistic about future employment opportunities in health care settings for health education specialists. With changes in the medical care system rapidly occurring, the increased emphasis on cost-cutting measures, and movement toward more managed care, it is likely that prevention will take a higher profile in the future. As these changes occur, health education specialists will be the best prepared professionals to assume responsibility for helping individuals adopt healthy lifestyles.

## A Day in the Career of a Health Care Setting Health Education Specialist

Mary's day begins at 8:30 A.M., when she arrives at the hospital, picks up her mail, and proceeds to her office. She is the only health education specialist employed by this large metropolitan hospital, but she does have a secretary/assistant who works closely with her to carry out the duties of the position.

At 9:00 A.M. Mary has to attend the weekly staff meeting. This is a meeting with all department heads at the hospital. Much of the agenda does not concern Mary directly,

## Box 7.5 Practitioner's Perspective: Health Care Educator

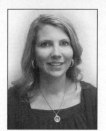

NAME: Carrie Wilcox, RN, M.S.

CURRENT POSITION/TITLE: Community Health Educator

EMPLOYER: Jay County Hospital

DEGREE/INSTITUTION/YEAR: B.S./M.S. Ball State University, 2001–2002; A.S.N. Ivy Tech 2007

MAJOR(S): Health Science and Nursing

(Reprinted by permission of Carrie Wilcox)

**Job responsibilities:** I have a number of job responsibilities in my role as Community Health Educator for Jay County Hospital. I am responsible for teaching diabetes education, congestive heart failure education, and smoking cessation classes to members of our community. I also provide this type of education to patients admitted to the hospital during their stay. I created a wellness program that was implemented in our local high school to teach students the importance of making healthy lifestyle choices. I also serve as the facilitator for a childhood weight management program entitled *Stop Taking On Pounds*. Lastly, I coordinate community health awareness events for the hospital.

**How I got my job:** The position was posted in my local newspaper. The requirements for the job included being a registered nurse, experience in community health, and interest in diabetes. I possessed all three qualities. As part of my health science education, I interned with the Diabetes Prevention Program on the Tohono O'odham Indian Reservation in Sells, Arizona. This experience made me a prime candidate for this position to deliver diabetes education to a population in a rural community.

**What I like most about my job:** I love the variety of my work. Every day is different and there is a great deal of opportunity for creativity. Program development allows me to assess a population, determine their needs, and plan a program to meet such needs. I have freedom in this planning process and am able to make connections with other community members as a result of such programs.

**What I like least about my job:** Working at a small, rural hospital limits the resources available for programs. Funding is always an issue that has to be considered before starting a project. In addition to funding, personnel resources are limited, so I carry the entire responsibility for my work. I am expected to provide education both inside and outside of the hospital, which can be challenging at times.

**How my work relates to the responsibilities and competencies of a health education specialist:** My job as Community Health Educator requires me to constantly assess the needs of the community. From this assessment, I plan, implement, and evaluate health education/promotion programs. When working with patients admitted to the hospital, I must assess their learning levels and readiness to change to provide the most effective health education/promotion resources. I serve as a resource for health education/promotion to our community and hospital as a whole. I also coordinate health education/promotion services between Jay County Hospital and the community.

**Recommendations for those preparing to be health education specialists:** I would strongly suggest choosing internships that allow you some valuable hands-on experience with program planning. Developing health education/promotion programs is the heart of your responsibility as a health education specialist. Gaining experience and becoming comfortable with assessing patient/population needs, developing a program to meet these needs, and evaluating the outcomes is vital in

**Box 7.5 Practitioner's Perspective**    Continued

preparing you for future employment. Also, create a portfolio of the projects you complete both in the classroom and in your internship experiences to share with potential employers in an interview. Proof of your ability to provide effective health education/promotion and develop needs-appropriate programs will speak volumes to a potential employer. Finally,

get involved. Eta Sigma Gamma was a wonderful experience for me as a health science student and allowed me to take leadership within my field of study. There are many opportunities on campus to participate in health education/promotion-related activities. Be proactive and get involved in a club or organization you believe in.

but it is important for her to know what is going on in all departments. At today's meeting, it was decided to have an open house for the public to see the newly renovated obstetrics wing of the hospital. Mary is given the responsibility of planning and advertising this event.

At 10:00 A.M. Mary has an appointment with the administrative head of the Cardiac Rehabilitation Program at the hospital. The purpose of the meeting is to begin planning the development of two brochures that will eventually be distributed to all cardiac rehabilitation patients. One brochure will be on stress-management strategies, and the other on different types of dietary fat. They brainstorm ideas, and Mary agrees to develop a rough draft of the content of the brochures for the administrative head to review prior to their next meeting. They will also discuss graphics, layout, and production at the next meeting.

At 11:00 A.M. Mary leaves the hospital to drive to one of the local malls. The mall has decided to conduct a three-day health fair, and the hospital has agreed to be a co-sponsor of the event. Today is a planning meeting for all of the agencies and businesses that will participate. In addition to serving on the planning committee, Mary is responsible for setting up the hospital's display and coordinating nurses and physicians to work in several screening stations. During the health fair, Mary will be at the hospital's booth all day, handing out materials, answering questions, and promoting the hospital's community outreach health promotion programs.

After lunch, Mary returns to the hospital around 1:00 P.M. and spends the next two hours working on the hospital's health and wellness newsletter. As a public service and to promote the hospital, Mary is responsible for developing a newsletter every other month that is mailed to all households in the hospital's immediate service area. Each edition of the newsletter features one department in the hospital and contains several additional articles about health and wellness. Mary writes much of each newsletter, using information she obtains from the Internet and from a variety of health journals and newsletters to which she subscribes. She designs and formats the newsletter with a desktop publishing program she has on her computer. She marvels at how important good writing skills are to her position.

At 3:00 P.M. Mary leads a weight-loss support group for hospital employees. Most of the participants are nurses and housekeeping staff from either the first or second shift. At each session, participants weigh in, share their experiences over the previous week, and listen to a thirty-minute presentation designed to enhance their weight-loss program. Mary is responsible for each week's presentation. In addition, she provides participants with healthy recipes, exercise tips, motivational incentives, and recognition awards.

After class, Mary returns phone calls, answers e-mails, and ties up loose ends until it is time for her to go home at 5:00 P.M. It is not unusual for Mary to take some work home in the evenings or on weekends. Tonight, however, Mary must return to the hospital at 7:30 P.M. to teach a stress-management class for the community. The stress class is part of the hospital's ongoing community outreach program. Each month a different health topic is taught, and Mary is responsible for either teaching the class or lining up the instructor for the class.

## Additional Responsibilities

Health education specialists working in health care settings are involved in numerous and varied activities. The actual responsibilities can differ greatly from one health care setting to another. Planning, implementing, and evaluating programs and events are certainly major tasks. Health education specialists may also be involved in grant writing, one-on-one or group patient education services, publicity, public relations, employee wellness activities, and various collaborative efforts with other hospital staff, community agencies, or departments of public health.

Administration is a major responsibility of many health education specialists working in hospitals. They are often hired as managers, directors, or coordinators of programs. Hospitals often adopt a "team" approach to health education/promotion, in which doctors, nurses, physical therapists, and other health specialists are all part of the team. Health education specialists plan and coordinate the programs and serve as resources for the other team members, who actually present the programs. In this type of position, the health education specialist provides little direct client service (Breckon, Harvey, & Lancaster, 1998). (See **Table 7.9**.)

**Table 7.9** Advantages and disadvantages of working in a health care setting

| Advantages |
| --- |
| • Job responsibilities are highly varied and changing. |
| • There is increased credibility due to the health care connection. |
| • There is usually a high community profile. |
| • Health education specialists work with multiple groups of people. |
| • Wages and benefits are good. |
| • There is a high degree of self-satisfaction. |

| Disadvantages |
| --- |
| • Health education/promotion may have low status and low priority within health care settings. |
| • Health education specialists must continually justify the program's value. |
| • Jobs are difficult to obtain. |
| • Turf issues over educational responsibilities can develop. |
| • Hours may be long and irregular. |
| • Some medical doctors may be difficult to work with. |

## Health Education/Promotion in Colleges and Universities

Colleges and universities are another source of employment for health education specialists. Within the college setting, there are typically two types of positions that health education specialists hold. The first is an academic, or faculty, position, and the second is a health education specialist in a student health service or wellness center.

As a faculty member, the health education specialist typically has three major responsibilities: teaching, community and professional service, and scholarly research (Hayden, 2007). The amount of emphasis on each of these major responsibilities is dependent on the institution. In very large research institutions, faculty may spend most of their time writing grants and conducting research. In smaller four-year colleges, teaching may be the major responsibility. In addition to the major responsibilities, faculty may be asked to advise students, serve on committees, coordinate or lead student groups, attend professional conferences, and accept administrative duties.

The minimum qualification for working as a faculty member in the college/university setting is usually a doctoral degree in health education/promotion. Though some junior colleges and small four-year schools may hire faculty with only a master's degree, most tenure track positions require a doctorate. In addition, depending on the position for which one is applying, it may be necessary to have had prior experience or academic training in school health, public/community health, or worksite health promotion. Holding or being eligible for a Certified Health Education Specialist (CHES) credential is often listed as a preference or requirement for faculty positions.

For a health education specialist in a university health service or wellness center, the major responsibility is to plan, implement, and evaluate health education/promotion programs for program participants (see **Box 7.6**). In some universities, the program participants are students, while in others it is the faculty and staff. Often both groups are responsible for programming. In addition to program planning, the health education specialist may be responsible for maintaining a resource library; one-on-one advising with students; developing and coordinating a peer education program; speaking to residence hall, fraternity, and sorority groups; conducting incentive programs; and planning special events.

The minimum qualifications for working in a university health service or wellness center typically include a bachelor's or master's degree in health education/promotion. A master's degree is usually preferred. Students interested in working in this setting are advised to work as volunteers or consider completing a practicum or internship in the campus wellness center while an undergraduate. Many universities have peer education programs in which undergraduate students are trained by the professional health education specialist to conduct programs for their peers. This type of experience is invaluable, whether or not a student is subsequently employed in a university health service or wellness center. It would also be a good idea to obtain the CHES credential for work in this area.

## International Opportunities

Health education/promotion professionals may wish to consider working in foreign countries for all or a portion of their careers. There is great need for professionals with health education/promotion skills in many developing countries. These positions often

### Box 7.6 Practitioner's Perspective    University Wellness Center

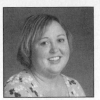

(Reprinted by permission of Jodi Brawley)

NAME: Jodi Brawley, M.S., CHES

CURRENT POSITION/TITLE: Health Educator

EMPLOYER: Boise State University

DEGREE/INSTITUTION/YEAR: Master's of Science, California Polytechnic State University, San Luis Obispo, 1999

MAJOR: Kinesiology, Exercise Science and Health Promotion

**How I obtained my job:** After seven years working in a variety of health promotion positions, I decided I wanted a job in higher education. Having lived in California all my life, I was open for a change. I found the position on a national job recruiting Web site. After being offered the position, I relocated to Boise, Idaho. Four years later, I am very pleased with my choice to move.

**How I utilize health education/promotion in my job:** The health education/promotion tools that are intrinsic to my daily work are planning, designing, and evaluating health promotion outreach programs that meet the needs of our students and staff. I also use learning outcomes for all programs and outreach as a way to keep focused on the educational purpose for all events.

**What I like most about my job:** I thoroughly enjoy supervising the Wellness Works Peer Education internship program. I have the opportunity to mentor students as Peer Educators, watching them develop as young professionals while coordinating health promotion events and educational campaigns. The Peer Educators program deals with a variety of health topics including fitness and nutrition, body image and eating disorders, stress, sleep, sexual health, back health, and depression and anxiety. It is a great experience watching these student leaders grow and make a lasting impact on our campus and in the lives of our students.

**What I like least about my job:** Every job has its downside. My least favorite aspect of my current job is not having enough resources to provide the services needed on our campus. Staff and funding are often limited, although there is additional need for services, and only so much can be done with the resources available. In an ideal world there would be adequate professional staff and a sufficient budget to help all the students and staff meet their health and wellness goals.

**Recommendations for those preparing to be health education specialists:** I highly encourage students to participate in an internship program. Internships are a great opportunity to experience various work environments and apply classroom knowledge to real-life settings. Health education/promotion can vary diversely from work place to work place, so the more internships you can do, the greater likelihood you will find a setting that you enjoy and can flourish in.

**The role of health educators/health promotion specialists in the future:** The future is ours to create. Health care continues to be a hot topic, and as the population ages, the role of the health education specialist will continue to grow. Health education specialists are going to be called upon to work with individuals for behavior modification programs, develop and support public policy, and influence changes that create healthy environments for people to live, work, and play.

require special dedication, as the living and working conditions may be more challenging than those experienced in the United States. For those so inclined, however, the rewards in terms of personal satisfaction and accomplishment can be tremendous. Further, the experience gained by planning, implementing, and evaluating health promotion and education programs in foreign countries can be invaluable to one's professional development.

Working in developing countries often requires the health education specialist to examine different health problems and to try different approaches. For example, instead of helping people reduce high-fat, high-cholesterol diets, as in the United States, the health education specialist may be helping people deal with problems of starvation, malnutrition, and parasitic and bacterial infections. Instead of dealing with heart disease and lung cancer, the health education specialist in a developing country may be facing schistosomiasis, diarrhea, and ascaris and tapeworm infections.

Consider the case of Sofia. Sofia was working as a community health education specialist for the health department in a rural community of about two thousand people in a developing country. The water source for this community consisted of several large ponds. These ponds were the only source of drinking water and were also used for bathing, clothes washing, and care of animals. Many people were getting sick with severe diarrhea, and there had been several deaths among the elderly and very young. To alleviate this problem, it was decided to develop an educational campaign to get people to boil their water prior to consumption. Sofia was given the responsibility for developing this campaign. There were no local newspapers or radio stations, and no billboards, and many of the people could not read. After consulting with local leaders, it was decided that the best way to spread the information would be to use a "mobile communication system." This was accomplished by hooking up an old stereo system to a car battery and driving around the community, broadcasting information about the importance of boiling water. In addition, Sofia set up several demonstrations around the community about how to boil water effectively. These sessions were also advertised via the "mobile communication system."

As can be seen from Sofia's experience, health education specialists working in foreign countries must be able to develop creative, innovative programs to solve identified health problems. Most often, these programs must be low-cost, easily developed and implemented, acceptable to the social norms of the community, and available to all aspects of the public. It is imperative that these programs be developed in conjunction with the local people being served. It is also helpful when programs are sponsored by organizations seen as credible by the priority population.

One of the best ways to begin a career in international health is to volunteer with the Peace Corps. Health education/promotion professionals are in demand by the Peace Corps, and students should begin the application process early in their senior year. Many colleges and universities are visited by Peace Corps recruiters every year, and talking to one of these Peace Corps volunteers is a good place to start. Faculty members on your campus may have been former Peace Corps volunteers, and talking to these individuals can provide valuable insight into the Peace Corps experience.

There are many advantages to volunteering with the Peace Corps. The Peace Corps provides volunteers with some of the best language and technical training in the world. Each Peace Corps volunteer is granted a monthly allowance for housing, food, clothing, and miscellaneous expenses. Free dental and medical care are provided, as well as free transportation to the placement setting and twenty-four vacation days per year. Deferment of federal student loans is also possible while serving in the Peace Corps. After completing the two-year experience, volunteers are given a post-service readjustment allowance of $7,425. They are also given preference for federal jobs and have enhanced scholarship and assistantship opportunities at many major colleges and universities (Peace Corps, 2010). In addition, a successful Peace Corps experience may serve as a stepping stone to paid positions in other international health organizations (see **Table 7.10**).

**Table 7.10**  International health organizations

| |
|---|
| National Council for International Health |
| American Association for World Health |
| World Health Organization (WHO) |
| Pan American Health Organization |
| U.S. Agency for International Development (A.I.D.) |
| CDC Coordinating Office for Global Health |

The Centers for Disease Control and Prevention is expanding its presence overseas. This may create future opportunities for health education specialists. "CDC is committed to ensuring that people around the world will live safer, healthier, and longer lives through the achievement of its Global Health Goals: Global Health Promotion, Global Health Protection, and Global Health Diplomacy" (CDC, n.d.).

## Nontraditional Health Education/Promotion Positions

In addition to the traditional settings for health education/promotion that have been described in this chapter, there are a variety of nontraditional jobs that health education specialists may wish to consider. These positions may or may not carry the title of health education specialist. In some cases, they require the health education specialist to use the skills and competencies in different or unique ways. Further, it is often necessary for health education specialists to sell themselves to get these positions, as the persons doing the hiring may be unfamiliar with the skills and training of a health education specialist.

Given health education specialists' knowledge of health and fitness, sales positions related to health are a real possibility. Pharmacy sales, fitness equipment sales, and the sales of health-related textbooks are all areas in which health education specialists have found employment. Life and health insurance are two additional options to consider in the area of sales.

By emphasizing the communication competencies that are part of the professional training in health education/promotion, the health education specialist may seek employment in journalism, TV, or radio. Many television stations have a regular health or medical reporter who does feature stories on health-related issues. Newspapers may have a health column that could and should be written by a health education specialist. Writing articles for health-related Web sites or actually developing Web sites for health-related organizations are other possibilities (see **Box 7.7**). Again, it is necessary for health education specialists to sell themselves to obtain these positions. Taking elective classes or minors in media, communications, and journalism and doing one's internship in these settings also may assist those interested in this career field.

Health education specialists should always be alert to unique job opportunities, many of which may not even carry the title of health education specialist. One health education specialist, for example, was hired by a state mental hospital as a "Teacher II." His job was to provide drug education to patients who had a history of drug problems and sex education to patients who had a history of sex problems. The remainder of his work schedule involved tutoring patients in math and science who were studying to obtain their high school general equivalency diploma.

## Box 7.7 Practitioner's Perspective — Nontraditional Health Education/Promotion Positions

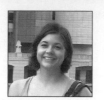

(Reprinted by permission of Nicole Nichols)

NAME: Nicole Nichols

CURRENT POSITION: Content & Editorial Director; Resident Fitness Expert

EMPLOYER: SparkPeople, Inc. (SparkPeople.com and BabyFit.com)

DEGREE, INSTITUTION, MAJOR: B.S.Ed., University of Cincinnati, 2005, Health Promotion & Education with Exercise & Fitness Emphasis

**Current job responsibilities:** As the primary content developer and editor for SparkPeople.com and BabyFit.com, it's my responsibility to create and manage all of the content on our Web sites. SparkPeople.com is the fastest growing health site on the Web and covers a wide variety of health, nutrition, fitness, and weight loss topics, while BabyFit.com helps women have healthier pregnancies and babies by focusing on good nutrition and prenatal exercise.

"Content" can mean a wide range of things for both sites. It's my job to either create the content by writing it myself, or by hiring and managing freelancers or health experts for certain projects. I write and edit articles, create interactive quizzes and assessments, conduct polls, review products and books, write instructions for our exercise demos, create online workout videos, summarize current research studies that apply to our members, and write and manage our thirteen different daily and weekly e-newsletters. While this type of content focuses on general health, fitness, and nutrition, it's also my responsibility to proof, edit, and sometimes write other pieces of content on the sites—like instructions for using the site, member surveys, announcements, technical FAQs, company press releases, and promotional pieces for other magazines and newspapers.

While content creation and management makes up the bulk of my job, I'm also involved with our Community Message Boards as a Resident Fitness Expert. When members ask questions about weight loss, exercise, nutrition, and more, I can answer their questions and point them to other helpful resources. Lastly, I create and manage our unique employee wellness program, which we call the SparkPeople Adventure. It entails daily, weekly, and monthly nutrition and fitness goals that everyone must meet in order to earn a year-end bonus.

**Health education/promotion responsibilities I use most in my job:** Although my job is nontraditional, I use a lot of the core responsibilities of a health education specialist on a daily basis:

- Assess Needs: I have to assess the needs of the members of our site in order to create content that is appealing and helpful to them. After all, we want them to return to the site and reach their goals. I can assess these needs by conducting polls or surveys, and by skimming the message boards to see the types of questions that are asked most often.

- Plan and Implement Effective Programs: When I find the needs of our members, I brainstorm topics to meet those needs and come up with the most effective way of educating members on a topic, whether it be an article, a quiz, or an indepth guide. I'll either write the content myself, or assign it to one of our in-house experts or freelancers as a way of "implementing" the program.

- Evaluate Program: Because members can easily contact us via e-mail or message boards, they are able to ask additional questions, point out errors, or give feedback about the content on the site. This lets me know whether the content is doing well, or if I might need to revisit it.

- Act as a Resource: This is probably what I do most. By writing and generating content, I'm taking the steps to find accurate, reliable, and helpful information that members

| **Box 7.7** Practitioner's Perspective | Continued |

can use. All of our content is backed by research and is medically accurate. If and when generally accepted guidelines on fitness, nutrition, and health change, then I also need to react and update our resources on the site. Regarding message boards, I have to know when I'm qualified to answer questions on certain topics, or when another expert (or resource) is needed, and be able to point people in the right direction.

**How I got my job:** In college, I knew that I wanted to be a health and fitness writer, so I took additional courses in journalism and copyediting. I obtained a part-time job at the college newspaper, writing health articles. That led me directly to SparkPeople, because one of their employees saw my work and asked me if I'd want to write for them as a freelancer. After I wrote my first article, they contacted me for an interview, and hired me on the spot. I worked as the assistant editor part-time while in school and got a full-time job offer upon graduation.

**What I like most about my job:** I love knowing that each day my efforts are directly helping and educating people. Since we're a small company, I can work independently and make decisions without waiting for the approval of others. This way, I'm much more efficient and able to get a lot accomplished. I feel fortunate that staying on top of current health trends and news is part of my job, and that I help people interpret that information and apply it to their own lives to become healthier. Making the workout videos is one of my favorite tasks—and getting free products and books from other companies who hope we'll mention or use their stuff is a fun perk. My co-workers and our company culture are also pluses. Everyone is passionate about doing their job well so SparkPeople and BabyFit can help millions of people around the world.

**What I like least about my job:** I'd say the only downside to my job is the lack of face-to-face contact with the people I am educating. Although my work is online and can potentially help more people than most health professionals can expect to reach with traditional health programs, I do it all from behind a desk, without any real interactions with these people.

Recommendations for students preparing to be health education specialists: I have what many people would consider to be a fun job with an excellent company. And the reason I am here today, especially so early in my career, is directly related to my undergraduate work and experience. Whether you hope to write for a magazine or Web site, or just want to get the best job possible, I believe these points are keys to success:

- Take your classes seriously and really learn the material. I have to apply things that I learned in college on a daily basis—I'm expected to know certain things so that every piece of content on our site is accurate, safe, and easily understood. No matter where you work, you'll need to be an "expert" on something. A high GPA is a highlight on a resume that might help you land that first job.

- Get work experience in the field. This will help you narrow down what you want to do as a career, and help you stand out against the competition. Try a variety of part-time jobs and volunteer opportunities while in college.

- Work to improve your writing and communication skills. No matter what health education/promotion job you get, you'll have to write and speak well to be taken seriously and increase your credibility.

- Network. Get to know your professors, your boss, and other professionals in the field. Attend events that will expand your network and join professional associations. After all, you never know who might recommend you or tell you about a job opportunity.

- Find your passion. Whether it's a type of work (like writing, in my case), or a particular area in the health field, it's important to care about the nature of your work. That makes you more effective in your job, and makes your job more rewarding.

## Landing That First Job

At first, it may seem unusual to discuss landing one's first job while still in an introductory course, but this is the best time to consider the issue of future employment. There are several actions students can take during their college years to enhance their chances of obtaining employment. By following the suggestions made in this section, a student will be far ahead of those who wait until the end of their degree program to address these issues.

No matter what the setting in which a health education specialist hopes to eventually work, landing the first job can be a frustrating experience. Students often find themselves in a dilemma. Employers want their new employees to have had "experience," but where are students supposed to get experience if they can't get hired? There are several possible answers to this question. One way to gain experience is to obtain part-time or summer employment in one's preferred health education/promotion setting. Typically, there are many more students looking for this type of employment than there are employment situations. Should such an opportunity be available, however, it is an excellent way to gain experience prior to graduation. Another way to obtain experience is to volunteer time in the chosen health education/promotion setting. Most professional health education specialists working in the field are more than willing to accept and use the volunteer time of health education/promotion students. In addition to experience, volunteering also begins the important process of **networking.** Networking involves establishing and maintaining a wide range of contacts in the field that may be of help when looking for a job and in carrying out one's job responsibilities once hired.

Some health education/promotion programs now offer **service learning** opportunities to their students (Cleary et al., 1998). Organized service learning opportunities provide course credit for students to work with a community agency to meet an identified community need. They provide hands-on, practical, real-world experience that students cannot obtain from the classroom. They are also beneficial in broadening one's professional network, which is so important in the health education/promotion field. Take advantage of as many service learning opportunities as possible. The experience and networking gained through service learning can give new health education/promotion professionals a tremendous advantage in the job market.

Carefully planning internships and practicums can help students obtain their first professional position (see **Box 7.8**). Required field experiences are often the best way to obtain practical experience in one's chosen setting. Students should consider what they would like to be doing five years after graduation and select an experience that closely matches that goal. Often students are hired by the agency after completing their practicum or internship experience.

In addition to obtaining experience, students should strive to obtain an excellent academic record. When there is heavy competition for an open position, one of the first strategies in making hiring decisions is to examine grade point average. This is not to say that the person with the highest grade point average is always the best person or will always get the job. But, when there are fifty applications for one job, grade point average is an easy way to begin limiting the field.

Develop a well-organized, professional-looking portfolio. A **portfolio** is a collection of evidence that enables students to demonstrate mastery of desired course or program

## Box 7.8 Practitioner's Perspective: Student Internship

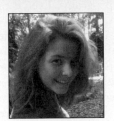

NAME: Melinda Hershey

INTERNSHIP LOCATION: Kampala, Uganda and Bwindi, Uganda

INTERNSHIP ORGANIZATION: Conservation Through Public Health (CTPH)

DEGREE/INSTITUTION, AND GRADUATION DATE: B.S. - The University of Cincinnati, Health Promotion and Education, Public/Community Health Concentration; September 2010

(Reprinted by permission of Melinda Hershey)

**Internship placement:** I was interested in pursuing a career in international health and decided that I wanted to explore health promotion issues in Africa. I did an online search for organizations in Africa that dealt with health and came across CTPH. The organization studies the relationships between human and animal diseases in Uganda.

**Internship description:** My major responsibility during this internship was to conduct health interviews within two separate parishes in the Bwindi community. I explored the hygiene and sanitation standards within the community and advised community members on how to better their health by improving their hygiene and sanitation practices. I also asked questions about family planning awareness and explained to community members the connection between smaller families and better overall health. In addition, I spoke with key community members such as hospital administrators and school principals to learn about the pressing health issues in their communities. I also created brochures and flyers to create awareness about health issues, including an Anthrax epidemic in nearby Queen Elizabeth National Park.

**Pros and cons of my internship:** I really enjoyed the fact that I was able to experience my internship in Uganda. It was truly a learning experience and allowed me to compare and contrast the health issues of the United States with the health issues of Africa. It was also an extremely culturally rich experience for me and

I learned so much about an entirely different group of people. However, working in Africa is much different than working in the United States. Sometimes you have to really fend for yourself and work independently on your own projects with very little guidance, which was a lesson in perseverance for me. Overall, I am glad that I chose to do my internship in Uganda because it opened my eyes to what it's like to work in a different country.

**Internship importance:** Participating in this internship was extremely important in helping me determine my future career. I came to Uganda thinking that I wanted to do international development work for the rest of my life. However, working there made me realize that I have so many other interests, like environmental health and women's empowerment. I came out of this experience with a whole new perspective on what I want my life's work to be, which turns out to be much different than I had initially imagined.

**Recommendations for health education/promotion students:** When you're looking for an internship, do your research. What do you want to get out of the experience? Is it really going to help you determine your future career? Don't just pick an internship because it's easy, close by, and convenient. Pick one that you think is going to help you both professionally and personally; this is your chance to explore the field before you jump into a real job, so make it count!

outcomes. In health education/promotion, the responsibilities, competencies, and sub-competencies should be emphasized. Many health education/promotion programs now require portfolios as part of their professional preparation programs. Even if the portfolio is not required, students should develop a portfolio on their own. Thompson and Bybee (2004) note that a portfolio is a "living document that is ever-changing with the increasing depth of knowledge and experience of the individual" (p. 52). They go on to identify five basic elements that should be included in any portfolio: (1) table of contents, (2) resume, (3) education and credentials, (4) samples of work, and (5) references. The samples of work could include such exhibits as student papers or course projects, audio- or videotapes of students giving a presentation, analyses of student work by professors and/or outside reviewers, student goal statements, reflections, and summaries (Cleary & Birch, 1996, 1997). Students may also want to consider developing the portfolio in an electronic format instead of the more traditional notebook or binder. In addition to providing more flexibility in the way exhibits are presented and displayed, an electronic format also provides the opportunity to showcase one's creativity and to demonstrate technology skills to potential employers (McKenzie, Cleary, McKenzie, & Stephen, 2002). Imagine the impact on a prospective employer when a new health education specialist provides a well-developed, attractive portfolio.

Your resume is extremely important in obtaining your first job. The resume is your advertisement for yourself. It is the first item of yours that most prospective employers will see. It will create a first and lasting impression of you. What you include in the resume and how you present the information may make a difference in whether or not you are hired. You should start now to involve yourself in experiences that will look good on your resume. As you develop your resume make sure that there are no spelling or grammar errors. One former student actually lost a job opportunity due to three spelling errors on her resume. The more specific you can be in describing your accomplishments on the resume, the better. Jeff Brizzolara, a health education specialist and Chief Clinical Officer for Viverae Health Care, has some suggestions on how to be more specific; these can be seen in **Table 7.11**.

Beyond the portfolio and resume, consider what certifications are going to be important in landing your first job and carefully plan to make sure they are awarded either prior to graduation or as soon after graduation as possible. All professional health education specialists should pursue the Certified Health Education Specialist (CHES)

**Table 7.11** Resume—Words of wisdom

| Out-of-Date Resume (Overused Cliches) | More Effective Resume (Be Specific—Provide Examples) |
|---|---|
| Results Oriented | Describe a problem that you solved |
| Team Player | Describe a team project you were part of and the results |
| Excellent Communication Skills | Demonstrate how your communication skills produced meaningful results |
| Strong Work Ethic | Provide an example of how you went "above and beyond" to produce results |
| Meets or Exceeds Expectations | Explain how you were recognized for your effort/work |

*Source:* Jeff Brizzolara, PhD, MPH, MBA. Chief Clinical Officer, Viverae Health Care, Inc. Used by permission.

credential. In the future, this may be a prerequisite for many health promotion and education positions. Other certifications should be obtained depending on work setting and need.

Get to know your faculty. They are a great source of information about jobs and how to compete for them successfully. Often employers contact faculty directly, asking for the names of students who might be interested in a particular position. But unless a faculty member knows a student by name and knows that the student is in the job market, there is little the faculty member can do.

Most colleges and universities have placement centers that provide a variety of services to students, including help in developing an effective resume. They may also assist by maintaining a list of job openings, providing workshops or handouts on interviewing skills, and establishing reference files for students. It would be a good idea to contact the placement center well before graduation to determine when and how to access its services.

A final suggestion is to join one or more of the professional associations (see Chapter 8). Employers are typically impressed when they see that a young professional has been a member of a professional association and perhaps has attended one or more professional meetings. "Professional meetings and conferences are filled with opportunities. . . . Where else can you find hundreds, even thousands, of education professionals from all over the world coming together to share cutting-edge knowledge through presentations, sessions, workshops, socials, and other events, than at professional meetings and conferences?" (Dixon-Terry, 2004, p. 16). If your campus has a chapter of Eta Sigma Gamma, the professional health education/promotion honorary, try to get involved. Eta Sigma Gamma recognizes high academic achievement, provides opportunities to obtain valuable leadership experience, and allows students to plan, implement, and evaluate various service projects and social activities.

In addition to the aforementioned suggestions, one caution is in order. Be careful what you place on social networking websites such as Facebook and Twitter. Prospective employers are savvy and often will look online to see what additional information they can find about you. "Susan Masterson, a recruiter with TeamHealth in Knoxville, TN, said, using social networking sites is a strategy that anyone in recruiting, whether it be physicians or otherwise, needs to incorporate in their plan. It's here. It's here to stay" (Dolan 2009). Health education/promotion internship site supervisors have even looked online before accepting a student for internship. One author of this text actually received a letter from a prospective employer indicating that he had not hired a particular student due to offensive content he found online. Further, he admonished the program to caution students about what they include online. Students' posting questionable information on line seems to be a somewhat common practice. According to an *AMNews* article, in one study 60 percent of U.S. medical schools surveyed reported incidents of students posting unprofessional content on line (Dolan, 2009). What is questionable content is difficult to define. Certainly pictures involving sex, alcohol, or drugs are not appropriate, but anything that causes doubt should be removed. Students should also restrict who can be friends and can access their information as much as possible.

Students who follow the aforementioned suggestions will be better positioned to obtain initial employment in the health promotion and education profession. This is a good time to be a health education specialist, and the future looks even brighter than the present. According to the U.S. Department of Labor Bureau of Labor Statistics

(2010a), the number of health education specialists will need to grow from the current 66,200 to a projected 78,200 by the year 2018—an 18 percent increase. Floyd and Allen (2004) noted, "As the field of health education continues to expand, the number and type of careers will continue to expand. Health education professionals must be willing to implement innovative and quality school and non-school programs for an increasingly diverse population in increasingly diverse settings. The future of health education is here" (p. 36).

## Excelling in Your Health Education/Promotion Career

Landing a job is merely the first step in becoming a successful health education specialist. Once you have the job, it is critical that you excel in the job. This is important for two reasons. First you must excel to demonstrate that you are an important and contributing member of the organization that hired you and to enhance your career potential. Second, you need to excel to help further the health education/promotion profession. Your work reflects on all health education specialists and may determine whether your organization or other organizations will hire more health education specialists in the future.

What does it take to excel in health education/promotion? Obviously, one must demonstrate the ability to meet the competencies and sub-competencies of a health education specialist, but one must also meet the standards of a good employee. Numerous authors writing about careers in health education/promotion have elaborated on what is needed to excel as an employee in a health education/promotion position. In talking about how to excel in a voluntary health agency position, one author wrote, "Completing your tasks and projects on time, under budget, and with minimum problems is your most obvious goal, but do not underestimate the value of attitude, spirit, and the ability to work under pressure and with difficult people. A positive, can-do attitude, a willingness to learn new and different skills on the job, and the ability to work in an environment that values teamwork is a 'must'" (Daitz, 2007, pp. 5–6). Other authors writing about working in health and medical care note, "Being successful means meeting and exceeding the expectations of the job and showing initiative in achieving organizational goals" (Totzkay-Sitar & Cornett, 2007, pp. 9–10). In discussing federal health education/ promotion positions, Howze (2007) said, "With any job, success requires continually showing how you add value to the organization. For example, many federal agencies are struggling to find workers with language skills, so consider becoming fluent in a second language" (p. 13). And finally, if you are trying to excel in a public health department position (see **Box 7.9**), "Become known as a high achiever/performer and a good team player. Make a positive and lasting impression on your supervisor as well as upper level managers with whom you may have contact through your assignments. Anticipate what needs to be done" (Hall, 2007, p. 17).

The aforementioned quotes clearly indicate that, regardless of the setting, you must go beyond simply meeting the minimum expectations of the job to being a good employee and a good health education specialist. To excel you must go the extra mile and do the unexpected as well as the expected. You need to be a good "people person," demonstrate a positive attitude, and be willing to learn and take on new tasks. These are the things that will separate you from other employees and establish you as a truly outstanding health education specialist.

**Box 7.9 Practitioner's Perspective** | Employer of Health Education Specialists

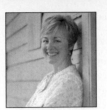

(Reprinted by permission of Stacy Wegley)

NAME: Stacy Wegley, M.S., ACSM

CURRENT POSITION/TITLE: Director Health Promotion & Education

EMPLOYER: Hamilton County Public Health

DEGREES/INSTITUTIONS/YEAR: Bachelor's of Science: Consumer Science— Nutrition Ohio University—1993; Master's of Science: Exercise Science and Health Studies, Miami University—2003

**Employment history:** I currently serve as the Director of Health Promotion & Education for Hamilton County Public Health (HCPH). I have degrees in nutrition and exercise science and a passion for empowering individuals and communities to live their healthiest. I worked for three years between my undergraduate and graduate degrees for the Women, Infants, and Children program (WIC). My focus for a service-oriented career was cemented in this work. After graduate school, I began my employment with public health and without a formal degree in community health. I embraced each opportunity to learn about public health and population-based health education/ promotion strategies. I have since worked with my agency to grow health promotion and education from myself as sole health educator, to a division of eleven, including two supervisors.

**Job responsibilities:** My current responsibilities are focused on building and executing a health promotion and education strategic plan for the residents and communities served by HCPH. This includes an ongoing review of data to determine greatest need, seeking funding for implementation, determining evaluation needs, reporting findings, grant development and administration, and staff and partner recruitment, retention, and leadership, among others.

**How I develop a job description:** Health educator job descriptions at HCPH are focused on the seven areas of responsibility of a health educator. In addition, there are often professional skills such as problem solving and public health notations for serving as a resource in an emergency that are also included in the job description.

**What I look for when reviewing applications:** When looking for health promotion and education candidates, a professional cover letter and resume make a strong first impression. A clean, well written, error-free document is key. Beyond this initial review, candidacy is strengthened by internship or other work or volunteer-related experiences. I look for active descriptions of job or volunteer responsibilities. It is my goal to best match candidate experience with the position roles. I understand that it is often difficult to gain work experience when you have no experience and am very open when a candidate can communicate how professional skills are transferred from one situation to another.

**What I look for in an interview:** Interviews are far more than just answering the questions. A successful interview begins with preparing to talk about your experiences related to the position available. To accomplish this, invest the time to find out what you can about the organization you're interviewing with, the specific department and the projects or staff. Talk with professors, colleagues, or others who may have interned or partnered with the organization. The more you know, the better prepared you'll appear and the better you will be able to link your experiences to the desired job skills.

An interview with HCPH will be focused on experience-based questions. As your potential supervisor, I'm interested in your analytical skills, communication style, professional knowledge, personal goals, and potential fit with the organizational culture.

**Box 7.9 Practitioner's Perspective**     Continued

The general process for an employment search at HCPH begins with a traditional first interview. After the first interviews are completed, candidates of interest are often asked back to present on a defined topic to a larger panel of colleagues. Prior to a job offer, additional screenings such as background checks and drug testing may also apply.

The health education/promotion network is quite broad, yet very connected. Assume that any work, intern, or volunteer experience you have will be part of the information another potential employer will have available in their decision making. I often contact people I know who have worked with a potential candidate in the past. Also, note that employers may choose to do an Internet search to learn more about you as a potential candidate. Make information found via a Google search another opportunity to relay your professional skills, volunteer activities, and professional judgment.

**Final thoughts:** This is an amazing time to be a health educator. There is greater evidence about how to create and support significant population-based health outcomes, increased resources for accomplishing this important work, and increased community-generated demand. There are growing opportunities for the types of organizations and health-specific topics where our skill sets can be applied and growing opportunities for career advancement as a health educator. One of the challenges and greatest joys of my work is the constant of change. Each change has created an opportunity to increase my knowledge, expand my skills, and demonstrate my competencies. Be proactive, flexible, and embrace the constant of change so that you may pursue your passion to serve.

## SUMMARY

There are many settings in which a health education specialist can seek employment. In this chapter, we have discussed in detail health education/promotion positions in schools, public/community health agencies, worksites, health care facilities, colleges and universities, and international settings. In addition, we have examined the potential for employment in nontraditional settings and have considered what introductory-level undergraduate students can do to help themselves obtain their first job. Finally, we discussed what it takes to be successful in a health education/promotion position.

## REVIEW QUESTIONS

1. Identify four major settings and two nontraditional settings in which health education specialists are employed.
2. Compare and contrast the roles and responsibilities of health education specialists working in schools, public/community health agencies, worksites, and health care facilities. How are all of these settings similar? How are they different?

3. What is the difference between a position funded with hard money and a position funded with soft money? Which position is preferable and why?

4. Explain why it might be said that health education/promotion has never reached its real potential in the health care setting. What factors have kept health education/promotion positions at a minimal level in this setting?

5. What is networking and why is it important in health education/promotion?

6. What can introductory-level health education/promotion students do now that might help them land their first job after graduation?

## CASE STUDY

Marla has a B.S. degree in health education/promotion and is CHES certified. For the past five years, since graduating from college, she has been working as a health education specialist for a private vendor who then contracts with companies to offer health education/promotion and fitness services to their employees. During this time the vendor has placed her at three different corporations. All three corporations have been extremely satisfied with her services and the vendor/employer has also given her positive evaluations.

Recently Marla has become dissatisfied with her position. She feels that her $29,000 annual salary is too low, and she gets no retirement, dental, vision, or pharmacy benefits. With her current employer, there is no opportunity for promotion, and raises are small and infrequent. She has two very specific goals for the future. One, she wants to continue working in health education/promotion, but she is open to working in any setting. Two, she wants to earn a higher salary and have better benefits. If you were advising Marla, identify options you could suggest. What things could she do to make herself more marketable? What additional education or professional development does she need? What does she need to do in terms of networking? What types of positions and settings should she be considering? Outline a plan for Marla in the next 12 months that will help her to realize the two goals she has established.

## CRITICAL THINKING QUESTIONS

1. Select any health education/promotion setting and give specific examples of how a health education specialist working in that setting would need to utilize all seven responsibilities of a health education specialist (i.e., when thinking about assessment at the worksite setting, a health education specialist might have to assess the health needs of employees, assess the current health behaviors of employees, assess how responsive employees would be to a given health promotion program, assess upper management support for a given program, etc.).

2. If you were in a position to hire a new health education specialist, what qualities, traits, and experiences would you look for in making your hiring decision? Compare this with the qualities, traits, and experiences you currently possess. Make a list of things you could do to enhance your marketability prior to graduation.

## ACTIVITIES

1. Select the one setting you think you would most like to work in. Develop a short essay describing why you prefer this setting to other health education/promotion settings and what you think you will need to do to land a job in that setting.

2. Visit a health education/promotion professional who works in the setting in which you would most like to be employed. Develop a job description for this person's position that explains the qualifications and responsibilities needed for the job.

3. Examine the classified ads of a major-city Sunday newspaper. Circle in red those jobs you find that specifically ask for a health education specialist. Next, look through the same classified ads and circle in blue those that do not ask for a health education specialist but require competencies and skills similar to those of a health education specialist.

4. Interview someone who is responsible for hiring health education specialists. Find out what that person looks for in a letter of application, a vita, and a personal interview.

5. Contact the placement office at your institution. Determine what services it offers and when these services should be accessed.

## WEBLINKS

1. http://www.bls.gov

   U.S. Bureau of Labor Statistics

   Go to this Web site and run a search for "health education specialists." Review the various documents you find to determine workforce size, average salaries, states with most health education specialists employed, states with highest average salaries, metropolitan areas with highest average salaries, and other important information about health education specialists.

2. http://www.peacecorps.gov/index.cfm

   Peace Corps

   This Web site provides information about the Peace Corps, what volunteers do, where the Peace Corps is active, benefits of Peace Corps service, how to become a Peace Corps volunteer, and much more.

3. http://www.welcoa.org/freeresources/index.php?category=8

   Wellness Council of America

   This page indexes a number of free worksite health promotion resources that are available and can be easily downloaded in PDF format.

4. http://www.cdc.gov/nccdphp/dnpao/hwi/programdesign//index.htm

   Centers for Disease Control and Prevention's Healthier Worksite Initiative

   This page provides access to a number of resources to help one plan, implement, and evaluate worksite wellness programs.

5. **http://www.csuchico.edu/cjhp/5/2/index.htm**

   California State University, Chico

   This is the URL for Volume 5, Issue 2 of the *Californian Journal of Health Promotion*. Once there, go to the article written by Byrd, Hoke, and Gottlieb titled "Integrating Health Education into Clinical Settings." This is an excellent article that describes a successful use of health education specialists in a clinical setting.

6. **http://www.csuchico.edu/cjhp/2/1/index.htm**

   California State University, Chico

   This is the URL for Volume 2, Issue 1 of the *Californian Journal of Health Promotion*. Once there, go to the article by Eleanor Dixon Terry titled "Attending Professional Health Education Meetings: What's In It for the Student and New Professional." Click on the page numbers to download the article in an Adobe Acrobat format. This is an excellent article with good advice for students or new professionals attending their first professional health education/promotion meeting.

7. **http://www.acha.org/Publications/Guidelines_WhitePapers.cfm**

   *American College Health Association*

   Once at this website, click on the button to download the PDF document titled "Guidelines for Hiring Health Promotion Professionals in Higher Education." Compare yourself against the guidelines and recommendations presented in this document. While this document was designed specifically for health education specialists working in college or university wellness programs, many of these guidelines and recommendations would be appropriate for employers in other settings.

## REFERENCES

Allensworth, D., & Kolbe, L. (1987). The comprehensive school health program: Exploring an expanded concept. *Journal of School Health, 57,* 409–412.

American College of Sports Medicine. (2003). *ACSM's worksite health promotion manual.* Champaign, IL: Human Kinetics.

American School Health Association. (2010). What is school health? Retrieved September 6, 2010, from http://www.ashaweb.org/i4a/pages/index.cfm?pageid=3278

Association of Schools of Public Health (2010). Careers in public health. Retrieved September 6, 2007, from http://www.whatispublichealth.org/careers/index.html

Breckon, J., Harvey, J. R., & Lancaster, R. B. (1998). *Community health education: Settings, roles, and skills for the 21st century.* Gaithersburg, MD: Aspen Publishers, Inc.

Byrd, T. L., Hoke, M. M., & Gottlieb, N. H. (2007). Integrating health education into clinical settings. *California Journal of Health Promotion, 5* (2): 18–28.

Centers for Disease Control and Prevention (CDC). (2010a). *About Us: Division of Adolescent and School Health.* Retrieved August 31, 2010 from: http://www.cdc.gov/HealthyYouth/about/index.htm

Centers for Disease Control and Prevention (CDC). (2010b). *Coordinated school health program.* Retrieved September 6, 2010, from http://www.cdc.gov/HealthyYouth/CSHP/

Centers for Disease Control and Prevention (CDC). (n.d.). *Career opportunities in global health.* Retrieved September 12, 2009, from http://www.cdc.gov/search.do?action=search&queryText=Career+Opportunities+in+Global+Health&x=0&y=0

Chapman, L. S. (2006). Fundamentals of worksite wellness. *Absolute Advantage, 5* (4), 3–23.

Chenoweth, D. H. (2007). *Worksite health promotion.* 2nd ed. Champaign, IL: Human Kinetics.

Cleary, M. J., & Birch, D. A. (1996). Using portfolios for assessment in the college personal health course. *Journal of Health Education, 27* (2), 92–96.

Cleary, M. J., & Birch, D. A. (1997). How prospective school health education specialists can build a portfolio to communicate professional expertise. *Journal of School Health, 67* (6), 228–231.

Cleary, M. J., Kaiser-Drobney, A. E., Ubbes, V. E., Stuhldreher, W. L., & Birch, D. A. (1998). Service learning in the "third sector": Implications for professional preparation. *Journal of Health Education, 29* (5), 304–311.

Daitz, S. J. (2007). Health education careers at nonprofit voluntary health agencies. *Health Education Monograph, 24* (1), 4–6.

Dixon-Terry, E. (2004). Attending professional health education meetings: What's in it for the student and new professional? *California Journal of Health Promotion, 2* (1), 16–21.

Dolan, P. L. (2009). Social media behavior could threaten your reputation, job prospects. *AMNews.* Retrieved October 13, 2009, from http://www.ama-assn.org/amednews/2009/10/12/bil21012.htm

English, G. M., & Videto, D. M. (1997). The future of health education: The knowledge to practice paradox. *Journal of Health Education, 28* (1), 4–7.

Fisher, C., Hunt, P., Kann, L., Kolbe, L., Patterson, B., & Wechsler, H. (2003). Building a healthier future through school health programs. In *Promising practices in chronic disease prevention and control: A public health framework for action.* Atlanta: Department of Health and Human Services.

Floyd, P. A., & Allen, B. J. (2004). *Careers in health, physical education and sport.* Belmont, CA: Wadsworth-Thompson Learning, Inc.

Hall, J. Y. (2007). Entering and navigating a health education career in the local public sector. *The Health Education Monograph, 24* (1), 15–17.

Hayden, J. (2007). A health education career in higher education. *The Health Education Monograph, 24* (1), 23–28.

Howze, E. H. (2007). Health education jobs in the federal government. *The Health Education Monograph, 24* (1), 11–14.

Jalloh, M. G. (2007). Health education careers in schools. *The Health Education Monograph, 24* (1), 18–22.

Joint Committee on Health Education and Promotion Terminology. (2001). Report of the 2000 Joint Committee on Health Education and Promotion Terminology. *American Journal of Health Education, 32* (2), 89–104.

Joint Committee on National Health Education Standards. (2007). *National Health Education Standards: Achieving Excellence.* 2nd ed. Atlanta: American Cancer Society.

Kaiser Family Foundation. (2010). *U.S. health care costs: Background brief.* Retrieved September 11, 2010, from http://www.kaiseredu.org/topics_im.asp?imID=1&parentID=61&id=358

McKenzie, J. F., Cleary, M. J., McKenzie, B. L., & Stephen, C. E. (2002). E-portfolios: Their creation and use by pre-service health education specialists. *International Electronic Journal of Health Education, 55,* 79–83.

McKenzie, J. F., Neiger, B. L., & Thackeray, R. (2009). *Planning, implementing, & evaluating health promotion programs.* 5th ed. San Francisco: Pearson Benjamin Cummings.

McKenzie, J. F., Pinger, R. R., & Kotecki, J. E. (2008). *An introduction to community health.* Boston: Jones & Bartlett.

Miller, B., Birch, D., & Cottrell, R. R. (2010). Current status and future plans for undergraduate public/community health education program accreditation. *American Journal of Health Education, 41* (5), 301–307.

Naidoo, J., & Wills, J. (2000). *Health promotion: Foundations for practice.* 2nd ed. Edinburgh, Scotland: Bailliere Tindall.

National Commission for Health Education Credentialing. (2010). *Health education profession.* Retrieved September 6, 2010, from http://nchec.org/credentialing/profession/

Peabody, K. L., & Linnan, L. A. (2007). Careers in worksite health promotion. *The Health Education Monograph, 24* (1), 29–32.

Peace Corps. (2010). *Peace Corps: What are the benefits?* Retrieved September 11, 2010, from http://www.peacecorps.gov/index.cfm?shell=learn.whyvol.finben

Rubleski, J. (2007). Embracing workplace wellness. *Absolute Advantage, 6* (5), 30–33.

Society for Public Health Education (SOPHE). (2010). *What does health care reform do for prevention and wellness?* Retrieved September 5, 2010, from http://www.sophe.org/advocacy_matters.cfm

Thompson, S. E., & Bybee, R. F. (2004). Professional portfolios for health education specialists and other allied health professionals. *California Journal of Health Promotion, 2* (1), 52–55.

Totzkay-Sitar, C., & Cornett, S. (2007). Health education options in health and medical care. *The Health Education Monograph, 24* (1), 7–10.

U.S. Department of Health and Human Services. (2000a). *Healthy People 2010: Introduction.* Retrieved September 9, 2010, from http://www.healthypeople.gov/document/html/uih/uih_1.htm

U.S. Department of Health and Human Services. (2000b). *Healthy People 2010* (Conference Edition, in Two Volumes). Washington, DC.

U.S. Department of Health and Human Services. (September 2003). *Prevention makes common "cents."* Retrieved September 11, 2010, from http://aspe.hhs.gov/health/prevention/

U.S. Department of Labor Bureau of Labor Statistics. (2010a). *Occupational Outlook Handbook, 2010–2011 Edition.* Retrieved September 12, 2010, from http://www.bls.gov/oco/ocos063.htm#projections_data

U.S. Department of Labor Bureau of Labor Statistics. (2010b). *Occupational Employment and Wages—May 2009.* Retrieved September 6, 2010, from http://www.bls.gov/oes/

Wellness Council of America. (2006). Planning wellness: Getting off to a good start—part 1. *Absolute Advantage, 5* (4). Retrieved September 11, 2010, from http://www.welcoa.org/freeresources/index.php?category=8

# Agencies/Associations/Organizations Associated with Health Education/Promotion

## CHAPTER OBJECTIVES

After reading this chapter and answering the questions at the end, you should be able to:

- Define each of the following terms and give several examples of each: *governmental health agency, quasi-governmental health agency, nongovernmental health agency.*
- Briefly describe the levels of governmental agencies and provide several examples of each.
- List and explain the four primary activities of most voluntary health agencies.
- Explain the purpose of a professional association/organization.
- Identify the benefits derived from membership in a professional organization.
- Identify the primary professional associations/organizations and coalitions associated with health education/promotion.
- Describe the process by which a person can become a member of a professional association/organization.
- Describe what the National Commission for Health Education Credentialing, Inc. is and briefly describe its mission and purpose.

There are many health agencies, associations, and organizations with which health education specialists interact. Most of these agencies/associations/organizations were created to help promote, protect, and maintain the health of individuals, families, and communities. For many health education specialists, these agencies/associations/organizations will be places of employment. These groups regularly hire health education specialists to plan, implement, evaluate, and coordinate their educational efforts. Health education specialists not employed by these groups will find them to be valuable sources of up-to-date information and materials. This chapter classifies the agencies/associations/organizations into three major categories: governmental, quasi-governmental, and nongovernmental. Because information on most of these agencies/associations/organizations that support the efforts of health education/promotion is available elsewhere (e.g., McKenzie, Pinger, & Kotecki, 2012) and because this text was written primarily as an introduction to the profession, the primary emphasis of this chapter is on the professional health education associations/organizations.

## Governmental Health Agencies

**Governmental health agencies** are health agencies that have authority for certain duties or tasks outlined by the governmental bodies that oversee them. For example, a **local health department** has the authority to protect, promote, and enhance the health of people living in a specific geographical area. It is given this authority by the county, city, or township government that oversees it. Governmental agencies, which are primarily funded by tax dollars (they may also charge fees for services rendered) and managed by government employees, exist at four governmental levels: international, national, state, and local (city and county). **Table 8.1** provides examples of governmental agencies and their governing bodies.

## Quasi-Governmental Health Agencies

**Quasi-governmental health agencies** (see **Figure 8.1**) are so named because they possess characteristics of both governmental health agencies, and of nongovernmental agencies. They obtain their funding from a variety of sources, including community fund-raising efforts such as the United Way, special allocations from government bodies, fees for services rendered, and donations. They carry out tasks that are often thought of as services of governmental agencies, yet they operate independently of governmental supervision.

Probably the best known quasi-governmental health agency is the **American Red Cross (ARC)**. It was founded in 1881 by Clara Barton as an outgrowth of her work during the Civil War. Today, the ARC has several "official" responsibilities given to it by the federal government, such as providing relief to victims of natural disasters (Disaster Services) and serving as the liaison between members of the active armed forces and their families during family emergencies (Services to the Armed Forces and Veterans). The ARC also provides many nongovernmental services such as its blood drives and safety services classes such as water safety, first aid, and CPR.

**Table 8.1**    Governmental agencies and their governing bodies

| Level/Agency | Governing Body |
| --- | --- |
| **International Level** | |
| World Health Organization (WHO) | United Nations (UN) |
| Pan American Health Organization (PAHO) | An independent agency |
| **National Level** | |
| Centers for Disease Control and Prevention (CDC) | U.S. government, Department of Health and Human Services (HHS) |
| Food and Drug Administration (FDA) | U.S. government, Department of Health and Human Services (HHS) |
| **State Level** | |
| State health department | Individual state governments |
| State environmental protection agency | Individual state governments |
| **Local Level** | |
| Local health department (LHD) | City, county, or township governments |
| Local school district | Local school boards |

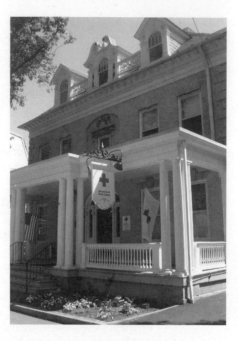

**Figure 8.1** The American Red Cross is one of the best examples of a quasi-governmental agency.
(James F. McKenzie)

## Nongovernmental Health Agencies

**Nongovernmental health agencies** operate, for the most part, free from governmental interference as long as they comply with the Internal Revenue Service's guidelines for their tax status (McKenzie et al., 2012). They are primarily funded by private donations, or, as is the case with professional and service groups, membership fees. The nongovernmental agencies can be categorized into the following subgroups: voluntary, philanthropic, service, religious, and professional.

### Voluntary Health Agencies

**Voluntary health agencies** (see **Figure 8.2**) are some of the most visible health agencies in a community. Voluntary health agencies are an American creation and grew out of unmet needs in communities. When governmental or quasi-governmental agencies were not in place to meet the needs of communities, interested citizens came together to form voluntary agencies. Such was the case with the American Cancer Society, the American Heart Association, the American Lung Association, the Alzheimer's Association, and the First Candle (formerly SIDS Alliance). The number of voluntary agencies seems endless, with agencies for about every disease and part of the body impacted by a disease or an illness. Most voluntary agencies have four primary purposes: (1) raise money to fund research and their programs, (2) provide education to both professionals and the public, (3) provide service to individuals and families affected by the disease or health problem, and (4) to advocate for beneficial policies, laws, and regulations that impact the work of the agency and in turn the people it is trying to help. Some of these organizations obtain their money from community fund-raising efforts like the United Way, but most raise their money through writing successful grant proposals, carrying out specific special

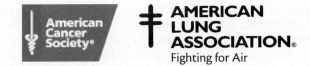

**Figure 8.2** Two of the largest voluntary health agencies are the American Cancer Society and the American Lung Association.

(The American Cancer Society logo is reprinted by permission of the American Cancer Society. Logo of the American Lung Association, courtesy of the American Lung Association).

events (i.e., dance-athons, golf outings), conducting door-to-door solicitation or direct mail campaigns, and other means of receiving donations.

## Philanthropic Foundations

**Philanthropic foundations** play an important role by funding programs and research on the prevention, control, and treatment of diseases and other health problems. *Philanthropy* means "altruistic concern for human welfare and advancement, usually manifested by donations of money, property, or work to needy persons, by endowment of institutions of learning and hospitals, and by generosity to other socially useful purposes" (Random House, 2010, ¶ 1). Philanthropic foundations differ from voluntary health agencies in two primary ways, but many will accept charitable contributions. First, they were created with an endowment and, thus, do not have to raise money. Second, they are able to finance long-term projects that may be too expensive or risky to be funded by other agencies. Examples of some philanthropic foundations that have supported work by health education specialists are the Ford Foundation, the Robert Wood Johnson Foundation, and the Rockefeller Foundation.

## Service, Fraternal, and Religious Groups

Many different service, fraternal, and religious groups have also been important to health education specialists. Even though none of these groups has the primary purpose of enhancing the health of a community, they often get involved in health-related projects. It is not uncommon for health education specialists to interact with these groups as part of community coalitions or when they are seeking resources to fund or enhance their programs. Examples of service and fraternal groups (and their health-related projects) include the Fraternal Order of the Police (food and clothing donations for the needy), Lions (Lions Quest and preservation of sight), Shriners (children's hospitals), and American Legion (community recreation programs).

Religious groups have also contributed to the work of health education specialists' projects, both on a global level (e.g., the Protestants' One Great Hour of Sharing, the Catholics' Relief Fund, and the United Jewish Appeal) and on a local level (e.g., food pantries, sleeping rooms, soup kitchens).

## Professional Health Associations/Organizations

As noted at the beginning of this chapter, the primary focus of this chapter is the professional health associations/organizations. The mission of **professional health associations/ organizations** is to promote the high standards of professional practice for their respective profession, thereby improving the health of society by improving the people in the profession (McKenzie et al., 2012). The mission is carried out by advocating for the profession; keeping the members up-to-date via the publication of professional journals, books, and newsletters; and providing the members with an avenue to come together at professional meetings. At these meetings, members have the opportunity to share and hear the new research findings, network with fellow professionals, and find out more about the latest equipment and published materials in the field. In addition, professional associations/organizations provide their members with benefits such as reduced rates on various types of insurance, participation in tax-deferred annuity programs, discounts (annual national conventions, car rental, eye wear, long-distance telephone calls, publications, travel), job placement, and a variety of other associated items (see **Box 8.1**).

---

**Box 8.1**    BENEFITS OF JOINING A PROFESSIONAL ASSOCIATION/ORGANIZATION AS A STUDENT MEMBER

- Opportunity to interact, collaborate, and network with other professionals in the profession
- Opportunity to meet and interact with health education/promotion students and faculty from other colleges and universities
- Develop professional colleagues
- Have a professional identity
- Professional guidance and mentoring
- Leadership development
- Learn more about how the profession and the association/organization operate
- Keep up to date on happenings in the profession and new health information
- Opportunity to participate in the association's/organization's electronic listserv, e-newsletters, Web chats, Webinars, and e-learning communities
- Advocacy alerts and updates
- Opportunity to grow professionally and personally while being supported and encouraged by others
- Be exposed to current research and pedagogy of the profession through meeting attendance and reading the publications of the association/organization
- Make professional contacts for future practicums, internships, or jobs
- Get connected to job banks
- Opportunity to make a presentation at a professional meeting
- Opportunity to serve the profession through an association/organization
- Discounted registration fees for professional meetings and publications
- If certified, opportunity to earn continuing education contact hours (CECHs) for recertification of the Certified Health Education Specialist and Master Health Education Specialist credentials and other licensures

*Source:* Adapted from Society for Public Health Education, Inc. and from Young & Boling (2004).

Professional associations/organizations are member driven and composed, for the most part, of professionals who have completed specialized education and training and who are eligible for certification/licensure in their respective professions. These associations/organizations are funded primarily by membership dues, but it is becoming more common for these associations/organizations to seek grant funds (*soft money*) to help promote their missions. Most of these associations/organizations hire staff for day-to-day operations, but the officers of the associations/organizations are usually elected professionals.

In the remaining portions of this chapter, we present information on the national professional associations/organizations that help promote the health education/promotion profession. The reader should also be aware that many of these national associations/organizations have affiliates and other related groups at the regional and/or state level. For example, the American Public Health Association is a national organization, but there are also state associations such as the Ohio Public Health Association, or the Indiana Public Health Association. In addition, there are also some state-only organizations that are not affiliated with any national organization. (Ask your instructor if there are any such organizations in your state.) Often it is these regional or state affiliates/organizations that health education/promotion students become members of first because of their proximity to campus, opportunities to get involved in the professional organization, less expensive membership dues, and local networking benefits. **Table 8.2** and Appendix C contain information about the following organizations.

**Table 8.2**   Information about key professional associations/organizations

**The American Academy of Health Behavior**
*Address*:
17 Indian Creek Drive
Rudolph, OH 43462
Telephone and Facsimile: 419/760-6020
*Internet*: http://www.aahb.org

**American Alliance for Health, Physical Education, Recreation and Dance (AAHPERD)**
*Address*:
1900 Association Drive
Reston, VA 20191-1598
*Telephone*: 800/213-7193; 703/476-3400
*Facsimile*: 703/476-9527
*Internet*: http://www.aahperd.org/index.cfm

**American Association for Health Education (AAHE)**
*Address*:
1900 Association Drive
Reston, VA 20191
*Telephone*: 800/213-7193 and 703/476-3437
*Facsimile*: 703/476-6638
*Internet*: http://www.aahperd.org/aahe

**Table 8.2**    (*continued*)

**American College Health Association (ACHA)**
*Address*:
891 Elkridge Landing Road, Suite 100
Linthicum, MD 21090
*Telephone*: 410/859-1500
*Facsimile*: 410/859-1510
*Internet*: http://www.acha.org

**American Public Health Association (APHA)**
*Address*:
800 I Street, NW
Washington, DC 20001
*Telephone*: 202/777-APHA (2742); 202/777-2500 (TTY)
*Facsimile*: 202/777-2534
*Internet*: http://www.apha.org

**American School Health Association (ASHA)**
*Address*:
4340 East West Highway, Suite 403
Bethesda, MD 20814
*Telephone*: 301/652-8072
*Facsimile*: 301/652-8077
*Internet*: http://www.ashaweb.org

**Eta Sigma Gamma (ESG)**
*Address*:
2000 University Avenue
Muncie, IN 47306
*Telephone*: 800/715-2559; 765/285-2258
*Facsimile*: 765/285-3210
*Internet*: http://www.etasigmagamma.org

**International Union for Health Promotion and Education (IUHPE)**
*Address*:
42 Boulevard de la Libération
93103 Saint-Denis Cedex, France
*Telephone*: 33 1 48 13 71 20
*Facsimile*: 33 1 48 09 17 67
*Internet*: http://www.iuhpe.org

**Society for Public Health Education, Inc. (SOPHE)**
*Address*:
10 G Street, NE, Suite 605
Washington, DC 20002
*Telephone*: 202/408-9804
*Facsimile*: 202/408-9815
*Internet*: http://www.sophe.org

**Table 8.2**    (*continued*)

| **National Wellness Institute, Inc. (NWI)** |
| --- |
| *Address*: |
| 1300 College Court |
| PO Box 827 |
| Stevens Point, WI 54481 |
| *Telephone*: 715/342-2969 |
| *Facsimile*: 715/342-2979 |
| *Internet*: http://www.nationalwellness.org |

**The American Alliance for Health, Physical Education, Recreation and Dance**    The American Alliance for Health, Physical Education, Recreation and Dance (**AAHPERD**) is an alliance of five national associations (American Association for Physical Activity and Recreation [AAPAR], American Association for Health Education [AAHE], National Association for Girls and Women in Sport [NAGWS], National Association for Sport and Physical Education [NASPE], National Dance Association [NDA]), six district associations (Central, Eastern, Midwest, Northwest, Southern, and Southwest), and a research consortium. (Note that the district associations comprise AAHPERD members located in the states represented by these parts of the country. Also, states have an affiliate organization of AAHPERD—for example, the Ohio Association of Health, Physical Education, Recreation and Dance. A professional can be a member of both the state and national organizations, or just one or the other.) AAHPERD is several generations of professional organizations removed from its beginning in 1885, when "Dr. William G. Anderson invited a small group of professionals to meet with him to discuss mutual interests and concerns related to physical training. The purposes of the embryo association, resulting from this meeting, were simply stated: to disseminate knowledge, to improve methods, and to bring those interested in the subject into close relationship with each other" (Anderson, 1985, p. 94). The association continued to grow and turned into the American Physical Education Association (APEA) in 1937. In that year, the APEA "accepted an invitation from the National Education Association (NEA) to merge with its School Health and Physical Education Department to become an NEA Department with three divisions: health, physical education, and recreation" (Anderson, 1985, p. 1). The merger resulted in the formation of the American Association for Health and Physical Education. The word *recreation* was added to the title in 1938, creating AAHPER. In the mid-1960s, the NEA began to feel pressure, because of a challenge from the American Federation of Teachers, to become more active in the welfare movement for teachers. This challenge made the NEA look more closely at its focus. It was supporting thirty departments that had members of their own, most of which were not members of the NEA (Anderson, 1985). In 1968, the NEA changed its "bylaws regarding their departments: to remain a department, all its members had to join the NEA: one alternative was to become an affiliated organization, still identified with NEA and paying a small fee for rent and services; another choice was to become an autonomous associated organization paying the full costs of services rendered by NEA" (Anderson, 1985, p. 95). In 1968, AAHPER chose the former. "This status continued until September 1, 1975, when another NEA bylaws change discontinued this affiliated relationship and AAHPER became completely disassociated from NEA" (Anderson, 1985, p. 95). AAHPER added *dance* to its title in 1979 (Anderson, 1985).

Though all the associations in AAHPERD are associated with the promotion of healthy lifestyles, the one most directly related to the discipline of health education is the American Association for Health Education. Therefore, it will be the only one discussed here.

The **American Association for Health Education (AAHE)** is a new name (since July 1, 1996) for an older organization, the Association for the Advancement of Health Education (also AAHE). The Association for the Advancement of Health Education evolved from the School Health Division of AAHPER when the AAHPER was reorganized in 1973 (Nolte, 1985). Membership in AAHE is open to current, retired, and student (preparing for careers as) health education specialists and health promotion specialists regardless of their work setting. Current membership is at approximately 6,500 members. The mission of AAHE is to advance "the profession by serving health educators and other professionals who strive to promote the health of all people through education and other systematic changes" (AAHE, 2010a, slide 3).

The AAHE produces several publications that health education specialists find very useful. AAHE has two *peer-reviewed journals* (a journal in which other professionals in the field decide what is published and what is not). The *American Journal of Health Education (AJHE)* is a bimonthly publication that is available in both print and online versions. Most of the articles published in the *AJHE* are research articles, but the journal also publishes commentaries, and has a special column for community, care setting, and worksite initiatives. Two of the articles in each issue are designated as continuing education articles, so Certified Health Education Specialists and Master Certified Health Education Specialists can earn Category I credits toward recertification by reading and answering questions about the articles. The second AAHE journal is *The International Electronic Journal of Health Education (IEJHE)*. It was first available in 1997 and was the first Web-based peer-reviewed journal for health education, promotion, and behavior. The *IEJHE* provides a complete text of articles ranging from research to theory-based manuscripts. In addition, the *IEJHE* maintains a series of interviews with legends from the profession. AAHE also provides an e-newsletter called *InfoSource*. It is distributed twice a month and contains information on upcoming meetings, new releases from various organizations and agencies, information on new research findings and surveys, and much more (AAHE 2010c, ¶ 5).

In recent years, AAHE has been involved in several activities of note:

- The American Association for Health Education offers four networking communities that focus on communicating and creating relationships with individuals in the health education/promotion profession (AAHE, 2010b). The networking sites include AAHE4ME (for university students majoring in health education), the Health & Wellness Teaching Community (for instructors of college-level personal health classes), AAHE on Ning (for all professional members of AAHE), and AAHE on Twitter (for all who want to follow AAHE).

- AAHE is recognized as a multiple event provider of health education continuing education contact hours (CECHs) by the National Commission for Health Education Credentialing (NCHEC). This designation allows AAHE to offer CECHs for Certified Health Education Specialists (CHES) and Master Certified Health Education Specialists (MCHES) through the *American Journal of Health Education* and other special publications, and for participation in the annual AAHPERD/AAHE National Convention.

- The SOPHE/AAHE Baccalaureate Program Approval Committee (SABPAC) is a joint committee of SOPHE and AAHE responsible for directing the SAPBAC

Program Approval process, which is a voluntary credential for undergraduate professional programs in community health education.

- AAHE has been an active partner with three other professional associations and the American Cancer Society in the creation of the *National Health Education Standards* (ACS, 2007). The standards were developed to assist in the creation of health-enhancing behaviors in children in all grades—pre-K through grade 12. Now in their second edition, the standards are used to guide school health curriculum development.

- The National Council for Accreditation of Teacher Education (NCATE) has allowed AAHE to be the professional health education association/organization responsible for reviewing folios submitted to NCATE by colleges and universities when they are seeking NCATE accreditation for their teacher education programs.

**American Public Health Association**   The **American Public Health Association (APHA)** "is the oldest, largest, and most diverse organization of public health professionals in the world" (APHA, 2010a, ¶ 1). The APHA was founded in 1872 "as a result of the public health movement to combat yellow fever and other diseases in the 1870s" (APHA, n.d., p. 3). The mission of APHA is to "improve the health of the public and achieve equity in health status" (APHA, 2010a, ¶ 7). The Association works toward this mission by providing public health leadership and collaborating "with partners to convene constituencies; champion prevention; promote evidence-based policy and practice, and advocate for healthy people and communities" (APHA, 2010a, ¶ 7).

Membership in the APHA is open to professional, student/trainee, and retired health workers, as well as consumers who are interested in supporting the mission of the association. Currently, the more than 50,000 members come from over 50 occupations in public health. Once individuals become members, they have the opportunity to select one or more of the subgroups of the organization—called Sections and Special Primary Interest Groups (SPIGs). The basic organization unit of the APHA is the Sections. The 27 Sections "represent major public health disciplines or public health programs. These sections are designed to allow members with shared interests to come together to develop scientific program content, policy papers in their areas of interest or fields of practice, provide for professional and social networking, career development and mentoring" (APHA, 2010b, ¶ 1). SPIGs are open groups "of self-selected APHA members sharing a common occupational discipline or program area interest and electing no primary Section affiliation" (APHA, 2010b, ¶ 2). More specifically, these subgroups propose policy statements, advise on publications, provide testimony and reports, help develop the content and structure of annual meetings, and assist in APHA governance (APHA, n.d.). The sections most closely related to health education are (1) Public Health Education Section, which formed in 1922 and in 1991 changed its name to Public Health Education and Health Promotion Section, and (2) School Health Education Section, which formed in 1942 and in 1980 changed its name to School Health Education and Services Section. The Public Health Education and Health Promotion section "promotes the advancement of the health promotion and education profession and provides a forum for public health educators and those involved in health promotion activities to discuss ideas, research, and training; promotes activities related to training public health professionals" (APHA, 2010b, ¶ 1), whereas the School Health Education and Services section "focuses on development and improvement of health services, health education programs, and environmental conditions in schools, colleges, and early childhood care settings; advances public health in all school settings" (APHA, 2010b, ¶ 1).

The primary publication of APHA is the *American Journal of Public Health (AJPH)*. This peer-reviewed journal is published monthly. A typical issue of the *AJPH* includes editorials, commentaries, book reviews, job announcements, notification of upcoming meetings, and authoritative articles in both general and specialized areas of research, policy analysis, and program evaluation of public health. Areas covered in the articles include the environment, maternal and child health, health promotion, epidemiology, administration, occupational health, education, international health, statistics, and more. The association also publishes *The Nation's Health* ten times per year. This newspaper includes reporting on current and proposed legislation, policy issues, news of actions within the federal agencies and Congress, and special features. The publication also includes association news, job openings, and information on upcoming conferences. In addition to the *AJPH* and *The Nation's Health*, the APHA also publishes books and other media on a variety of public health topics. Examples include the best-selling titles *Control of Communicable Disease Manual* (Heymann, 2009) and *Case Studies in Public Health Practice* (Coughlin, 2010). The most recent addition to the APHA's publications is its online newsletter called *Inside Public Health*. This "e-newsletter communicates important activities and announcements to Association members" (APHA, 2010c, ¶ 8).

There are other professional health associations that have a more focused mission. Some of those include the American College Health Association (ACHA), the American School Health Association (ASHA) (see **Figure 8.3**), the National Wellness Institute,

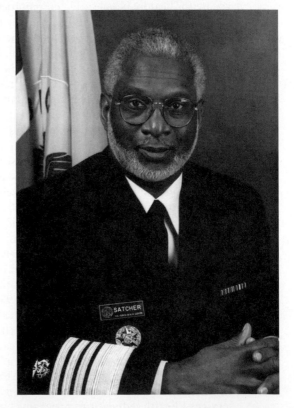

**Figure 8.3** David Satcher, MD, PhD, who was a former Surgeon General, Director for the Centers for Disease Control and Prevention, and Administrator of the Agency for Toxic Substances and Disease Registry, addressed the membership of the ASHA in 2010. Annual professional conventions are an important benefit of membership in a professional organization.

*Source:* U.S. Public Health Service

Inc. (NWI), the Society for Public Health Education, Inc. (SOPHE), and the American Academy of Health Behavior.

**American College Health Association**   The **American College Health Association (ACHA)** was founded originally as the American Student Health Association in 1920. In 1948, the name of the association was changed to its current name. ACHA's mission is to "provide advocacy, education, communications, products, and services, as well as promote research and culturally competent practices to enhance its members' ability to advance the health of all students and the campus community" (ACHA, 2010a, ¶ 1). The association has three distinct types of memberships. One is for institutions of higher education. Currently, there are more than 900 such members. ACHA also serves more than 2,800 individual members who are interested in college health—that is, the health of college students. Included in the members are administrators, physicians and physicians' assistants, nurses and nurse practitioners, health education specialists, pharmacists, dentists, support staff who care for this special group of young adults, and students who are dedicated to health promotion on their campus. Most of these individual members are associated with the health service facilities on their respective campuses. The third type of membership is called sustaining members. This group is made up of nonprofit and for-profit associations, organizations, and corporations that are interested in being more connected with the college health field (ACHA, 2010b).

Like some of the other associations/organizations, the ACHA also has subgroups. "ACHA is divided into 11 regional affiliate organizations. Each affiliate organization is governed by its own elected affiliate officers, who provide guidance and leadership to members and help forge strong partnerships with colleagues on the state or regional level. ACHA members receive concurrent membership in the affiliate organization at no additional cost" (ACHA, 2010a, ¶ 2). In addition, ACHA has nine membership sections, which are defined by the disciplines of college health. The Health Education Section, now called the Health Promotion Section, was formed in 1958.

ACHA publishes several newsletters, numerous health information brochures, and other special publications. It has a members-only newsletter that is available online at the Association's Web site. The professional journal of the ACHA is the *Journal of American College Health*. It is published bimonthly and is the only journal devoted entirely to the health of college students. The journal publishes articles encompassing many areas of college health, "including clinical and preventive medicine, health promotion, environmental health and safety, nursing assessment, interventions, and management, pharmacy, and sports medicine. The journal regularly publishes major articles on student behaviors, mental health and healthcare policies, and includes a section for discussion of controversial issues" (ACHA, 2010c, ¶ 4).

**American School Health Association**   The **American School Health Association (ASHA)** began on October 27, 1927, as the American Association of School Physicians (see **Figure 8.4**). It began to use its current name in 1936 (ASHA, 1976). The mission of the ASHA "is to build the capacity of its members to plan, develop, coordinate, implement, evaluate, and advocate for effective school health strategies that contribute to optimal health and academic outcomes for all children and youth" (ASHA, 2010a, ¶ 1).

Membership in the association is comprised of individuals and institutions with an interest in the health and well-being of school-aged children and youth. The ASHA is a multidisciplinary organization with more than 2,000 members. Included in its membership

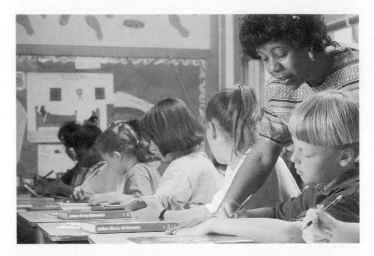

**Figure 8.4** The American School Health Association focuses on the health of the school-aged child.

(Will & Deni McIntyre/Photo Researchers)

are administrators, counselors, dentists, health education specialists, physical educators, school nurses, and school physicians who advocate for high-quality coordinated school health programs. With membership in the ASHA comes the opportunity to join subgroups of the association called sections and councils. These subgroups allow members to interact with others who have the same school health interests. Examples of a few of the councils are health behaviors, international and cross-cultural health, school health instruction and curriculum, food and nutrition education, and sexuality education.

The ASHA has several publications. They include the *Journal of School Health*, which is published ten times per year; "The Pulse," a newsletter that is published online for members and provides the latest news and analysis of the ASHA; and a variety of other resources for school health personnel. Another publication that can be ordered from the ASHA is *Tell Me About AIDS*. It is a developmentally appropriate Grades K-6 curriculum that was created to help establish a foundation for effective prevention education that begins before youth are likely to engage in risky behaviors (ASHA, 2010b).

The *Journal of School Health* is recognized widely and "is committed to communicating information regarding the role of schools and school personnel in facilitating the development and growth of healthy youth and healthy school environments. This focus on healthy youth pre-K to Grade 12 and healthy school environments encompasses a variety of areas including health education; physical education; health services; nutrition services; counseling, psychological, and social services; healthy school environment; health promotion for staff; and family/community involvement" (ASHA, 2010b, ¶ 2). The readership of the *Journal* includes administrators, educators, nurses, physicians, dentists, dental hygienists, counselors, social workers, nutritionists, dietitians, and other health professionals. These individuals work cooperatively with parents and the community to achieve the common goal of providing children and adolescents with a coordinated school health program to promote health and to improve learning.

**National Wellness Institute, Inc.**   The **National Wellness Institute (NWI)**, founded in 1977, "was formed to realize the mission of providing health promotion and wellness professionals unparalleled resources and services that promote professional and personal growth" (NWI, 2010a). The mission of NWI "is to serve the professionals and organizations that promote optimal health and wellness in individuals and communities" (NWI, 2010b, ¶ 2). The mission is accomplished by:

- Identifying quality resources
- Providing quality continuing education and resources
- Promoting opportunities for life-long learning
- Providing new and innovative professional development programs
- Developing effective educational lifestyle assessments
- Serving professionals and organizations that promote health and wellness (NWI, 2010b, ¶ 2).

There are two types of membership in NWI, individual and organizational. The organizational membership is for entities like corporations or institutions such as colleges and universities. Within the individual membership category, one can have a student, core, or core plus membership. With membership comes a number of publications. They include four online publications: *Ask The Experts,* a bimonthly publication that answers NWI member questions on a preselected topic; *Wellness Management,* a quarterly newsletter that includes information about successful programs, programming tips, resources, research, events, career opportunities, professional development, and more; *Wellness News You Can Use,* a collection of downloadable, reproducible consumer-oriented short articles, quotes, and flyers for use in newsletters, payroll stuffers, and promotional pieces; and *Health Promotion Practitioner,* a bimonthly newsletter published by Health Enhancement Systems that provides innovative and practical ideas in a concise, easy-to-apply style. For those who are core plus members, the peer-reviewed *American Journal of Health Promotion* is also provided bimonthly (NWI, 2010c).

One of the most visible components of the NWI is its National Wellness Conference, held each July in Stevens Point, WI. It is open to members and nonmembers alike, and is a unique conference because it is a week of immersion into a wellness experience.

**Society for Public Health Education, Inc.**   The Society of Public Health Educators (SOPHE), founded in 1950, is the only professional organization devoted exclusively to public health education and health promotion. In 1969, the organization changed its name to the **Society for Public Health Education, Inc. (SOPHE)**. The mission of the SOPHE "is to provide global leadership to the profession of health education and health promotion and to promote the health of society" (SOPHE, 2010a, ¶ 2). At the national level, SOPHE's membership includes about 4,000 professionals from throughout the United States and many foreign countries. Members work in a variety of places, including K–12 schools, universities, medical/managed care settings, corporations, voluntary health agencies, international organizations, and federal, state, and local government. There are currently twenty-one SOPHE chapters covering twenty-nine states (SOPHE, 2010a) (see **Box 8.2**). Like several of the other associations/organizations, SOPHE members have the opportunity to associate with one or more smaller working groups. In SOPHE the smaller groups are called Communities of Practice (CoP). CoPs "promote continuing

## Box 8.2 Practitioner's Perspective — Professional Association (Indiana Society for Public Health Education)

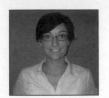

NAME: Leslie Gray, B.S., CHES

CURRENT POSITION/TITLE: Health Coach

EMPLOYER: Principal Wellness Company

DEGREE/INSTITUTION/YEAR: B.S., Ball State University, 2007

MAJOR: Health Science

(Reprinted by permission of Leslie Gray)

**Job Responsibilities:** I'm required to provide one-on-one telephonic health coaching to at-risk individuals. These individuals have completed a health screening provided by their employer. An individual would qualify for the health coaching program if one or more risks were "flagged," such as high blood pressure, blood sugar, high body mass index (BMI), or abnormal triglycerides or cholesterol levels. As a health coach, it's my responsibility to reach out to these individuals to educate, encourage, and support healthy behavior changes in the areas of exercise, nutrition, weight loss, smoking cessation, and stress management. A health coach is very similar to a sports coach, in the sense that the coach challenges, encourages, and guides the participants towards the goal of better health. During a coaching session, I will use various techniques to move a participant towards healthy changes. Some tools I use are: the Transtheoretical model, motivational interviewing techniques, up-to-date health information, and life experiences to relate and encourage healthy choices. My department also provides resources and information on various health topics we feel would be beneficial to use during coaching sessions. At the closing of a coaching session, which typically last 10–15 minutes, I schedule for a follow-up session to continue where we left off. We would continue this process until the participant has completed all of his/her coaching sessions.

**How I obtained my job:** I found this position through an online job posting using the Website www.indeed.com. I applied for two positions within the company, a Health Coach and a Health Screening Specialist. After my interviews, it was decided I would fit best as a Health Coach because I had more experience with consultations and I held the Certified Health Education Specialist (CHES) credential.

**What I like most about my job:** I love hearing from my participants that I've helped them move towards living a healthier lifestyle, whether they've made large or small changes. It's an amazing feeling to know that I can help change people for the better. I find my motivation from each and every participant. It reminds me why I do what I do and it helps keep my passion alive.

**What I like least about my job:** The least enjoyable part of my position is the ever-growing workload. Because of lower than expected sales of our wellness products and the resulting layoffs, the health coaches are carrying more work than normal. Thus, I'm seeing a higher rate of burnout and frustration among my co-workers.

**The impact of Indiana Society for Public Health Education (InSOPHE):** Currently, I'm the Communications Director for InSOPHE. I obtained my position through the nomination process and membership vote. It has been an invaluable experience for me. When I first pursued this volunteer position I felt underqualified, because I only had a year and a half of professional experience and a bachelor's degree. However, the new and former board members have been extremely welcoming and it's been a pleasure growing and developing in this position. I would highly encourage involvement as a member within this or a similar organization for several reasons—networking,

**Box 8.2 Practitioner's Perspective** **Continued**

growth and development, and continuing education opportunities. InSOPHE also offers several workshops each year at a discounted rate for members, which helps me to maintain my CHES credential. The workshops have also provided networking opportunities where I've met other health education specialists who have become my mentors. If you have extra time on your hands, I strongly encourage you to take your membership with a professional organization a step further and serve on a committee or the board. Since joining the organization and serving on the board, I have found new interests and passions for health and it has shaped me into a well-rounded health education specialist.

**Recommendations for those preparing to be health education specialists:** My internship experience paved the way to finding my current job. I completed my internship for a small health clinic where our services were contracted out to a gas and electric company in Northwest Indiana. I gained invaluable experience developing incentivized wellness programs for the employees, conducting evaluations of existing and preexisting wellness programs, assessing and analyzing biometric results from a company-wide health screening, developing and implementing individualized fitness programs, revamping all of the marketing material, helping plan and implementing a company health fair, and conducting bone density scans with one-on-one consultations about the importance of bone health.

I would also encourage you to become CHES certified. This certification opened several doors for me, professionally and personally. It has allowed me to differentiate myself from other health science graduates and confirm my ability to carry out the responsibilities of a health education specialist. It has provided me with several development and continuing education opportunities to maintain my certification as well as helped me develop my interests in the health field. I've attended workshops and training addressing sports nutrition, smoking cessation, stress management, urologic health, health literacy, health communications, and heart health.

Not only was I able to learn about specific health issues from the workshops, I also learned the importance of networking with other health education specialists with different preparation and work experiences.

---

education, networking, information exchange and advocacy among SOPHE members interested in specific topics and/or work settings. Members share a similar role or a passion about a health topic or area of practice and a desire to exchange ideas, resources, research, or solutions to common problems. In addition to networking roundtables at SOPHE Midyear and Annual Meetings, all CoPs maintain listservs throughout the year to encourage dialogue and exchange" (SOPHE, 2010b, ¶ 10).

SOPHE has four primary publications. They include two peer-reviewed journals, *Health Education and Behavior* and *Health Promotion Practice*, and two newsletters called "News & Views" and "News U Can Use." *Health Education and Behavior*, published bimonthly, is a well-respected journal that is aimed primarily at the dissemination of research findings, but a typical issue also includes perspective papers, practice notes, book reviews, and SOPHE-related information. *Health Promotion Practice* is published quarterly and is "devoted to the practical application of health promotion and education. The journal is unique in its focus on critical and strategic information for professionals engaged in the practice of developing, implementing, and evaluating health promotion and disease prevention programs" (SOPHE, 2010d, ¶ 4). "News & Views" "features spotlights on members, updates on the latest happenings in the health education profession, as well as news from SOPHE chapters, committees, and ambassadors. In an effort to 'go green,' this newsletter is posted in the Member Communities Section online six times a year. Along with its electronic posting, it is printed and delivered to National SOPHE members' homes twice a year" (SOPHE, 2010d, ¶ 2). "News U Can Use" is a weekly electronic newsletter that includes news items, new resources, funding opportunities, and job openings.

Over the years, SOPHE has had a good working relationship with the APHA. SOPHE holds its annual meeting the weekend prior to the APHA annual meeting in the same city as the APHA. Like several of the other associations/organizations, the annual meeting of SOPHE provides opportunities to share and receive the most recent research findings, to earn continuing education contact hours, to participate in its job bank service, and to network with other professionals.

In addition to the above-mentioned items, SOPHE has been involved in some other special projects. Some examples include:

- An annual health education advocacy summit at which health education specialists receive training in advocacy techniques and get to apply their new knowledge on a trip to Capitol Hill in Washington, DC, to discuss health-related issues with staffers from key legislative subcommittees and representatives of their congressional districts

- An annual mid-year scientific conference in the spring, which focuses on a topic of special interest to those in the health education/promotion disciplines

- Partnership in the SOPHE/AAHE Baccalaureate Program Approval Committee (SABPAC) (see p. 267).

- SOPHE also has taken the leadership for and partnered with a number of other organizations and agencies on several health promotion initiatives and professional development programs that are consistent with the mission and goals of SOPHE. At the time this book was written SOPHE was involved in projects dealing with injury prevention, environmental health, school health, health disparities, emergency preparedness, and accreditation of academic health education programs (SOPHE, 2010c).

**International Union for Health Promotion and Education**   Though all of the professional associations/organizations noted already in this chapter have members from countries other than the United States, there is one professional association that is truly worldwide: the **International Union for Health Promotion and Education (IUHPE)**. There are approximately 2,000 members worldwide. The IUHPE, founded in 1951 in Paris, is a global association with a mission "to promote global health and to contribute to the achievement of equity in health between and within countries of the world" (IUHPE, 2010a, ¶ 1). More specifically, the IUHPE has five major goals:

- "Greater equity in the health of populations between and within countries of the world;

- Effective alliances and partnerships to produce optimal health promotion outcomes;

- Broadly accessible evidence-based knowledge and practical experience in health promotion;

- Excellence in policy and practice for effective, quality health promotion; and

- High levels of capacity in individuals, organisations and countries to undertake health promotion activities" (IUHPE, 2010a, ¶ 1).

Because IUHPE is a worldwide organization, it is organized through eight regional offices: (Europe [IUHPE/EURO], Latin America [IUHPE/ORLA], North America [IUHPE/NARO], Northern Part of the Western Pacific [IUHPE/NPWP], Southeast Asia [IUHPE/SEARO], Southwest Pacific [IUHPE/SWP], Africa [IUHPE/AFRO], and Eastern Meditenanean [IUHPE/EMRO]). Because of the travel distance and the expense involved, the IUHPE only holds a total international conference once every three years. The most recent one was held in Geneva, Switzerland, in July 2010. The IUHPE has a "family" of journals. The official membership journal, which is published quarterly, is *Global Health Promotion* (formerly called *Promotion & Education*). "It is a multilingual journal, which publishes authoritative peer-reviewed articles and practical information for a world-wide audience of professionals interested in health promotion and health education" (IUHPE, 2010b, ¶ 2). All IUHPE members receive a print copy of *Global Health Promotion* and have access to an electronic version as well. In addition, members can purchase, at a reduced rate, any of the other six journals (*Critical Public Health, Health Promotion International, Health Education Research, International Journal of Mental Health Promotion, International Journal of Public Health,* or *International Journal of Prisoner Health*) published by IUHPE (IUHPE, 2010b).

**American Academy of Health Behavior**  The **American Academy of Health Behavior (AAHB)** is a professional organization unlike those presented so far in this chapter. Founded in 1997, the AAHB, or just *The Academy*, as it is referred to, is a society of researchers and scholars in the areas of health behavior, health education, and health promotion. *The Academy* "was created to improve the stature of health educators by supporting and promoting quality health behavior, health education, and health promotion research conducted by health educators" (Werch, 2000, p. 3). The mission of *The Academy* "is to serve as the 'research home' for health behavior scholars and researchers whose primary commitment is to excellence in research and the application of research to practice to improve the public's health" (AAHB, 2010a, ¶ 2). More specifically, *The Academy's* goals are:

"1. Establish financial solvency and security of The Academy to assure high quality and efficiency of the Academy.

2. Foster development and dissemination of knowledge through sponsorship of scientific meetings, symposia, and publications.

3. Increase member participation to improve the Academy.

4. Recognize outstanding achievements in the areas of health behavior, health education, and health promotion research.

5. Increase national/international influence of the Academy.

6. Encourage collaborative research efforts.

7. Influence health policy and allocation of resources within agencies, private foundations, and universities.

8. Foster the research career of young scholars" (AAHB, 2010a, ¶ 4).

Individuals must apply for membership in *The Academy* and acceptance is based upon one's area of academic preparation and level of scholarly activity. The specific qualifications for membership are listed on *The Academy's* Web site (see Table 8.2). The official journal of *The Academy* is the *American Journal of Health Behavior*. In a typical issue of this bimonthy publication, readers will find a number of data-based research articles along with articles on research techniques, uses of technology for research, biographical sketches of members of *The Academy*, and book reviews. In January 2010, the *American Journal of Health Behavior* changed from being published in a print format to an electronic (online) only format (AAHB, 2010b).

**Eta Sigma Gamma**   Founded in 1967, **Eta Sigma Gamma** (ESG) is the national health education honorary. The idea for the organization was born when three professors from Ball State University, Drs. William Bock, Warren E. Schaller, and Robert Synovitz, were on their way to a professional conference and were talking about the need for an honorary for the discipline. Their discussion led to the formation of the organization, which has had, from its very beginning, the primary purpose of furthering the professional competence and dedication of individual members of the health education/promotion profession (ESG, 1991). The ideals of the honorary are symbolized in its seal. The seal (see **Figure 8.5**) "is divided into four equilateral triangles, each carrying a symbol. A lamp of learning is in the center triangle, surrounded by an open book representing teaching, a microscope signifying research, and an outstretched hand representing service. These three elements form the basic purposes of the organization and profession; teaching, research, and service. The unifying element of these purposes is symbolized by the lamp of learning, since it is through the learning process that each purpose is achieved" (ESG, 1991, p. 2).

As noted in Table 8.2, the national office of Eta Sigma Gamma is located in Muncie, Indiana, on the campus of Ball State University in the Department of Physiology and Health Science. This is also where the Alpha Chapter (the first chapter of the honorary) is located. As of August 2010, there have been 123 chapters installed on university/college campuses throughout the United States (see Appendix C). Chapters are awarded to colleges/universities based on a review and vote by the National Executive Committee of Eta Sigma Gamma on an application prepared by personnel at the petitioning college/ university. From its beginnings, Eta Sigma Gamma has focused on the student members. It is while individuals are either undergraduate or graduate students that most people join the honorary. Membership is open to those who have a major or minor in health education and a grade point average equivalent to at least a *B*–. In fact, students can achieve membership only by affiliating through a collegiate chapter. Through their affiliation with the collegiate chapters they are eligible to apply for the awards and scholarships of the honorary. Professionals active in the discipline of health education/promotion and holding a degree can affiliate through the Chapter-At-Large (ESG, 1991) (see **Box 8.3**).

**Figure 8.5** Seal of Eta Sigma Gamma

*Source*: National Office of Eta Sigma Gamma, 2000 University Ave., Muncie, IN 47306. Used with permission.

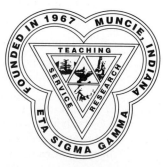

## Box 8.3 Practitioner's Perspective | Professional Association (Eta Sigma Gamma)

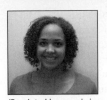

(Reprinted by permission of Janet Kamiri)

NAME: Janet Kamiri

CURRENT POSITION/TITLE: Recent graduate

EMPLOYER: N/A—job hunting

DEGREE/INSTITUTION/YEAR: B.A., Ball State University, 2010

MAJOR: School Health Education

MINOR: Oboe Performance

**Becoming a health science major:** When I started my undergraduate program, I was sure I was going to be a music teacher. I soon realized that even though I was passionate about music, it was not my professional calling. I began the search for a new major by taking career aptitude tests, talking to career counselors, and searching online for an answer. I finally asked myself, "What courses am I enrolled in that excite me? What courses have I taken that I have really enjoyed?" My favorite class in high school was health. I was currently enrolled in a personal health course at Ball State University and always found myself sharing what I learned in class with my friends. I set up an appointment to meet with a professor in the health science department to discuss options in health education. I enrolled in an introductory course for the next semester and was exposed to a variety of options in the field of health education. I decided health science would be my new major, with an emphasis on education in the school setting. I felt that this would be the ideal setting for me to help others.

**Getting involved in health education:** I wanted more from my education than just academics. I wanted to interact with people who had similar interests, develop professional relationships, make myself more marketable, and learn through real life, hands-on activities. I wanted to grow personally and professionally and make the most of my time at the university.

A few of my professors suggested that I look into joining Eta Sigma Gamma. In my first semester as a school health major, I attended meetings, interacted with the members, and participated in chapter events. I found that the students involved in Eta Sigma Gamma were serious and passionate about the field. They were actively applying their skills in a nonthreatening social environment. These students were creating a niche for themselves and a community to be a part of, which was especially beneficial at a large university where it is easy to get lost.

During my time as a student member of the Alpha Chapter of Eta Sigma Gamma, I was involved in many different projects and events on campus and in the community. On campus, we strengthened our program planning and implementation skills working on projects such as hosting an alcohol education program during *Spring Break Safety Week* and sponsoring activates during *Safer Sex Week* to educate students on safer sex practices and the importance of HIV awareness and testing. In the community, we cleaned our section of the highway through the Adopt-a-Highway organization, sponsored activities at the local Boys and Girls Club, and volunteered at a food bank. We also co-sponsored a "March for Babies" walk through the March of Dimes Foundation and hosted a breast cancer research fundraiser. These activities were not hypothetical. Rather, we were directly involved in improving peoples' health just as professional health education specialists are.

I served on the Executive Committee for the Alpha Chapter in the positions of Vice-President and President. Through these two positions, I gained valuable leadership skills, improved my organizational and planning skills, and learned how to balance details within the big picture.

## Box 8.3 Practitioner's Perspective   Continued

Being a member of Eta Sigma Gamma also opened other doors for me. I attended a national student leadership conference, which helped improve my effectiveness not only as a leader on campus, but also as a teacher in the classroom. I also applied for a travel grant through Eta Sigma Gamma. This grant helped make it possible for me and another chapter member to attend the national meeting for Eta Sigma Gamma. At the meeting, we learned what other students were doing on their campuses and in their communities and gained valuable preprofessional advice from current health education specialists.

**Completing an internship/student teaching:** As a school health major, student teaching was required. I was fortunate, however, also to complete an internship with St. Vincent Health (a hospital system in the Indianapolis, IN area). These two experiences boosted my confidence in interacting within the professional world and broadened my skill set. I was able to integrate skills and educational approaches from two different health education settings. In both roles, I collaborated with other professionals, planned and implemented instruction, and evaluated and analyzed the effectiveness and the impact of my work.

**Recommendations for those preparing to be health education specialists:** First, get involved. Opportunities for personal and professional advancement are readily available for people who are willing to go beyond their academic course work. Being involved on campus and in professional associations such as Eta Sigma Gamma allows you to apply what you learn in the classroom to practical situations and provides you with more opportunities to interact with professors and students at your university as well as with professionals and students from all over the country. Preprofessional involvement in the field increases your marketability and better prepares you for a job as a health education specialist.

Second, develop relationships with leaders in the field. Find a professor with whom you connect with and create a mentor/mentee relationship with them. Professors have a wealth of knowledge about the field, a willingness to share advice that they want to share, and connections to opportunities that can benefit you both personally and professionally. Also, do not be afraid to approach professionals at conferences, especially if their work interests or inspires you. Taking the initiative to seek out information and opportunities and to build professional relationships will only benefit you in the future.

Third, do not be afraid to stand out. Working your hardest is not only personally rewarding, but also can open many doors. Dedication and passion increase your opportunities to effect positive change and improve the lives of the people you work with.

Eta Sigma Gamma regularly produces three publications: its journal, *The Health Educator; The Health Education Monograph Series*; and "The Vision," an online newsletter. Each of these publications is distributed twice a year. Like the publications of the other associations/organizations, these publications include the current works of the professionals in the field. However, unlike the others, only individuals who are current members of Eta Sigma Gamma can write articles for *The Health Educator* and *The Health Education Monograph Series*. Another unusual characteristic of the publications of Eta Sigma Gamma is that one entire issue of the *Monograph Series* each year is composed of articles written only by student members. This is another indication that the honorary is very concerned about the preservice professional.

**Associations for Directors**   There are two other professional groups that have ties to health education. They are the (1) Directors of Health Promotion and Education and (2) Society of State Directors of Health, Physical Education, and Recreation. Unlike all the other professional groups discussed, membership in these organizations is tied to one's employment. The individuals who belong to these organizations are employees of their respective state/territorial/Indian Health Service departments of health or education. There are two types of membership available in the Directors of Health Promotion and Education (DHPE)—voting membership and associate membership. The number of DHPE voting members is limited. "Voting members are designated by the State Health Officer in each state health department. They represent the directors for health education and health promotion units and programs in state health agencies, US federal districts and territories, and the Indian Health Service areas (IHS) or their equivalent. For states, territories and IHS areas where no such designations exist, voting members shall be appointed by the state, territorial or IHS area health official" (DHPE, 2010, ¶ 1). "Associate membership is open to public health educators in state and local health departments, and community-based organizations; Indian Health Service staff; administrators and faculty of schools of public health; and health educators in other organizations" DHPE, 2010, ¶ 1). The primary functions of the **Directors of Health Promotion and Education (DHPE)**, which was formed in 1946, are to work to enhance the health education standards in public health agencies and to provide a means by which its members have an opportunity to network with one another.

This association is also an affiliate of the Association of State and Territorial Health Officials (ASTHO) which is the association for those who oversee state and territorial health departments. You can obtain more information about DHPE by contacting any state or territorial department of health, or by logging on to the DHPE Web site (see the URL for this Web site in the Web Links at the end of the chapter).

The Conference of State Directors of Health, Physical Education, and Recreation, which later changed its name to **Society of State Directors of Health, Physical Education, and Recreation (SSDHPER)**, was founded in 1926 and is "a professional association whose members supervise and coordinate programs in health, physical education, and related fields within state departments of education. Associate members are those who are interested in the goals and programs of the Society who do not work within a state education agency" (SSDHPER, 2010, ¶ 1). The mission of the SSDHPER is "to have a significant and enduring effect on the health, achievement, and life success of children and youth through school health education and physical education within a co-ordinated school health approach. The Society utilizes strategic advocacy, creative partnerships, state-of-the-art professional development, and timely identification of resources to enhance the leadership capacity of its members" (SSDHPER, 2010, ¶ 2).

You can obtain more information about SSDHPER by contacting any state department of education or the SSDHPER Web site (see the Web Links at the end of the chapter).

**Coalitions**    Because of the large number of professional health education/promotion associations, there are times when there is a need to have a common voice for the profession. To help provide such a voice, coalitions of health associations/organizations have been created. The most prominent coalition is the Coalition of National Health Education Organizations, USA.

The **Coalition of National Health Education Organizations, USA (CNHEO)** is a nonprofit federation of organizations dedicated to advancing the health education/promotion profession. It is comprised of representatives (delegates and alternates) from nine national associations/organizations that have identifiable health education specialist memberships and ongoing health education/promotion programs. The associations/organizations included are the American College Health Association, Health Education Section; the American Public Health Association, Public Health Education and Health

Promotion Section; the American Public Health Association, School Health Education and Services Section; the American School Health Association; the American Association for Health Education; Directors of Health Promotion and Education; Eta Sigma Gamma; the Society for Public Health Education, Inc.; and the Society of State Directors of Health, Physical Education, and Recreation. For many years there were only eight members of the CNHEO. The number increased to ten members with the addition of Eta Sigma Gamma in 1999 and the American Academy of Health Behavior (AAHB) in 2003. However, since that time AAHB has discontinued its membership, so currently there are nine member organizations in the coalition.

The CNHEO was formed on March 1, 1972, after a series of three meetings in 1971 and 1972 to determine the feasibility of such an organization. The primary mission of the coalition is "the mobilization of the resources of the Health Education Profession in order to expand and improve health education, regardless of the setting" (CNHEO, 2010a, ¶ 1). The work of the CNHEO is financed by funds obtained from coalition member organizations, public and private agencies, and contributions and gifts from individuals. Over the years, the working relationship of the member organizations has been outlined in the *Working Agreement of the CNHEO*. Also included in this document are the purposes of the coalition (CNHEO, 2006, ¶ 2).

1. To strengthen communications among the member organizations as well as between the health education profession and policy-makers, other professions, and consumers

2. To develop, implement, and evaluate a shared vision and strategic plan for health education and the health education profession

3. To educate policy-makers on the need for federal and state public policies that support healthy behaviors and healthy communities

4. To collaborate on common issues, problems, and concerns related to health education

5. Increase the visibility of the health education profession and its member organizations

Unlike the other organizations and groups discussed in this chapter, the CNHEO functions with no paid staff members or permanent location. "The CNHEO carries on business by means of e-mail communication, monthly conference calls, and periodic face-to-face meetings during member organization conferences. Through these means it has made significant progress in addressing its purposes and priorities" (Capwell, 2004, p. 13). Since its inception, the CNHEO has operationalized its purposes in a number of ways, contributing to the growth of the profession. Below is a list of some of the recent activities and accomplishments in which the CNHEO has been involved. (Note: Some items in this list are discussed in greater detail in other chapters of this book when they apply to the content of that chapter.)

- Creation of position papers on topics of importance to the profession, e.g., preparation of elementary school teachers in the area of health education, and the strengthening of health education in the public health arena.

- Mobilization of health education professionals seeking to add the Standard Occupation Classification (SOC) of *health educator* to the "List of Community and Social Service Occupations" by the United States Department of Labor, Bureau of Labor Statistics (USDOL, 2009) (see Chapter 2).

- Cosponsoring two invitational conferences in 1995 (NCHEC & CNHEO, 1996) and 2002 (CNHEO, 2003) to examine the status and future of the health education/promotion profession. These conferences led to the creation of goals and recommendations for the profession for the 21st century, and commitments by member organizations to lead or assist in addressing the recommendations (CNHEO, 2003). (See Chapter 10 for more on the future of health education/promotion.)

- Creation of a unified "Code of Ethics for the Health Education Profession" (see Chapter 5 and Appendix A).

- Cosponsoring the annual National Health Education Advocacy Summit that began in 1998. The purpose of the Summit is to increase the capacity of health education specialists to engage in effective advocacy for a common health education/promotion agenda. At the Summit attendees receive policy advocacy training and make legislative visits to educate congresspersons on priority issues in health education (CNHEO, 2010b).

- Support of the *Health Education Advocate* Web site. "The mission of the *Health Education Advocate* is to provide a central, timely source of advocacy information related to the field of health education and health promotion" (CNHEO, 2010b, ¶ 1). (See Web Links at the end of this chapter for the URL of the Web site.)

More information about CNHEO can be obtained by contacting the office of any of the member organizations or by logging on to the CNHEO Web site. The URL for this site is presented in the Web Links at the end of the chapter.

## Joining a Professional Health Association/Organization

Becoming a member of a professional organization is not difficult. With the exception of a few of the associations/organizations previously noted (CNHEO, the American Academy of Health Behavior, Eta Sigma Gamma, and DHPE and SSDHPER), membership in a professional organization can be obtained by completing an application form (available from any of the organizations, included in many of the official publications, or found at the organization's Web site [see Table 8.2]) and sending the money with the desired length and category of membership (different rates apply to different types of membership—for example, student, professional, retired) to the association/organization of choice. Most individuals join a professional association/organization for a year at a time. Some associations, however, provide multiple-year memberships at a reduced rate or even a lifetime membership. In general, the cost of a membership in a state or regional association/organization is separate from and less than a membership in a national association/organization. If you are interested in joining a state or local association/organization, you can usually contact its national office to find out whom to contact locally.

## The Certification Body of the Health Education/Promotion Profession: National Commission for Health Education Credentialing, Inc.

The National Commission for Health Education Credentialing, Inc. (NCHEC, pronounced N-check) is unlike any other organization that has been discussed in this chapter. It is not a professional organization that health education specialists join, but rather the organization responsible for the individual credentialing of health education specialists, thus it has no members. The history of the development of NCHEC was presented in Chapter 6, while the information presented here is to give the reader an understanding of how NCHEC operates.

"The mission of NCHEC is to enhance the professional practice of Health Education by promoting and sustaining a credentialed body of Health Education Specialists. To meet this mission, NCHEC certifies health education specialists, promotes professional development, and strengthens professional preparation and practice" (NCHEC, 2010d, ¶ 1). The charge of NCHEC "is to develop and administer national competency-based examinations; develop standards for professional preparation; and promote professional development through continuing education for health education professionals" (NCHEC, 2010d, ¶ 2). Four boards and the NCHEC staff carry out the work of NCHEC. The boards include the Board of Commissioners [BOC], the Division Board for Certification of Health Education Specialists, the Division Board of Professional Development, and the Division Board for Professional Preparation and Practice. The four boards meet monthly via conference calls and have one or two face-to-face meetings each year.

The BOC, which is comprised of 11 commissioners, is the governing board and the board responsible for all NCHEC activities (NCHEC, 2010d). The three division boards address the three activities noted in NCHEC's mission statement: certification, professional development, and professional preparation. Those who hold either the Certified Health Education Specialist (CHES) or the Master Certified Health Education Specialist (MCHES) credential elect the directors and commissioners of the various boards, with the exception of one. The lone exception is the public member of the BOC, who is appointed by the BOC after a call for nominations. In addition, the elected directors and commissioners are volunteers and must hold an active CHES or MCHES credential (NCHEC, 2010d).

The primary responsibility of the Division Board for Certification of Health Education Specialists (DBCHES) is to create the two examinations of NCHEC—the Certified Health Education Specialist (CHES) exam and the Master Certified Health Education Specialist (MCHES) exam. More specifically, DBCHES, which is composed of 13 directors, along with the guidance of Professional Examination Services (PES) assures a periodic review and evaluation of certification and examination processes; recommends policies and procedures for administering the CHES and MCHES examinations; writes the examination questions; creates the exams; determines the pass point (i.e., minimum score on the examinations required to obtain the certification), and ensures that NCHEC's competency testing meets acceptable standards (NCHEC, 2010d).

The work of the Division Board for Professional Development (DBPD), which is composed of seven directors, is to oversee the recertification and annual renewal procedures for the two credentials (NCHEC, 2010d). "More specifically, the DBPD recommends policies and procedures related to the designation of continuing education providers, recertification and the annual renewal of CHES and MCHES; recommends fees for recertification, annual renewal and provider designation; and assures that the processes are monitored and periodically evaluated" (NCHEC, 2010d, ¶ 3).

The Division Board for Professional Preparation and Practice (DBPPP), which is also composed of seven directors, is responsible for promoting professional preparation (NCHEC, 2010c). "More specifically, the DBPPP works with colleges, universities and accrediting agencies to improve professional preparation programs and promote best practices in health education settings; and monitors and updates the certification application and eligibility review process" (NCHEC, 2010d, ¶ 3).

The CHES examination was given for the first time in 1990. The first MCHES examination was offered in 2011. Both examinations are offered twice a year—one in April and one in October—at 126 locations around the country and in Puerto Rico. The examinations are each 165 questions long and candidates have 3 hours to complete the exam. The eligibility criteria to take the examinations are presented in **Box 8.4**.

---

**Box 8.4** ELIGIBILITY CRITERIA TO SIT FOR THE CHES AND MCHES EXAMINATIONS

**CHES Examination**

Eligibility to take the CHES examination is based exclusively on academic qualifications. An individual is eligible to take the examination if he/she has:

A bachelor's, master's or doctoral degree from an accredited institution of higher education; AND one of the following:

- An official transcript (including course titles) that clearly shows a major in health education, e.g., Health Education, Community Health Education, Public Health Education, School Health Education, etc. Degree/major must explicitly be in a discipline of "Health Education." OR
- An official transcript that reflects at least 25 semester hours or 37 quarter hours of course work (with a grade "c" or better) with specific preparation addressing the Seven Areas of Responsibility and Competency for Health Educators

http://www.nchec.org/exam/eligible/mches/

**MCHES EXAM ELIGIBILITY**

The MCHES exam eligibility includes both academic and experience requirements.

**Exam Eligibility**

- For CHES: A minimum of the past five (5) continuous years in active status as a Certified Health Education Specialist.
- For Non-CHES or CHES with fewer than five years active status AND five years experience:
  - A Master's degree or higher in Health Education, Public Health Education, School Health Education, Community Health Education, etc.,
  - OR a Master's degree or higher with an academic transcript reflecting at least 25 semester hours (37 quarter hours) of course work in which the Seven Areas of Responsibility of Health Educators were addressed.
  - Five (5) years of documented experience as a health education specialist

To verify applicants must submit:

1. Two verification forms from a current or past manager/supervisor, and/or a leader in a health education professional organization.

2. A current curriculum vitae/resume

In the verification form it must be indicated, and in the curriculum vitae/resume it must clearly be shown, that the applicant has been engaged in the Areas of Responsibility for at least the past five years (experience may be prior to completion of graduate degree).

http://www.nchec.org/exam/eligible/mches/

*Source:* The National Commission for Health Education Credentialing, Inc. (NCHEC). By permission.

NCHEC produces several different publications. "The *NCHEC News* is NCHEC's newsletter for all Certified Health Education Specialists" (NCHEC, 2010a, ¶ 1). It is published two to three times a year and is mailed to each current certification holder. Past issues of the newsletter are available online at the NCHEC Web site (NCHEC, 2010a). NCHEC also publishes documents that are useful for those working in professional preparation programs, those offering continuing education opportunities, and those individuals preparing to take either the CHES or the MCHES examination. Included in these publications are a historical account of the credentialing of health education specialists (Cleary, 1995); a companion guide for the examinations (NCHEC, 2010b), and the competency-based framework (NCHEC, SOPHE, & AAHE, 2010). As noted, this later publication is a joint publication of NCHEC and its publishing partners American Association for Health Education and the Society for Public Health Education. This document was generated from the findings of the Health Education Job Analysis—2010 (HEJA-2010) and has "implications for professional preparation, credentialing, and professional development of all health education specialists regardless of the setting in which they are employed" (NCHEC, 2010c ¶ 1).

More information about NCHEC can be obtained by contacting the NCHEC office (1541 Alta Drive, Suite 303, Whitehall, PA 18052-5642, Phone: (484) 223-0770, Toll-Free: (888) 624-3248, Facsimile: (800) 813-0727) or by logging on to the NCHEC Web site. The URL for this site is presented in the Weblinks at the end of the chapter.

## SUMMARY

This chapter discussed the various health agencies, associations, and organizations with which the profession of health education/promotion interacts. The agencies/associations/organizations were presented within three major categories: governmental, quasi-governmental, and nongovernmental. The primary emphasis of the chapter was to present information about a subcategory of the nongovernmental associations/organizations, the professional associations/organizations. Those discussed included the American Academy of Health Behavior; the American Alliance for Health, Physical Education, Recreation and Dance; the American Association for Health Education; the American Public Health Association; the American College Health Association; the American School Health Association; the National Wellness Institute, Inc.; the Society for Public Health Education, Inc.; the International Union for Health Promotion and Education; Eta Sigma Gamma; and associations for directors (Directors of Health Promotion and Education, and the Society of State Directors of Health, Physical Education, and Recreation). Also, information about a coalition—the Coalition of National Health Education Organizations, USA—and information on how to become a member of a professional association/organization was presented. The chapter concluded with an overview of the National Commission for Health Education Credentialing, Inc. and the eligibility criteria for taking the CHES or MCHES examination.

## REVIEW QUESTIONS

1. Define and explain the differences among the following types of agencies: *governmental health agency, quasi-governmental health agency, nongovernmental health agency.*

2. At what levels do governmental agencies exist? Provide an example of an agency at each level.

3. What are the four primary activities of most voluntary health agencies? Give an example of each.

4. What are the purposes of a professional association/organization?

5. What are the benefits derived from membership in a professional association/organization? Why should students become members?

6. What is the oldest and largest professional health association in the United States?

7. Name three professional health associations/organizations that focus their efforts on work settings for health education specialists. Name two other professional health associations/organizations that are not as focused on a work setting.

8. What is the name of the health education honorary? Where was it founded and where is the national office located? In general, where are the chapters of the honorary found?

9. What makes the American Academy of Health Behavior different from the other professional organizations/associations presented in this chapter?

10. What is a coalition? Name one health education coalition. What is the primary purpose of this coalition? What are some of the recent activities of the coalition?

11. How does a person become a member of a professional organization?

12. What is the National Commission for Health Education Credentialing, Inc.? How is it different from the other organizations presented in the chapter?

## CASE STUDY

Hilary has been employed by the XYZ voluntary health organization for almost a year now. The job has really gone well. She enjoys the work, likes her coworkers, and has been able to use much of what she learned during her health education/promotion professional preparation program. Just recently the organization received word that it had been awarded a $15,000 grant to conduct a health education/promotion program for a local senior citizens group on living a healthier life. Her supervisor, Ms. Denison, has given Hilary the responsibility to take the leadership for the project. One restriction on the use of the money is that the program must be planned by a representative group from local voluntary and governmental health education/promotion organizations. Therefore, Hilary's first task is to invite local groups to send a representative to the initial planning meeting. Hilary has set the goal of having seven different health voluntary and governmental agencies involved. If you were Hilary, which organizations would you invite to the initial meeting? Justify why you would select these seven.

## CRITICAL THINKING QUESTIONS

1. For a number of years, many practicing health education specialists have pushed for a single professional health education/promotion association that would bring together many of the existing associations (i.e., AAHE, ACHA, ASHA, SOPHE) so

that health education/promotion would have a single professional association voice. Would you be in favor of or against combining all the health education/promotion professional associations into a single association? Defend your response. As part of your response, indicate what you think are the strengths and weaknesses of your position.

2. In this chapter you have read about a number of different professional health education/promotion associations. Upon graduating from college few new professionals have enough money to join several different professional groups. Assuming that you have enough money to join one national professional group upon graduation, what association/organization would it be? Explain the reasoning you would use to select the one organization to join.

3. One of the major issues facing many professional health education/promotion associations is retaining members from year to year. Some members do not renew their membership because of cost. Others do not renew because they do not feel that they receive enough benefits. After conducting a membership survey, a professional health association has decided to revamp the benefits provided to members. Assume that you have been appointed as a student member to the executive committee of the professional association and that the president of the association has charged the committee with revamping the membership benefits package. Each member of the executive committee has been asked to create a list of benefits. What would be on your list? Explain why you selected each item.

4. Throughout this book you have been introduced to the work of health education specialists. This chapter focused on the different professional organizations of our profession. We also presented information on the National Commission for Health Education Credentialing, Inc. We stated that being a member of a professional organization is different than becoming certified as a health education specialist. Compare and contrast what you see to be the benefits of membership in a professional organization and becoming a certified health education specialist or master certified health education specialist. Aside from the financial costs, do you see any drawbacks of membership and certification?

## ACTIVITIES

1. Closely examine one professional health association/organization and write a two-page paper on the history of that association/organization.

2. Interview two health education/promotion faculty members at your school and ask them the following:
   - Do they belong to any professional health education associations/organizations?
   - If they belong, why?
   - What benefits do they see in belonging to them?
   - What association/organization would they recommend that you join?

3. Does your school have a chapter of Eta Sigma Gamma? If not, make an appointment with the department head/chairperson to inquire about the possibility of starting one on your campus.

4. Write a one-page paper using the following two sentences to start the paper: "If I could join one professional health association/organization, it would be _____. My reasons for choosing that association/organization are _____."

5. Visit the Web site of the Coalition of National Health Education Organizations (CNHEO) (http://www.cnheo.org). Once at the site, read the "21st Century" reports: (1) *The Health Education Profession in the Twenty-First Century Progress Report 1995–2001*, and (2) *Coalition of National Health Education Organization's 2nd Invitational Conference: Improving the Nation's Health Through Health Education—A Vision for the 21st Century*. After reading the reports, create your own list of five activities that you feel the profession should engage in during the next ten years to move the profession forward. Provide a brief (i.e., a couple of paragraphs) rationale for why you included each activity on your list.

## WEBLINKS

1. **http://www.astho.org**

   The Association for State and Territorial Health Officers (ASTHO)

   This is the Web site for the ASTHO, which is the national nonprofit organization representing the state and territorial public health agencies of the United States, the U.S. Territories, and the District of Columbia. Among other items, this site includes links to each of the state and territorial health departments.

2. **http://www.cancer.org/**

   American Cancer Society (ACS)

   This is the home page for ACS. The site presents the most up-to-date information on cancer, including treatment and prevention. The site also provides information about the ACS and the resources it can provide for cancer survivors and program planners.

3. **http://www.cnheo.org**

   Coalition of National Health Education Organizations (CNHEO)

   This is the home page for CNHEO. At the site, you will find information about all the member organizations, as well as the Coalition's mission, goals, *Working Agreement*, the "Code of Ethics for the Health Education Profession," and the "21st Century" reports.

4. **http://www.americanheart.org**

   American Heart Association (AHA)

   This is the home page for the AHA. It provides health education specialists with a wealth of information and materials about many of the cardiovascular diseases and stroke.

5. **http://www.lungusa.org**

   American Lung Association (ALA)

   This is the home page for the ALA. It provides a variety of information about various lung diseases, including asthma, chronic obstructive pulmonary disease (COPD), and lung cancer.

6. http://www.welcoa.org

The Wellness Councils of America (WELCOA)

This is the home page for the WELCOA. This site provides a variety of resources for those interested in worksite wellness programs.

7. http://www.cdc.gov/

Centers for Disease Control and Prevention (CDC)

This is the home page of the CDC. It includes information for the lay public (i.e., traveler's health and emergency preparedness) as well as information to assist health education specialists (i.e., health topics A–Z, CDC recommendations, *MMWR*, and special funded initiatives).

8. http://www.healtheducationadvocate.org/

Health Education Advocate

This is the homepage of the Health Education Advocate that is sponsored by the Coalition of National Health Education Organizations. This site provides up-to-date advocacy information for health education specialists, as well as links to other advocacy sites.

9. http://www.nchec.org

National Commission for Health Education Credentialing, Inc.

This is the home page for NCHEC. At this site you can find out more about the CHES and MCHES examinations, order publications to help you prepare for the examinations, and get up-to-date on individual credentialing.

(Note: See Table 8.2 for the URLs of the various professional associations/ organizations discussed in this chapter.)

# REFERENCES

American Academy for Health Behavior (AAHB). (2010a). *About AAHB*. Retrieved September 1, 2010, from http://www.aahb.org/AboutAAHB.html

American Academy for Health Behavior (AAHB). (2010b). *Publications*. Retrieved September 1, 2010, from http://www.ajhb.org/

American Association for Health Education (AAHE). (2010a). *About AAHE 2010*. Retrieved August 30, 2010, from http://www.aahperd.org/aahe/about/results.cfm

American Association for Health Education (AAHE). (2010b). *Professional networking*. Retrieved August 30, 2010, from http://www.aahperd.org/aahe/proNetworking/

American Association for Health Education (AAHE). (2010c). *AAHE publications*. Retrieved August 30, 2010, from http://www.aahperd.org/aahe/publications/

American Cancer Society (ACS). (2007). *National Health Education Standards* (2nd ed.). Atlanta, GA: Author.

American College Health Association (ACHA). (2010a). *About ACHA*. Retrieved September 1, 2010, from http://www.acha.org/About_ACHA/Who_We_Are.cfm

American College Health Association (ACHA). (2010b). *Membership*. Retrieved September 1, 2010, from http://www.acha.org/Membership/Membership_Categories.cfm

American College Health Association (ACHA). (2010c). *Publications*. Retrieved September 1, 2010, from http://www.acha.org/Publications/JACH.cfm

American Public Health Association (APHA). (2010a). *About us*. Retrieved on August 31, 2010, from: http://www.apha.org/about/

American Public Health Association (APHA). (2010b). *Member groups and state affiliates*. Retrieved on August 31, 2010, from: http://www.apha.org/membergroups/sections/

American Public Health Association (APHA). (2010c). *Publications & advertising*. Retrieved August 31, 2010, from http://www.apha.org/publications/

American Public Health Association (APHA). (n.d). *The American Public Health Association: Keeping public health in the public eye for more than a century*. Washington, DC: Author.

American School Health Association (ASHA). (1976). *History of the American School Health Association, 1926–1976*. Kent, OH: Author.

American School Health Association (ASHA). (2010a). *ASHA & school health*. Retrieved September 1, 2010, from http://www.ashaweb.org/i4a/pages/index.cfm?pageid=3277

American School Health Association (ASHA). (2010b). *Publications*. Retrieved September 1, 2010, from http://www.ashaweb.org/i4a/pages/index.cfm?pageid=3340

Anderson, G. (1985). AAHPERD from the beginning. *Journal of Physical Education, Recreation and Dance, 56* (4), 94–96.

Capwell, E. M. (2004). Coalition of national health education organizations. *California Journal of Health Promotion, 2* (1), 12–15.

Cleary, H. P. (1995). *The credentialing of health educators: An historical account 1970–1990*. Whitehall, PA: The National Commission for Health Education Credentialing, Inc.

Coalition of National Health Education Organizations (CNHEO). (2003). *21st Century Report*. Retrieved September 1, 2010, from http://www.cnheo.org/index.html

Coalition of National Health Education Organizations (CNHEO). (2006). *Working agreement*. Retrieved September 1, 2010, from http://www.cnheo.org/index.html

Coalition of National Health Education Organizations (CNHEO). (2010a). *About us*. Retrieved September 1, 2010, from http://www.cnheo.org/index.html

Coalition of National Health Education Organizations (CNHEO). (2010b). *Health Education Advocate*. Retrieved September 1, 2010, from http://www.healtheducationadvocate.org/

Coughlin, S. S. (2010). *Case studies in public health practice* (2nd ed.). Washington, DC: American Public Health Association.

Director of Health Promotion and Education (DHPE). (2010). *DHPE membership*. Retrieved September 1, 2010, from https://www.netforumondemand.com/eweb/StartPage. aspx?Site=dhpe&WebCode=HomePage&FromSearchControl=Yes

Eta Sigma Gamma (ESG). (1991, November). *Eta Sigma Gamma*. Muncie, IN: Author.

Heymann, D. L. (Ed.). (2009). *Control of communicable diseases manual* (19th ed.). Washington, DC: American Public Health Association.

International Union for Health Promotion and Education (IUHPE). (2010a). *About IUHPE*. Retrieved September 1, 2010, from http://www.iuhpe.org/index.html?page=5&lang=en

International Union for Health Promotion and Education (IUHPE). (2010b). *The IUHPE journal family*. IUHPE. Retrieved September 1, 2010, from http://www.iuhpe.org/index.html?page=18&lang=en

McKenzie, J. F., Pinger, R. R., & Kotecki, J. E. (2012). *An introduction to community health* (7th ed.). Sudbury, MA: Jones & Bartlett Publishers.

Miller, D. F., & Price, J. H. (1998). *Dimensions of community health* (5th ed.). Boston: WCB/McGraw-Hill.

National Commission for Health Education Credentialing, Inc., & Coalition of National Health Education Organizations, USA (NCHEC & CNHEO). (1996). The health education profession in the 21st century: Setting the stage. *Journal of School Health, 66* (8), 291–298.

National Commission for Health Education Credentialing, Inc. (NCHEC). (2010a). *The CHES bulletin*. Retrieved September 2, 2010, from http://www.nchec.org/news/bullet/

National Commission for Health Education Credentialing, Inc. (NCHEC). (2010b). *The Health Education Specialist: A companion guide for professional excellence* (6th ed.). Whitehall, PA: Author.

National Commission for Health Education Credentialing, Inc. (NCHEC). (2010c). *Health educator job analysis-2010: Press release*. Retrieved September 2, 2010, from http://www.nchec.org/news/what/#BM_NCH-MR-TAB2-169

National Commission for Health Education Credentialing, Inc. (NCHEC). (2010d). *Mission and purpose*. Retrieved September 2, 2010, from http://www.nchec.org/aboutnchec/mission/

National Commission for Health Education Credentialing, Inc. (NCHEC), Society for Public Health Education (SOPHE), & American Association for Health Education (AAHE). (2010). *A competency-based framework for health education specialists – 2010*. Whitehall, PA: Author.

National Wellness Institute (NWI). (2010a). *History*. Retrieved September 1, 2010, from http://www.nationalwellness.org/index.php?id_tier=2

National Wellness Institute (NWI). (2010b). *Mission*. Retrieved September 1, 2010, from http://www.nationalwellness.org/index.php?id_tier=2&id_c=24

National Wellness Institute (NWI). (2010c). *National Wellness Institute membership*. Retrieved September 1, 2010, from http://www.nationalwellness.org/index.php?id_tier=89

Nolte, A. E. (1985). Health education: An alliance commitment. *Journal of Physical Education, Recreation and Dance, 56* (4), 107–108.

Random House, Inc. (2010). Philanthropy. In *Dictionary.com Unabridged*. Retrieved August 30, 2010, from http://dictionary.reference.com/browse/philanthropy

Society for Public Health Education (SOPHE). (2010a). *About SOPHE*. Retrieved September 1, 2010, from http://www.sophe.org/about.cfm

Society for Public Health Education (SOPHE). (2010b). *Member communities*. Retrieved September 1, 2010, from http://www.sophe.org/community.cfm

Society for Public Health Education (SOPHE). (2010c). *Programs & initiatives*. Retrieved September 1, 2010, from http://www.sophe.org/programs.cfm

Society for Public Health Education (SOPHE). (2010d). *Publications & resources*. Retrieved September 1, 2010, from http://www.sophe.org/Publications_Resources.cfm

Society for Public Health Education, Inc. (n.d.). *Health education professional organizations and you* (a handout). Washington, DC: Author.

Society of State Directors of Health, Physical Education, and Recreation (SSDHPER) (2010). *About us*. Retrieved September 1, 2010, from http://www.thesociety.org/about.asp

U.S. Department of Labor, Bureau of Labor Statistics (USDOL). (2009). *Occupational outlook handbook, 2010–2011: Health educators*. Retrieved September 1, 2010, from http://www.bls.gov/oco/ocos063.htm

Werch, C. E. (2000). Editorial: What use, the American Academy of Health Behavior? *American Journal of Health Behavior, 24* (1), 3–5.

Young, K. J., & Boling, W. (2004). Improving the quality of professional life: Benefits of health education and promotion association membership. *California Journal of Health Promotion, 2* (1), 39–44.

## CHAPTER 9

# The Literature of Health Education/Promotion

## CHAPTER OBJECTIVES

After reading this chapter and answering the questions at the end, you should be able to:

- Describe the difference between a *primary*, a *secondary*, a *tertiary*, and a *popular press* literature source.
- Write an abstract or a summary of an article from a refereed journal.
- Use appropriate questions to critique a journal article.
- Become familiar with the most commonly used journals in the field of health education/promotion.
- Identify the most commonly used online computerized databases for finding health education/promotion information.
- Locate an article related to some aspect of health education/promotion using an online database.
- Conduct an Internet search for information about a health-related topic using one of the Web site URLs listed in the chapter.
- Critique the validity of the information obtained from searching a site on the Internet.

In her work as a health education specialist, Georgia administers a federally funded statewide center that distributes prevention information on alcohol, tobacco, and other drugs. Materials in the center include monographs containing the results of research studies on possible treatment protocols and prevention interventions; prevention and education materials from a variety of federal, state, and nonprofit agencies; information on evidence-based practice in both prevention and treatment; and an extensive video library. Almost daily, she and her staff receive requests for information from law enforcement agencies, legislators and organizational policy makers, community groups, school personnel, counselors, nonprofit organizations, treatment professionals, state agencies, churches, and individual patrons.

Over the past three or four years, more university health education/promotion students have been visiting to acquire materials for class projects, research studies, or potential thesis topics. These students often request Georgia or her staff to recommend the most up-to-date primary and secondary source materials and the most reputable Web sites related to substance abuse prevention.

After reading and digesting the information contained in this chapter, you should be able to address questions similar to those received by the staff of the center described above. Serving as a resource for health information is a critical skill that must be acquired by those practicing as health education specialists.

The amount of information about any given topic is growing at almost an exponential rate. Terms such as *information overload* and *information burnout* are being heard more and more. Arguably, the area in which information is growing fastest and in which there is tremendous public interest is health. People today seem obsessed with gathering information about such health topics as diet, exercise, stress management, vitamins, drugs, sexuality, depression, safety, disease, violence prevention, health care policies, health insurance options, and the cost of medical procedures or prescription drugs.

The increasing demand for information, coupled with the fact that information is being produced at an ever greater rate, creates added need for health education specialists (see **Box 9.1**). Two of the major responsibilities of a health education specialist, as discussed in Chapter 6, involve being a resource person for health information (Responsibility 6) and communicating to others about health education needs, concerns, and resources (Responsibility 7) (see **Figure 9.1**). In order to perform these tasks, the health education specialist must have the skills to find information, evaluate the source of the information to determine its credibility, disseminate the information to consumers through the appropriate channels, and explain the meaning of the information in an understandable manner. This chapter introduces prospective health education students to the most common sources of health-related information used by health education specialists. It also describes how to access the information from these sources. When searching for information, it is always wise to seek the assistance of a reference librarian should questions arise.

---

**Box 9.1 Practitioner's Perspective**    **Use of Health Literature**

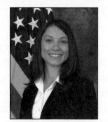

NAME: Stephanie Wheeler, B.S., CHES

DEGREE: B.S. in Health Promotion from Boise State University, 2004

CURRENT POSITION: Health and Wellness Center (HAWC) Health Educator

INSTITUTION: Minot Air Force Base, Minot, ND

EMPLOYER: Contract employee of the USAF

(Reprinted by permission of Stephanie Wheeler)

**How I obtained my job:** This position was obtained through sheer determination. At the time I applied, the company that held the central contract required a longer work history in the field than I possessed. After multiple contacts with the company (some may call it pestering) and going through extensive phone interviews, I was hired. Then the process of proving my abilities began.

---

**Box 9.1 Practitioner's Perspective**    **Continued**

**How I utilize health education and the literature in health in my job:** Perseverance is the key to health promotion. If one avenue does not lead the way to success, you must go back to the planning process and reevaluate. When a plan or program does not go as well as one would hope, there is no need to scrap the entire project. Take the pieces that worked well and build from them. Always go back to the original goal and make sure that it is a valid goal for both you and the population. One advantage to working for a military installation is that I have access to health data. At each chosen interval we can track changes to see if the desired outcome is surfacing. Additionally, we use surveys and sample groups to determine what was useful and what was not. Utilizing data from other studies can streamline efforts to what has worked for others and avoid their mistakes. While we all want our own ideas to be successful, it is ethically sound to research heavily before funding the plan. We have limited resources, which must be stretched maximally.

**What I like most about my job:** Seeing the joy of individuals and groups as they meet and exceed their goals is the best part of what I do. I love getting e-mails, phone calls, or visits from people telling me that they have learned from me and it has changed their life. Hearing newfound confidence in their voice and learning that they are sharing that information and enthusiasm with others are what health promotion is about.

**What I like least about my job:** Early in my career there was a particular point when I was contemplating whether or not I was making a difference. Often, we are planting the seeds without ever having the chance to see what the full harvest will yield. My mentor at the time asked me a question that seemed odd at the time. She asked me, "If your job was to make pigs fly and only one flew, would you have failed?" At the time, I recall thinking that it was a slightly silly question. Now I see her point. We cannot expect immediate results of our effort. We will not always see the return on investment (ROI). We must have faith that everything, every person, is worth our effort.

**Recommendations for those preparing to be health education specialists:** Anyone going into health education/promotion needs to have the ability to take criticism. Behavior change is difficult and sometimes painful. You may be the perceived source of pain! Criticism is opportunity for change for both me and my clients. Often, our greatest aggravation can become our stepping stone to the best success.

**The role of health education specialists in the future:** The future of HP means getting out into the community in a more assertive fashion. This does not mean that we will enter homes and exchange their cake for broccoli. However, the idea that providing information and hoping that people will show up to learn it is an old thought process. Rather than being entrenched in the medical community, health education specialists will be in more areas that the general population accesses such as grocery stores and shopping centers.

## Types of Information Sources

When accessing information, it is important to note whether the source is primary, secondary, or tertiary. **Primary sources** of data or information are published studies or eyewitness accounts written by the people who actually conducted the experiments or observed the events in question. A journal that publishes original manuscripts only after they have been read by a panel of experts in the field (referees) and recommended for publication is termed a **refereed or peer-reviewed journal**. Examples of primary sources are research articles written by the researcher(s); personal records (autobiographies);

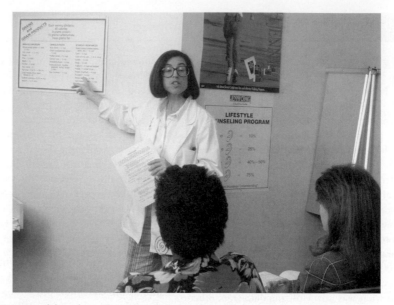

**Figure 9.1** Health education specialists often make presentations to community groups.

(Michael Newman/PhotoEdit)

podcasts or video/audio recordings of actual lectures (which may also be secondary sources depending on whether the information presented is the speakers' own work [primary] or a compilation of the works of self and others [secondary]); speeches, debates, or events; official records of legislative sessions or minutes of community meetings; newspaper eyewitness accounts; and annual reports.

Of note is the fact that some refereed/peer-reviewed journals now are published only in electronic format. These publications, known as **"open access" journals,** have articles that come in a variety of reader access levels. Some articles are immediately available to individual subscribers or subscribing institutions; others allow delayed access to articles for anyone with an Internet connection; and some of the publishing sites have a mixture of the two availability types. The "open access" designation means that the article is copyrighted but generally can be used more liberally than articles with more traditional copyrights. Databases such as BioMed Central (biomedcentral.com) are repositories of these types of journals, many of which are new and most of which utilize scientists who have been editorial board members on highly prestigious paper-based journals for their editorial review boards. The increased cost of paper-based journals and publishing company charges will undoubtedly expand the number of open access primary sources of information in the future.

**Secondary sources** are usually written by someone who was not present at the event or did not participate as part of the study team. The value of these sources is that they often provide a summary of several related studies or chronicle a history or sequence of events. The writers of secondary sources may also provide editorial comments or alternative interpretations of the study or event. Secondary sources often provide a bibliography of primary sources. Examples of secondary sources are journal review articles, editorials, and noneyewitness accounts of events occurring in the community, region, or nation.

Although refereed/peer-reviewed journals usually publish primary source articles, they occasionally contain secondary source articles. The types of secondary source articles most likely to be found in a refereed journal are articles summarizing the results of several studies, editorials, or positions deemed important enough (by a panel of expert reviewers) to be interesting and useful to those who read the journal.

**Tertiary sources** contain information that has been distilled and collected from primary and secondary sources. Examples include handbooks, informational pamphlets/brochures from governmental organizations (or hospitals, or national nongovernmental agencies such as the American Cancer Society or March of Dimes), almanacs, encyclopedias, fact books, dictionaries, abstracts, and other reference tools. At this stage, information from such sources is accepted as fact by the scientific community. The operative word in the preceding sentence is "fact." Information that has no documentation and is laced with opinion or intended for marketing a service or product is not considered a tertiary source; publications of that type are classified as popular press sources.

A fourth source of health information, **popular press publications,** is probably the most difficult to check for credibility. Popular press publications range from weekly summary-type magazines (e.g., *Time, Newsweek, U.S. News & World Report*) and newspaper supplements (e.g., *Parade*) to monthly magazines (e.g., *Reader's Digest, Better Homes and Gardens, Esquire*) and tabloids (e.g., *The Star*). At times, any of these may be a primary source of information (as in an interview). Most often, however, they are secondary sources at best. Often, articles in the popular press include opinions or editorials that express the bias of the author or the editor of the publication. Popular press articles should be heavily scrutinized as to the source of the information before being cited as authentic and accurate.

Before concluding this discussion, it is important to note that, with the exception of open access journals, no Web site references were included in the literature types described above. This is because Web sites are generally not refereed. Just about anyone can publish an article on the Web without an impartial reader or group of readers reviewing it beforehand. To be sure, Web pages are often wonderful sources of information, but they can just as often be replete with bad information. A discussion of methods to determine the accuracy of information on the Web is included later in this chapter. Sorting through the maze of health information can be a daunting task, even for the most skilled health education specialist. In order to equip the health education specialist for assuming the responsibilities of providing and disseminating information, several tasks need to be mastered. The next several sections of this chapter are designed to provide background for the student in: (1) identifying the components of a research article; (2) critically reading a research article; (3) ascertaining the accuracy of the information in articles that are non-research based or are from secondary or popular press sources; (4) writing an abstract or a summary of a journal article; (5) identifying and locating primary and secondary sources most commonly used by health education specialists using indexes, abstracts, and computerized databases; and (6) retrieving health-related information on the Internet.

## Identifying the Components of a Research Article

A research article usually begins with an abstract, which is a brief description of the study's results. The abstract describes the research questions that were tested, outlines the study design, and lists one or two major findings from the study. The abstract is meant to communicate essential information, so that readers will know whether the study has information related to the topic they are interested in. An example of an abstract (Normand and Osborne, 2010) follows:

> A healthy diet is a key ingredient to good health and can help prevent a number of adverse health conditions. Although many people can describe a healthy diet, they often cannot accurately report the nutritional content of their own diets. In this study, daily dietary feedback consisting of recommended daily nutrient values accompanied by estimated calorie and fat data of daily food purchases was provided to four college undergraduates. The estimated calories and percentage of calories from fat data were based on records of participant purchases at university dining establishments. The introduction of daily dietary feedback resulted in the students purchasing fewer calories and fewer calories from fat per day. (p. 183)

The introduction section, which sometimes is divided into subsections, follows the abstract. Its purpose is usually threefold: (1) to give readers a more detailed description of the research question(s) or hypotheses being tested; (2) to review related literature; and (3) to explain the need for or the significance of the study. This section communicates the rationale behind the researchers' decision to conduct the study.

The methodology section comes directly after the introductory material. In this section, there is usually a description of (1) the research design used, (2) the subjects who took part in the research, (3) the instruments used to gather the information necessary to answer the research questions, and (4) any administrative procedures involved in conducting the research, such as methods used to select the subject, gather the data, or protect the rights of the subject.

Following the methodology section are the results and discussion sections. The results section gives the research findings by describing the results of the statistical procedures used in analyzing the data (in the case of studies involving quantitative methods—methods involving the analyses of numerical data) and provides an overall answer to the research questions or hypotheses that were described in the introductory section. The discussion section provides a forum for the researcher to interpret the conclusions and meanings and to comment on the implications of the data analyses. In addition, the researcher often includes a narrative about the limitations of the study and makes recommendations for further research on the topic.

## Critically Reading a Research Article

The volume of articles on any single health topic continues to escalate. It is important to be able to evaluate the information for accuracy and saliency from sources of all types. Research articles serve as primary sources of valuable information for health education specialists. Beginning students in the field of health education/promotion are not expected to be able to immediately understand every nuance in a research article. It is essential, however, to begin to frequently read scientific reports and journal articles to become familiar with their style. Often, pre-formulating generic questions suitable for critiquing any study can help when evaluating study results. Following is a sequence of questions found to be of help when such an evaluation is necessary. The list is adapted from *Studying a Study and Testing a Test: How to Read Medical Evidence* (Riegelman, 2005).

1. Were the goals/aims of the study defined in a clear manner?
2. Were the research questions/hypotheses clearly stated?

3. Was the description of the subjects clear? Did the article state how the subjects were recruited?

4. Were the design and location of the study described clearly?

5. Were the data collection instruments described?

6. Were reliability and validity reported for the instruments?

7. Did the results directly address the research questions/hypotheses?

8. Were the conclusions reasonable in light of the research design and data analyses performed?

9. Were the findings extrapolated to a population that is similar to the population studied?

10. Were the study implications meaningful to the population you serve?

The final test comes when students can read an article and begin to view themselves in the position of a reporter who has the task of describing the study, its findings, and its limitations to an audience in no more than five minutes. People who can restate study findings and limitations in their own words have accomplished much in becoming critical consumers of scientific and nonscientific literature as well as better resources for others.

## Evaluating the Accuracy of Non-Research-Based Sources

As with journal articles that are research based, it is important to be able to evaluate whether or not the information presented is reliable, regardless of the source. Cottrell (1997) conducted a search for instruments that could assist him in teaching his students to assess the accuracy of information found in almost any type of journal or magazine. The questions that emanated from the results of his search include the following:

1. What are the author's qualifications? Does the person have an academic degree in the field being written about? (A note of caution—a degree does not make someone absolutely qualified, but it provides evidence that suggests the person is qualified.)

2. What is the style of presentation? Look for health information written in a scientific style of writing, not a style that uses generalities or testimonials.

3. Are references included? A well-written article provides references to the primary sources used. Be aware when someone is writing about another person's research, as that individual may be interpreting the results in a different way than the author did.

4. What is the purpose of the publication? Be aware of publications, news or otherwise, that contain advertisements designed to sell items discussed in the articles.

5. What is the reputation of the publication? Is it refereed? Professional journals are good sources of information. Popular press publications can sometimes have poor information related to health issues.

6. Is the information new? When reading for the first time, be skeptical. Information must be validated over time. New information is newsworthy but may not be valid.

It is important to realize that becoming a skeptical, critical consumer of printed health information is an important first step in being seen by others as credible. In order for the public to use the expertise and training of health education specialists to a greater degree, the health education specialist must develop a reputation for providing accurate and current information.

## Writing an Abstract or a Summary

Another valuable skill when reading and interpreting health-related literature of any kind (primary, secondary, tertiary, or popular press) involves learning to write an abstract or a summary of an article (see **Figure 9.2**). Although abstracts and summaries are both short forms of describing a research study, the major differences lie in the extent of the content. Abstracts are short (usually 150–250 words). They are written to identify the purpose of the research, the study questions, the methods used by the researcher, and one or two major findings. Summaries, on the other hand, may be two to three pages in length and include all of the elements of the abstract. In addition, summaries are meant to reveal any secondary findings, to describe study limitations, and to provide a more detailed review of the researcher's conclusions and recommendations from the viewpoint of the summary's author.

It is recommended that beginning health education specialists practice writing both abstracts and summaries of the articles they read. Using this technique sharpens the ability of the health education specialist to discriminate between health-related articles that are of substance and meaning for health education/promotion and those that contain erroneous or misleading claims or information.

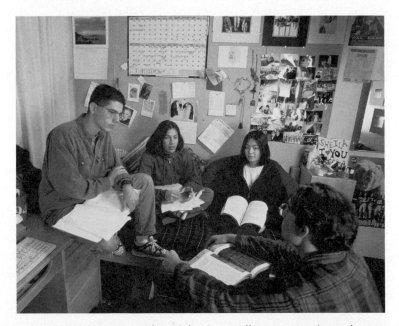

**Figure 9.2** Summarizing research articles in small group settings sharpens the ability to correctly interpret research findings.
(Mark Richards/PhotoEdit)

## Locating Health-Related Information

Health education specialists serve as major health information resource persons for many constituencies. It does not matter if they are employed in the school, the clinic, the worksite, or the community setting. In all cases, inquiries from a variety of people wanting to know about a health topic or wanting interpretation of the latest research findings are directed to health education specialists. Therefore, it is essential that the latter be knowledgeable about how to find the information requested. The next section identifies resources that health education specialists can use to locate information on health education/promotion and explains how to access the information.

### Journals

As has been previously mentioned, much of the information that health education specialists use to make decisions when planning, implementing, and evaluating health promotion programs can be found in journals that publish primary research articles and position papers about health topics and health programs. The following are examples of journals commonly used by health professionals. The list by no means includes all journals of benefit to the health education specialist.

1. *AIDS Education and Prevention.* An international journal designed to support the efforts of professionals working to prevent HIV and AIDS, *AIDS Education and Prevention* includes scientific articles by leading authorities from many disciplines, research reports on the effectiveness of new strategies and programs, debates about key issues, and reviews of books and video resources. In addition to discussing models of AIDS education and prevention, the journal covers a wide range of public health, psychosocial, ethical, and public policy concerns related to HIV and AIDS.

2. *American Journal of Health Behavior (formerly Health Values).* Articles accepted for publication feature research about the impact of personal behavior patterns, practices, and characteristics on health promotion. The journal emphasizes efforts at fostering a better understanding of the multidisciplinary nature of systems and individuals as they interface to impact behavior. Examples of successful multidisciplinary approaches to improving health at the community level are also included.

3. *American Journal of Health Education.* This journal is published by the American Association for Health Education. Most of the articles have broad application to the field of health education. Readers might find articles concerning opinions; original research on health issues and policies related to schools, communities or worksites; and methods and strategies for health instructional programs.

4. *American Journal of Health Promotion.* This journal features original research articles, the testing of health behavioral theory on selected populations, and program evaluation. It is an excellent source of articles related to worksite health promotion.

5. *American Journal of Health Studies (formerly Wellness Perspectives).* Articles target health promotion and wellness in the broadest sense. Readers will find selections on social and environmental support for health, health program planning strategies and evaluation methods, the testing of health behavioral theory, and opinions on the implications of health policy.

6. *American Journal of Public Health.* Published by the American Public Health Association, this journal features reports related to health research, program evaluations, and health policy analysis, as well as articles on special topics on the health of selected groups and communities.

7. *Evaluation and the Health Professions.* Articles generally focus on practitioner-friendly research related to the development, implementation, and evaluation of community-based health programs. Health care researchers and evaluators are provided with examples of state-of-the-art tools and methods for conducting meaningful evaluations.

8. *Family and Community Health.* Articles contain information and research on nutrition, exercise, health-risk appraisals, and the physical and emotional development of a variety of age groups. The overall goal of this journal is to publish articles that foster the role of self-care, family and community health care, and maintenance in the field of health promotion.

9. *Health Affairs.* This journal is published bimonthly and features health policy–related articles of national concern or interest. Of note is that this publication serves as a major source of primary research concerning health care coverage, health economics, health reform, and the impact of policy on the health of the populace.

10. *The Health Educator: The Journal of Eta Sigma Gamma.* Published by Eta Sigma Gamma, the health education honor society, this journal includes articles related to most health education/promotion topics in a variety of settings. Many of the studies and commentaries are submitted by undergraduate and graduate students in health education/public health programs.

11. *The Hastings Center Report.* This journal focuses on the ethical, social, legal, moral, economic, and religious tenets of health policy and health decisions.

12. *Health Education & Behavior (formerly Health Education Quarterly).* The official publication of the Society for Public Health Education, Inc. (SOPHE), its articles center on health behavior and education, case studies in health, program evaluation, and strategies to improve social and behavioral health. Each submission includes a commentary on the application of findings to the practice setting and a "perspectives" section, which presents commentary and insight into the complex world of health behavior.

13. *Health Education Research: Theory and Practice.* This publication features articles concerning health promotion program planning, implementation, and evaluation. An effort is made to publish articles that provide a mechanism to assist those in the field to apply the results of the studies.

14. *Health Promotion International.* The majority of research studies and commentaries are on issues related to health promotion in schools, clinics, worksites, and communities located outside the United States. To maintain a true international perspective, submissions describing spontaneous activities, organizational change interventions, and social and environmental development are uniquely featured as well.

15. *Health Promotion Practice.* A journal that publishes articles devoted to the practical application of health promotion and education in a variety of settings including community, health care, educational, worksite, and international. Articles featuring the best practices and their application to health policies that promote health and disease prevention are also a focal point.

16. *The International Electronic Journal of Health Education.* This journal published its first edition in January 1998. It features articles on nearly every aspect of health education, including school health, community health, worksite health promotion, the ethical implications of health education, and the philosophy of health education.

17. *The Journal of American College Health.* Published by the American College Health Association in cooperation with Heldref Publications, its articles are limited to those that relate to health promotion or health service provision in the college or university environment. This is the only journal written by college health professionals for college health professionals.

18. *Journal of Community Health.* This is an all-inclusive journal, with articles relating to the practice, teaching, and research of community health; preventive medicine; and analysis of delivery of health care services. Many articles focus on projects making an impact on the education of health personnel.

19. *Journal of Health Communication.* This peer-reviewed journal is published bimonthly. It presents the latest developments in the field of health communication, including research in risk communication, health literacy, social marketing, communication (from interpersonal to mass media), psychology, government, policy making, and health education around the world.

20. *Journal of Nutrition Education and Behavior.* The official publication of the Society of Nutrition Education, this journal publishes articles that are germane to the interface between nutrition education and behavior as practiced worldwide. It serves as a resource for anyone interested in nutrition education or diet and physical behavior.

21. *Journal of Rural Health.* Published by the Rural Health Association, this journal's articles focus on professional practice, research, theory development, and policy issues related to health in the rural setting.

22. *Journal of School Health.* Published by the American School Health Association, all material in this journal is related to the public or private school setting from pre-K through grade 12. Articles generally focus on children's health issues but may include information related to other aspects of coordinated school health programs, such as employee wellness.

23. *Global Health Promotion.* This is an official publication of the International Union for Health Promotion and Education (IUHPE), published by Sage Publications. Most issues are topical in nature (e.g., environmental health, population health, infectious disease prevention) and feature articles related to the application of public health and health promotion in countries around the globe. Articles are published in several languages.

24. *Public Health Reports.* The official publication of the Public Health Service, this journal reports findings from many avenues of research related to health services acquisition, health policy development, and health promotion at the community level.

## Indexes and Abstracts

**Indexes** and **abstracts** provide links to articles from many refereed/peer-reviewed journals, books, and research reports. An index references articles from journals, books, and reports pertaining to topics that fall under the subject headings for which the index was created (e.g., health behavior, physical activity, methamphetamine treatment, or corporate health education/promotion programs). An abstract provides somewhat similar information but also includes short summaries of the article's content in order to help the researcher determine whether the article contains the information she or he is seeking.

Although some indexes and abstracts can still be found in hard copy, many of them are migrating to online or electronic formats. The cost of publishing paper versions plus the ease of user access to online materials will undoubtedly create a situation in the near future where new editions of paper versions of either indexes or abstracts will no longer be available. *Index Medicus*, an abstract that has been printed for over a century, is an example of a publication that is no longer available in paper copy due to the high cost of printing the volumes. In its place, the National Library of Medicine and the National Institutes of Health have created a site (http://www.PubMed.gov) that combines the information formerly available in *Index Medicus* with many other sources to create a database that is accessible to anyone with a computer.

## Government Documents

The U.S. Government Printing Office (GPO) publishes volumes of materials of use to health education specialists. This section (adapted from the University of Akron library Web site [University of Akron, 2010]) is meant to provide a generic description of the types of documents that can be accessed in the government documents section of an academic library. Because each library has slightly different procedures for finding these documents, students are encouraged to communicate with the government documents librarian at their university for the specifics on locating documents. It should be noted that the U.S. Government is shifting away from issuing paper copies and is increasing the number of documents available online.

Government publications range from official documents including laws, court decisions, and records of congressional actions to the results of government-sponsored technical and scientific studies. Information on topics such as obesity, water treatment, or exercise can also be found in a government documents section.

Government documents are not organized under the same classification scheme as a traditional general collection. Instead, they are organized and shelved according to SuDocs (Superintendent of Documents) numbers. The SuDocs number is unique in that it has a colon. For example, A1:1 is an annual report from the Agriculture Department. Numbers of the documents are arranged alphabetically by agency, and the numbers are whole numbers, not decimals (e.g., HE 1.6 comes before HE 1.9). The letter that begins the SuDocs number signifies the publishing agency, as noted below:

A       Agriculture Department
C       Census Bureau
D       Department of Defense
E       Department of Energy
HE      Health and Human Services
X–Y     Congress

Government documents contain a storehouse of valuable and current information and should not be overlooked when seeking information on a health topic of interest. Most libraries have online search capabilities for government documents, so,

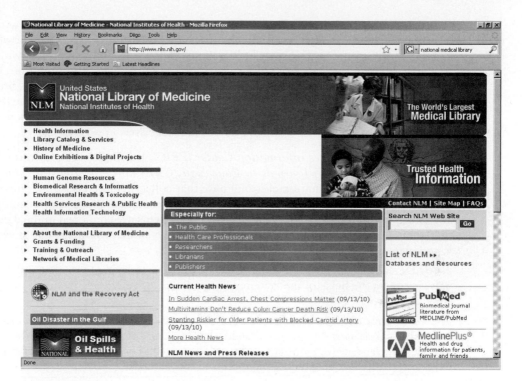

**Figure 9.3** Electronic databases such as the National Library of Medicine (NLM) provide ready access to information on a particular topic.

*Source:* The National Library of Medicine, National Institutes of Health. http://www.nlm.nih.gov.

as with many traditional sources of information, accessing them has become much less labor intensive.

## Electronic Databases

**Electronic databases** often provide a preferred alternative to manually searching indexes or abstracts (see **Figure 9.3**). As mentioned earlier, most, if not all, of the publishers of the hard-copy abstracts and indexes either have converted or are converting their documents to an online format. Much like an index or abstract, each database has a general subject area (e.g., medicine, education, psychology, community health). The electronic database provides access via the Internet. Computer searches using databases are significantly faster than manual searches, and they have the advantage of enabling the user to link several concepts together to provide focus for a search.

For example, if a person wanted to search for articles about "health behavior" and the influence of "health communication" on behavior, an electronic database would allow the user to enter both terms into the computer and connect them by placing the word *"and"* between them. The result will be to eliminate any articles that do not have both "health behavior" and "health communication" as key terms. Other terms can be used to further narrow a search to be as specific as desired. The main concern the computer database user faces is to accurately specify the key terms associated with the information desired, so the resulting list of references that is generated will be of use. Computerized searches require very little computer knowledge; however, it is always advisable to seek the assistance of a librarian when beginning to seek information. Users should also know that just because the information is readily available online, it is not free. Academic libraries spend thousands of dollars per year to ensure that students and faculty have access to the materials they need using such an expeditious methodology. The databases most used by health education specialists are:

1. *Educational Resources Information Center (ERIC).* It includes the previously mentioned *Current Index to Journals in Education (CIJE)* and *Resources in Education* (RIE). ERIC is an information clearinghouse that collects, sorts, classifies, and stores thousands of documents on topics pertaining to education and allied fields of study. An advantage to using ERIC is that many types of documents are contained in the database that are not journal articles—for example, proceedings of meetings, teaching strategies, lesson plans, commentaries, and policy documents.

2. *MEDLINE.* This is the premier biomedicine database indexing more than 3,000 journals. It covers the fields of medicine, nursing, dentistry, veterinary medicine, and preclinical sciences.

3. *ScienceDirect.* This is one of the largest full-text scientific databases in the world covering physical sciences, life sciences, health sciences, and engineering material. It indexes over 2,500 peer-reviewed journals and more than 11,000 books. Over 9.5 million journal articles and book chapters are contained in this database.

4. *Cumulative Index to Nursing and Allied Health Literature (CINAHL).* It contains more than 300,000 citations from 1983 until the present. It references journal articles and book chapters, pamphlets, audiovisuals, educational software, and conference proceedings in the areas of nursing, health education, health services, and health care administration.

5. *ETHXWeb.* This database covers ethical, legal, and public policy issues surrounding health care and biomedical research. Citations are derived from the literature of law, religion, ethics, social sciences, philosophy, the popular media, and the health sciences.

6. *Psychological Abstracts (PsycInfo).* This database is the analog of *Psychological Abstracts* in computerized form. As with all computer databases, narrowing a search to a specific topic can be accomplished more easily using *PsycInfo*.

7. *Ovid Healthstar.* Ovid Healthstar includes data from the National Library of Medicine's (NLM) MEDLINE and former HealthSTAR databases. As such, it contains citations of the published literature in health services, technology, administration, health policy, health economics, and research. It focuses on both the clinical and nonclinical aspects of health care delivery.

8. *PubMed.* A service of the National Library of Medicine that contains more than 17 million citations from MEDLINE and other life science journals for biomedical articles dating back over a half century. The database includes links to full text articles and other related resources.

9. *Physical Education Index.* This database includes references to more than 400 periodicals on physical education, health education, dance, physical therapy, and sports medicine.

# The Internet and the World Wide Web

Until a few years ago, it was possible only to dream about the day when health information would be readily available at home or at the office at the "touch of a button." Today, of course, that dream is a reality through the use of the Internet and the World Wide Web. The **World Wide Web** is an interactive information delivery service that includes a repository of resources about almost any subject imaginable. On the Web, documents that are related by subject area or place of origin are linked to each other, thus creating a web, or network, of materials. The Web relies mainly on **hypertext** as its means of interaction with users. Hypertext is nearly the same as regular text in that it can be searched, edited, and stored, but hypertext contains connections within the text to documents (in the form of printed matter, pictures, graphics, and/or sound) found on computers connected to each other around the globe. This integrated network of computers is known as the **Internet.**

In order to use the Web, a person must have access to a **browser.** The browser is a software package that can be installed on any computer with a graphical interface and can greatly simplify the ability to access information on the Web. Examples of commonly available browsers include Mozilla Firefox and Internet Explorer. Use of the browser involves entering a Web address, which usually starts with the characters "http://" (http stands for **hypertext transfer protocol**). Web addresses are known as URLs, or **Uniform Resource Locators (URL),** which are unique identifiers for a location on the global Internet much as the mailing address of your home is unique to where you live. The URL is composed of the Internet access protocol, the location, and the file—for example, "http://www.cdc.gov/mmwr/" is the URL for the **home page** of the CDC publication *Morbidity and Mortality Weekly Report* (MMWR). A home page is analogous to a combination of a cover and a table of contents in a book in that it names the site and directs the user to a list of information options available within the site. In the example, the "http://" is the Internet access protocol; the "www.cdc.gov" is the location; and "mmwr/" is the file.

Assume you are looking for the times, dates, and locations of some training sessions on certain aspects of health promotion that will be conducted by the Centers for Disease Control and Prevention (CDC). In order to find the information at the CDC Web site, you might open the Internet Explorer (or Mozilla Foxfire) browser by double-clicking on its icon on your computer desktop. Once the browser opens, you can get to the desired Web page in one of the following two ways:

- Place the cursor on the column labeled "File" at the top left-hand side of the screen. Click and hold down the mouse to reveal the menu that cascades down below "File." Move the cursor to "Open" and release. A dialogue box will appear on the screen that asks you to type in the address (URL) of the location you are seeking.

- You may also type the desired Web address (URL) into the horizontal space located at the top of your screen that displays the current URL.

In either case, type in "http://www.cdc.gov" (the URL of the Centers for Disease Control and Prevention), and the home page of the CDC will appear (as shown in **Figure 9.4**).

On the home page will be some buttons to click to find the information you are looking for. In addition, any blue wording on an organization's home page can be double-clicked with the mouse, and information related to the word or phrase that is

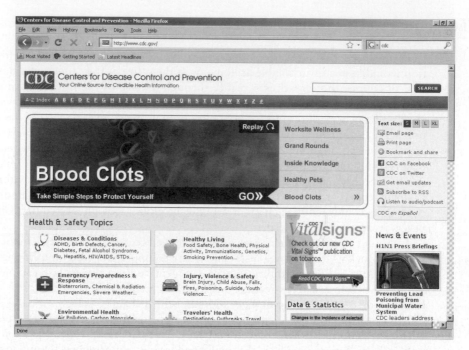

**Figure 9.4** Home page of the Centers for Disease Control and Prevention as found on the Internet

*Source:* Centers for Disease Control and Prevention. http://www.cdc.gov.

clicked will be provided. The blue wording denotes a topic or name that has been linked to another site to help the user access additional information about that topic.

Another method for locating information on the Internet involves using a **search engine.** Various search engines are available (e.g., Google, Yahoo, Bing, Ask, AOL Search, and Googlescholar). The advantage of using a search engine over typing in a URL (which is specific to one site) is that the search engine allows you to type in the name of the topic you want to find information about, and after a few seconds it identifies and lists several sites related to that topic. All the user needs to do to access the information from any of the listed sites is to click the pointer on the name of the site and it will appear. The search engines are usually located on the main search page of the browser or may be accessed by typing in their URL.

An example of the page for the Bing search engine can be found in **Figure 9.5**. Note that in this example the topic being searched for is "methamphetamine." After entering that phrase in the search box and clicking on "search" or pressing the Enter key on the keyboard, a list of sites related to "methamphetamine" will appear (see **Figure 9.6**). Click on any of the sites, and you will be transported to the page and information corresponding to that site.

Sometimes you may want to use a specific search engine. Because all of the search engines have nearly the same URL, the home page for any of the search engines can be readily accessed by typing in the specific Web address (URL) from the Internet Explorer "File" menu, as was demonstrated in the example using the Centers for Disease Control. For example, the URL for the Google search engine is http://www.google.com; for Yahoo, it is http://www.yahoo.com; and for Bing, it is http://www.bing.com. If the term

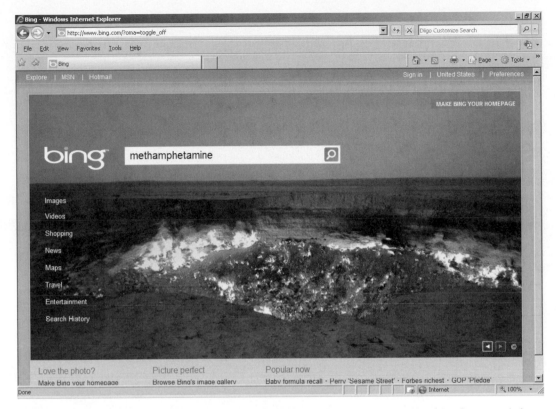

**Figure 9.5** Bing search engine page with "methamphetamine" entered in the search box

*Source:* Bing™ screenshot for search term "methamphetamine." © 2010 Microsoft. Used with permission from Microsoft.

you are searching for has more than one word (such as "sexually transmitted infections"), it is wise to use quotation marks around the term when it is entered into the box marked "search." This will let the search engine know that the exact phrase, as contained in the quotation marks, is to be used when seeking sites that match. If the quotation marks are not used, the search engine will find sites that contain all of the words in the query. However, at least some of the sites might not be relevant to the topic of interest (sexually transmitted infections in this case) since the words can appear in any order and at any place on the sites searched.

## Evaluating Information on the Internet

Earlier in the chapter, directions were given for evaluating the accuracy and validity of information from journal and popular press sources. Because of the massive amount of information available on the Internet and because nearly anyone who has a knowledge of HTML (**hypertext markup language,** the programming language used on the Internet) can publish on the World Wide Web, it is equally imperative that the health education specialist know how to evaluate information obtained via an Internet search. Kotecki and Chamness (1999) published an excellent article in the *Journal of Health Education* that featured a tool for evaluating a health-related Internet site. The information included in their

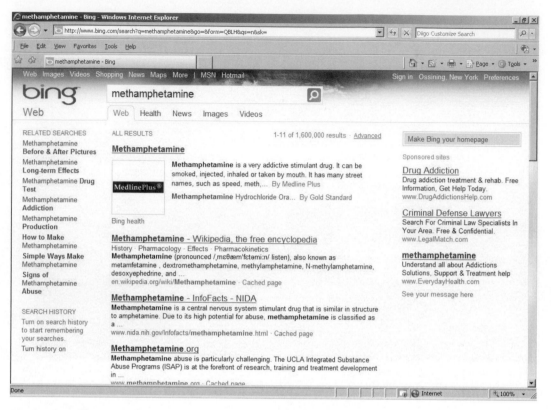

**Figure 9.6** Bing search results page with site matches to the search query for the term "methamphetamine"

*Source:* Bing™ screenshot for search results for "methamphetamine." © 2010 Microsoft. Used with permission from Microsoft.

article corresponds closely with that provided by T. J. Madden (personal communication, Albertson Library, Boise State University, August 2010), a reference specialist in the Albertson Library at Boise State University, and D. Britigan (personal communication, e-mail, April 2007), a librarian and doctoral student at the University of Cincinnati. These expert sources mention that the most important areas to consider when evaluating information retrieved on the Internet are:

1. *Content.* Material included has been verified or has survived a minimal screening or refereeing process. Sources are cited. Frequently, the addresses end in ".edu," ".gov," or ".org" if from a known professional organization.

2. *Authority.* The credentials of the authors are clearly presented. The authors' e-mail addresses and/or phone numbers are provided for contact.

3. *Publisher source.* This information should be unambiguous and clearly identifiable. It should be readily apparent who is sponsoring or otherwise representing the page. Care should be taken to determine whether the source originates from an advocacy group. If that is the case, make certain to check the facts against other sources (see criterion 6 below).

4. *References.* Have other pages used this site as a link to their own page?

5. *Documentation.* Documentation is consistently provided. The sources are important, because a source that lacks documentation often falls in the opinion or editorial category.

6. *Facts.* Are the facts consistent with information obtained from other sources? Be cautious of sites that have an address ending in ".com" as they are commercial sites and may be selling a product.

7. *Date of authorship or posting.* Be certain that the information obtained is as current as possible. Many Web sites and links are no longer upgraded, but the information on them might live indefinitely online if someone does not remove the site from the Internet or the site URL remains active.

## SUMMARY

This chapter has presented an overview on accessing and evaluating health-related information. An increasing demand for health information, coupled with the fact that the information is being produced at an ever greater rate, creates added responsibility for health education specialists. Two of the major roles of health education specialists as discussed in Chapter 6 involve being resource people for health information and communicating to others about health education/promotion needs, concerns, and resources. In order to perform these tasks, the health education specialist must have the skills to find information, must evaluate the source of the information to determine its credibility, and must disseminate the information through the appropriate channels to consumers. In addition, the health education specialist must be able to explain the information effectively. Becoming familiar with the tools found in this chapter is a necessity for all students wanting to enter the field of health education/promotion.

## REVIEW QUESTIONS

1. Describe the difference between primary, secondary, tertiary, and popular press sources.

2. How do an article abstract and an article summary differ in content?

3. What are the questions you should ask yourself when critiquing a journal article? What are the differences between the questions asked when evaluating a primary research article and those asked when evaluating a secondary source or popular press article?

4. What are five of the most commonly used journals in the field of health education/promotion? What types of information would you expect to find in each of the journals you named?

5. What advantage might the information from a government document have over another source on the same topic?

6. How does one go about evaluating information retrieved from the Internet?

7. In your own words, describe how to access information concerning "breast cancer" on the Internet. Try using at least two different search engines and compare the results.

## CASE STUDY

As a health education/promotion major, you have just finished studying about the Responsibilities and Competencies for Entry-Level Health Education Specialists (found in Appendix B of this text). During this unit the instructor invited a group of practicing health education specialists to the class to participate in a panel discussion on the validity of the various roles in the real-life practice of health education/promotion.

Following the presentation, each of the panelists offered to host two to three students from the class for four hours per week for three weeks at her/his place of work. This opportunity resulted from student questions to the panelists concerning their desire to transfer the classroom learning to the work setting. Several of the students expressed frustration at what they perceived to be the emphasis on theory and the lack of application in their courses and coursework. The panelists readily conceded that the twelve-hour block of time each student would spend at the worksite with them would not totally solve theory-practical application problems, but they hoped it might help the students to see that, at least in the case of the majority of the responsibilities and competencies, what they studied about in class was what the health education specialist was doing.

After a quick meeting between the instructor and the panel members, placement assignments were made for the students. Because of your interest in becoming a health education specialist in a clinical setting, you were assigned to a community health clinic to shadow a physician to see what kind of health education is given to patients.

On your first day, the physician to whom you are assigned requests that you accompany her into the examination room as she sees patients. During the first two hours, she sees three patients for colds/influenza, two patients for hypertension, one patient for emphysema, one patient for diabetes, one for a broken hand, and two teenage patients for sports physicals. After these appointments, she takes some time to visit with you and discuss your initial perceptions. During the conversation, she asks if you are aware of any good health education/promotion information sites for teens on the Internet. You promise to do some research on this question and bring the information on your next visit. What information do you think would be of benefit to teens? Which two or three sites would you recommend and why?

## CRITICAL THINKING QUESTIONS

1. Assume that all information about any topic is available on the Web. If that were true, would there be any need for health education specialists? Defend your answer.

2. Make a list of the five greatest advantages and the five greatest disadvantages of the Internet from your perspective. Assuming that your list reflects universal truths about the Internet, how might you persuade a noncomputer user to adopt computer use?

3. How does the availability of so much material online affect the use of a library?

4. Several health agencies have begun conducting workshops online designed to help practicing health professionals update their skills. Is there a type of health professional that this training would best suit? Provide a rationale for your answer.

5. If the Internet had been developed in the early 1900s, how might the U.S. health care system and the role of health education specialists differ from what they are today?

## ACTIVITIES

1. You are employed as a health education specialist in a district health department and have just received a call from a member of a local coalition wanting to know where to find some peer-reviewed studies that summarize the content and effectiveness of available school-based sexuality education curricula. Use an index to find a reference to an article that meets those criteria.

2. Was the article you located in activity #1 a primary or secondary source of information? Provide a rationale for your answer.

3. Using a database (CINAHL, MEDLINE, or ERIC), find a primary research article relating to traffic safety (e.g., the use of seat belts, air bags, road surfaces). Critique the article by applying the questions found in the "Critically Reading a Research Article" section of this chapter.

4. As a newly employed health education specialist in a hospital outpatient clinic, one of your jobs is to provide information to patients after they have seen the physician. Ms. X has just been diagnosed with coronary artery disease, and the physician has sent her to you to discuss the impact of lifestyle on her condition. Using the Internet, find several sources of information that you could give her to read that might assist you with the education process. Evaluate the accuracy of the information you retrieve.

5. Make a list of the health education journals described in this chapter that are available at your college/university library. For those journals not in your library's holdings, check with a librarian to determine if they are available through an online database, interlibrary loan, or some other exchange service.

## WEBLINKS

### EPIDEMIOLOGICAL AND STATISTICAL INFORMATION

1. CDC WONDER

   http://wonder.cdc.gov

   Wide-ranging online data for epidemiologic research—an easy-to-use, menu-driven system that makes the information resources of the Centers for Disease Control and Prevention (CDC) available to public health professionals and the public at large. It provides access to a wide array of public health information.

2. National Center for Health Statistics

http://www.cdc.gov/nchs/

NCHS is the nation's principal health statistics agency. Their Web site offers access to an extensive collection of health statistics intended to guide those working to improve public health.

3. Morbidity and Mortality Weekly Report (MMWR)

http://www.cdc.gov/mmwr/

MMWR is a weekly report prepared by the Centers for Disease Control and Prevention. State Health Departments report their findings to MMWR. The site offers access to studies and reports, and also provides useful information on a wide range of diseases.

4. U.S. Bureau of the Census

http://www.census.gov

The Web site of the U.S. Census Bureau allows the user to access specific data for his or her state, county, or city. View results from Census 2000 (and soon Census 2010) and access analytical reports on population change, race, age, family structure, and more.

## INFECTIOUS DISEASES

5. Centers for Disease Control and Prevention—Data and Statistics

http://www.cdc.gov/DataStatistics/

With the mission of preventing illness, disability, and death, the CDC conducts epidemic investigations, laboratory research, and public education programs to attempt to prevent and control diseases and disorders of all types.

## CHRONIC DISEASES

6. CDC Chronic Disease Prevention and Health Promotion

http://www.cdc.gov/chronicdisease/index.htm

This section of the CDC is dedicated to chronic diseases and provides links to a variety of helpful sites, including a diabetes public health resource and sites discussing heart disease, nutrition, and physical activity.

7. National Cancer Institute

http://www.nci.nih.gov/

The National Cancer Institute's Web site covers information on a variety of cancer topics, discussing treatment, prevention, research, and much more. The NCI supports prevention and treatment of cancer, rehabilitation, and continued care of cancer patients and their families.

8. American Diabetes Association

http://www.diabetes.org

The ADA provides diabetes research, scientific findings, information, and advocacy. The site contains helpful information for people with diabetes, their families, health professionals, and the public.

## DISEASE CONTROL AND PREVENTION

9. Substance Abuse and Mental Health Services Administration

   http://store.samhsa.gov/home

   This site features links to ordering government materials online that focus on professional and research topics, issues in the field of treatment, prevention, and recovery, and information on conditions and disorders.

10. Center for Substance Abuse Prevention (CSAP)

    http://prevention.samhsa.gov/

    CSAP is funded by the Substance Abuse and Mental Health Services Administration (SAMHSA) and is responsible for improving the access to and quality of substance abuse prevention services to the public. CSAP provides national leadership in the development of policies, programs, and services to prevent the onset of illegal drug use and underage alcohol and tobacco use, and to reduce the negative consequences of using substances.

11. Office of National Drug Control Policy (ONDCP)

    http://www.whitehousedrugpolicy.gov

    With the goal of reducing illicit drug use, substance abuse-related crimes, drug trafficking, and drug-related health problems, the ONDCP is working to establish a national strategy to fight these dilemmas. The site contains national priorities, annual reports, and a tremendous amount of drug information.

12. CDC's Division of HIV/AIDS Prevention

    http://www.cdc.gov/hiv/aboutDHAP.htm

    With a mission to prevent HIV infection and reduce the incidence of HIV-related illness, the CDC's Division of HIV/AIDS Prevention Web site provides useful information for those working in the health field. The site includes such topics as prevention tools, research, brochures, and fact sheets.

13. Medical Matrix

    http://www.medmatrix.org

    Medical Matrix is a peer-reviewed site that offers continually updated clinical medicine resources. The information is organized in such a way as to make searching for information more timely and efficient. Over 6,000 medical Web sites are listed.

14. Children's Safety Network

    http://www.childrenssafetynetwork.org

    The Children's Safety Network, funded by the Maternal & Child Health Bureau and the U.S. Department of Health and Human Services, provides technical assistance, training, and resources to MCH and other injury prevention professionals in an extensive effort to reduce the burden of injury and violence to our nation's children.

15. **Food and Drug Administration**

    http://www.fda.gov/Food/default.htm

    This site not only outlines national programs intended to increase food safety awareness, but it also contains information concerning the laws enforced by the FDA and provides helpful tips on preventing food-related illness.

16. **OncoLink**

    http://oncolink.com

    OncoLink, provided by the Abramson Cancer Center of the University of Pennsylvania, is the Web's first cancer resource. The site provides up-to-date cancer news and research. Locate information on the causes of cancer, screening and prevention, clinical trials, and other resources on cancer.

17. **Travelers' Health**

    http://www.cdc.gov/travel/

    Locate health information for specific destinations, stay up to date on outbreaks throughout the world, and learn how to avoid illness from food and water.

18. **CDC's Division of Tuberculosis Elimination**

    http://www.cdc.gov/tb/

    With the mission of "preventing, controlling and eventually eliminating tuberculosis from the United States," the Web site of the CDC's Division of Tuberculosis Elimination contains useful information to aid that mission. Learn all there is to know about TB, locate statistics on the occurrence of TB, and obtain education and training materials on TB.

19. **National Women's Health Information Center**

    http://www.4women.gov

    The National Women's Health Information Center, sponsored by the Department of Health and Human Services Office on Women's Health, provides health information for women across the country. It offers information on heart disease, body image, breastfeeding, screening and immunization schedules, and more.

20. **Men's Health Network**

    http://www.menshealthnetwork.org

    The Men's Health Network is an informational and educational organization recognizing men's health as a specific social concern.

21. **KidsHealth**

    http://www.kidshealth.org/

    KidsHealth is the largest and most visited site on the Web, providing doctor-approved health information about children from before birth through adolescence. Created by The Nemours Foundation's Center for Children's Health Media, the award-winning KidsHealth provides families with accurate, up-to-date, and jargon-free health information they can use.

22. **National Safety Council**

    http://www.nsc.org/

    The National Safety Council is focused on providing safety and health information in order to reduce the number of injuries and deaths from preventable accidents. Their Web site contains information on new policies and laws enacted to prevent unintentional injuries. It also provides statistics and helpful tips regarding this health topic.

23. **Community Tool Box**

    http://ctb.ku.edu

    The goal of the Community Tool Box is to support work in community health promotion and development. The Tool Box provides multiple pages of practical skill-building information on over 250 different topics related to community development. Topic sections include step-by-step instruction, examples, checklists, and related resources.

## NATIONAL AGENCIES

24. **CDC—Centers for Disease Control and Prevention**

    http://www.cdc.gov

    The Centers for Disease Control and Prevention is recognized as the leading federal agency for protecting the health and safety of the public, providing credible information to enhance health decisions and promote health. The Web site of the CDC includes a variety of helpful health and safety topics. The information covers everything from health promotion to vaccines to traveler's health. Data, statistics, publications, and products are also available.

25. **USDHHS—Department of Health and Human Services**

    http://www.hhs.gov

    The Department of Health and Human Services is the U.S. government's principal agency for health protection and the provision of human services. Its site is divided into health topics such as Safety & Wellness, Diseases & Conditions, and Families & Children. Readers can also use the Resource Locator and Reference Collections to find such things as health care facilities and publications.

26. **EPA—Environmental Protection Agency**

    http://www.epa.gov

    The EPA is focused on protecting human health and the environment by working for a cleaner, healthier environment. The site provides air quality reports, current environmental news stories, and tips on how the public can make the environment healthier. The QuickFinder allows fast and easy access to a variety of environmental topics.

27. **IHS—Indian Health Service**

    http://www.ihs.gov/

    Indian Health Service is the Federal Health Program for American Indians and Alaska Natives. IHS is focused on improving the health of these groups while attempting to ensure they have access to culturally acceptable health services.

28. **American Medical Association**

    http://www.ama-assn.org

    This Web site is divided into a section for physicians and medical students and a section for patients. The patient section allows the user to search for a doctor and obtain health information and resources. The physician section provides information on such topics as medical education, legal issues, and advocacy.

29. **National Institutes of Health (NIH)**

    http://www.nih.gov

    The Web site of the National Institutes of Health is loaded with a wide variety of great health information. It contains an A–Z index of health resources, a wealth of grant information, and a section dedicated to scientific resources.

30. **National Library of Medicine (NLM)**

    http://www.nlm.nih.gov/

    The Web site of the National Library of Medicine—part of the National Institute of Health. Excellent central source of current information on results of health research for the lay person, the practicing health professional, the health researcher, and health librarians. Updated daily.

## INTERNATIONAL AGENCIES

31. **WHO—World Health Organization**

    http://www.who.int/en

    The Web site of the World Health Organization is an incredible resource. The site includes a tremendous listing of pages, organized by health and development topics, that contain links to WHO projects, initiatives, activities, information products, and contacts.

32. **PAHO—Pan American Health Organization**

    http://www.paho.org

    The Pan American Health Organization, affiliated with the World Health Organization, focuses on a multitude of public health topics, with the mission of promoting health in the Americas.

## WEB-BASED MEDLINE SEARCH SYSTEMS

33. **PubMed**

    http://www.pubMed.gov/

    PubMed is a service of the National Library of Medicine. It includes literally millions of citations for biomedical articles going back to the 1950s. The citations are from MEDLINE and additional life science journals. PubMed includes links to many sites providing full-text articles and other related resources.

34. **Medscape from WebMD (free access to MEDLINE)**

    http://www.medscape.com/px/urlinfo

    Medscape allows the user to register for free access to MEDLINE, CME courses, medical journals, medical news, and more. Medline's database of medical abstracts may be searched by title or author.

35. National Library of Medicine

    http://www.nlm.nih.gov

    The National Library of Medicine (NLM), on the campus of the National Institutes of Health in Bethesda, Maryland, is the world's largest medical library. The Library collects materials and provides information and research services in all areas of biomedicine and health care.

36. MFedlinePlus

    http://medlineplus.gov

    Health professionals and the general public alike can easily access information on MedlinePlus that is accurate and up to date. MedlinePlus has extensive information from the National Institutes of Health and other trusted sources on over 650 diseases and conditions.

## PUBLIC HEALTH PRACTICE

37. Office of State, Tribal, Local and Territorial Support (CDC)

    http://www.cdc.gov/ostlts/index.htm

    This office resulted from a reorganization at the Centers for Disease Control and Prevention. The priority of the OSTLTS is to improve the capacity and performance of the public health system at all levels. The office works both within CDC and in the field to identify gaps, opportunities for collaboration, and the strategies needed to support growth and enhancement of public health work.

38. American Public Health Association

    http://www.apha.org

    The APHA is the world's largest and oldest organization of public health professionals. Useful sections include Continuing Education, Newsroom, and Science and Programs.

## STATE AND LOCAL PUBLIC HEALTH DEPARTMENTS

39. Association of State and Territorial Health Officials (ASTHO)

    http://www.astho.org/

    ASTHO is the national nonprofit organization representing the public health agencies of the United States, the U.S. Territories, and the District of Columbia, as well as the 120,000 public health professionals these agencies employ. ASTHO members, the chief health officials of these jurisdictions, are dedicated to formulating and influencing sound public health policy and to assuring excellence in state-based public health practice.

40. Health Resource Guide USA

    http://www.healthguideusa.com/index.htm

    Health Guide USA provides quick reference to a tremendous listing of health care–related resources throughout the United States. It provides locations of state and local health departments, as well as medical schools and medical licenses.

## GENERAL HEALTH INFORMATION

41. Bing

    http://www.bing.com

    Bing is an excellent keyword search engine and features videos, maps, and travel as well as desired information. With advanced settings and helpful tools, users can refine their searches and quickly access the most pertinent and useful health information.

42. Google

    http://www.google.com

    Google's keyword search engine is pop-up free and a great tool for finding anything on the Web. Visit "Google Help Central" to locate advice on advanced searches, access the Web Search Features, and check out the Google Services and Tools.

43. myOptumHealth.com

    http://www.myoptumhealth.com/portal

    Provides MD-reviewed information on a variety of health topics. The information is easy to understand and can be utilized by a health education specialist to research background information related to all aspects of health.

44. WebMD

    http://www.WebMD.com

    Site devoted to providing current and relevant consumer health information on a variety of topics. Medical facts are reviewed by physicians prior to posting.

45. Yahoo! Health

    http://www.yahoo.com/Health/

    Get in-depth coverage on a variety of health issues, including a directory of the most popular Web sites related to a particular health topic.

46. Mayo Clinic

    http://www.mayoclinic.com

    The Mayo Clinic offers a wealth of health information developed and reviewed by more than 2,000 physicians and scientists. The site also allows access to healthy living tools, such as a personal health card, and a first-aid and self-care guide.

47. Cal Berkeley Wellness Letter

    http://www.berkeleywellness.com

    The Wellness Letter relies on the expertise of the School of Public Health and other researchers at UC Berkeley, as well as other top scientists from around the world. It translates this leading-edge research into practical advice for daily living—at home, at work, while exercising, and in the market or health-food store.

48. Healthfinder®

    http://www.healthfinder.gov

    Healthfinder, developed by the Department of Health and Human Services, directs the user to various health resources depending on his or her needs. Resources include such things as online publications, clearinghouses, support groups, government agencies, and Web sites.

49. **NOAH: New York Online Access to Health (Bilingual Site)**

http://www.noah-health.org

NOAH provides access to full-text consumer health information in English and Spanish. From its list of a multitude of health topics and its comprehensive subject index, the user can easily obtain information of interest.

50. **USA.gov-Health**

http://www.usa.gov/Citizen/Topics/Health.shtml

The Health and Nutrition section of the U.S. Government's Official Web portal is filled with great health information. The Healthfinder link enables access to the "personal health tools" link, which features tools for calculating BMI and taking an online checkup. The site also features health topics for population groups and helps the user locate health services in his or her area.

51. **GrantProposal.com**

http://www.grantproposal.com

GrantProposal.com provides free resources for both advanced grant-writing consultants and inexperienced nonprofit staff. Many "helpful hints" are included that are proven to bring positive results in obtaining grants.

52. **Go Ask Alice!**

http://www.goaskalice.columbia.edu/

Go Ask Alice's Q&A database houses numerous health-related questions and answers. It is produced by Columbia University's Health Education Program.

53. **National Health Information Center**

http://www.health.gov/nhic

The National Health Information Center (NHIC) is a health information referral service. NHIC puts health professionals and consumers who have health questions in touch with organizations that are best able to provide answers.

## NEWS STORIES

54. **Reuters Health Products and Services**

http://www.reutershealth.com

Reuters is the premier supplier of health and medical news on the Internet. The Health eLine is a wonderful section for the general public.

55. **USA Today Health**

http://www.usatoday.com/news/health/default.htm

This section of *USA Today* provides some of the most current news stories related to health.

56. MedlinePlus—Health News by Date

    http://www.nlm.nih.gov/medlineplus/newsbydate.html

    The news section of MedlinePlus provides current health-related articles from the past 30 days from the New York Times Syndicate, Reuters Health Information, and others.

## HEALTH EDUCATION/HEALTH PROMOTION JOBS

57. HPCareer.Net

    http://www.hpcareer.net

    This is the official career resource site for the American Kinesiotherapy Association (AKTA), the Medical-Fitness Association (MFA), and the National Commission for Health Education Credentialing (NCHEC).

58. Rollins School of Public Health at Emory—Career Action Center

    http://www.sph.emory.edu/studentservice/career.html

    Includes sections entitled Public Health Employment Connection and Public Health Candidate Connection. Career Action Tip Sheets are also available.

59. American Alliance for Health, Physical Education, Recreation, and Dance (AAHPERD) CareerLink

    http://www.aahperd.org/careers/CareerLink.cfm

    CareerLink is AAHPERD's chief online employment resource for health and physical education, recreation, dance, and sport professionals. The site has sections meant for the job seeker and the employer.

## HEALTH POLICY

60. National Academy for State Health Policy

    http://www.nashp.org

    The National Academy for State Health Policy conducts policy analysis; provides training and technical assistance to states; produces informational resources; and convenes state, regional, and national forums. This site enables the user to access these services and the results of policy studies that have been completed.

61. The Heritage Foundation

    http://www.heritage.org

    This site provides access to well-written and well-documented health policy research and analysis papers in which the conclusions often reflect a more conservative perspective.

62. The Robert Wood Johnson Foundation

    http://rwjf.org/index.jsp

    The Robert Wood Johnson Foundation has a goal of funding projects that improve the health and health care of all Americans. This site features many of the foundation's policy papers, current and future studies, and projects that the foundation is or will consider funding. The organization is considered nonpartisan.

63. **The Henry J. Kaiser Family Foundation**

    http://kff.org/

    The Henry J. Kaiser Family Foundation is a nonprofit, privately operating foundation focusing on the major health care issues facing the nation. The foundation is an independent voice and source of facts and analysis for policy makers, the media, the health care community, and the general public.

64. **The Commonwealth Fund**

    http://www.commonwealthfund.org/

    This site contains policy briefs and full-text health policy papers that are well written and well documented and are often from a more liberal perspective.

65. **State Coverage Initiatives**

    http://www.statecoverage.org/

    The State Coverage Initiatives (SCI) program is a national initiative of The Robert Wood Johnson Foundation that works with states to plan, execute, and maintain health insurance expansions, as well as to improve the availability and affordability of health care coverage. The site includes the results of many states' initiatives to increase health insurance coverage for their residents.

## GENERAL

66. **Find articles**

    http://findarticles.com/p/articles/tn_health

    Provides free access to millions of articles from many top publications.

67. **Google Scholar**

    http://www.scholar.google.com

    This site provides another alternative to search through scholarly literature across many disciplines and sources, including theses, books, abstracts, and articles.

## REFERENCES

Cottrell, R. R. (1997). *A guide to evaluating a journal article.* Unpublished manuscript.

Kotecki, J. E., & Chamness, B. E. (1999). A valid tool for evaluating health-related WWW websites. *Journal of Health Education, 30* (1), 56–59.

Normand, M. P., & Osborne, M. R. (2010). Promoting healthier food choices in college students using individualized dietary feedback. *Behavioral Interventions, 25,* 183–190.

Riegelman, R. K. (2005). *Studying a study and testing a test: How to read medical literature* (5th ed.). Philadelphia, PA: Lippincott, Williams, & Wilkins.

University of Akron. (2010). *How to access government documents.* Retrieved on August 26, 2010, from http://www3.uakron.edu/ul/instruct/govdocs-access.html

## CHAPTER 10

# Future Trends in Health Education/Promotion

## CHAPTER OBJECTIVES

After reading this chapter and answering the questions at the end, you should be able to:

- Identify two settings in which health education specialists will practice in the next five years to a greater degree than they do today.
- Describe four major societal changes that will influence the practice of health education/ promotion this century.
- Explain how demographic changes in the United States will impact health education/ promotion delivery into the future.
- Delineate the major implications of credentialing for future health education specialists.
- Compare and contrast the roles of health education specialists in the four practice settings.
- Identify several reasons that health education specialists should be optimistic about future employment opportunities.
- Evaluate the role of the health education specialist in addressing the increasing costs of health care.

It is said that one of the few constants in life is change. Societal trends are having an increasing impact on the profession of health education/promotion. Health seems to be the current concern of the populace in the United States. With increasing numbers of citizens interested in health information, spiraling health care costs, a reliance on technology for information delivery and acquisition, rapidly changing demographic patterns, a heightened skepticism of the medical establishment, the passage of the Affordable Care Act (recent health care reform legislation), and a more interconnected world, the environment that will confront health education specialists in the future is vastly different from that of only a decade ago. These changes present the health education specialist with enormous opportunities. The focus of this chapter is to explore future developments in the discipline of health education/promotion and, we hope, to create a sense of excitement and anticipation about the challenges that lie ahead.

Imagine that you have just arrived in the United States from another planet. The year is 1980. Assume that the first thing you see is a one-hour television news program. Based solely on that program and the commercial messages during the station breaks, how would you describe the lives of people on the planet you are visiting? Now, transport yourself ahead to today and repeat the exercise. Although it is not the purpose of this chapter to dwell on comparative history, it is noteworthy that, in a brief, thirty-plus year span, the United States and many other countries have changed so dramatically as to be almost unrecognizable. Certainly, some of the problems faced by individuals, communities, and local, state, and federal governments are the same and the dress styles and modes of transportation have not changed much, but demographic and societal changes, some subtle and others not so subtle, have altered the landscape forever. Several of the aforementioned changes have profound implications for the way health education/promotion will be practiced as the twenty-first century enters its second decade.

The first section of this chapter discusses changing demographic patterns. Societal trends that are predicted to play a role in the practice of health education/promotion in future decades will be featured. Issues related to credentialing and preparation will be covered next. Using this information as a foundation, the chapter concludes by postulating about the impact of these changes for the health education specialist in the school, public health, worksite, and medical care settings. One caveat is in order prior to this discussion: Obviously, no one knows exactly what the future will hold. The information presented is meant to stimulate thinking about the role health education specialists will play from now until the years 2020–2030.

## Demographic Changes

Over the past thirty years, the population growth rate in the United States has increased at about 1 percent per year. Although this stable growth pattern is probably manageable for the long term, a more in-depth study of the **demographic profile**, the breakdown of the U.S. population by age group, sex, race, and ethnicity, shows a dramatically altered picture from that of just ten years ago. This consistently changing demographic profile—specifically, a greater percentage of minority residents and an ever aging population—has important implications for the future practice of health education specialists (see **Figure 10.1**).

### Minority Population Changes

Clark's (1994) comments, written midway through the last decade of the twentieth century, remain cogent today. She states, "We are undergoing a massive change in culture in our society. We are literally looking different as a nation and the conventional majority values and norms are being challenged as we become a more diverse, more ethnic, more integrated culture. Health educators have long prided themselves with working across cultures . . . The cultural changes are . . . greater than we have experienced previously" (p. 137).

It seems that the increased racial and ethnic diversity in the United States has several major causes. In the 1800s and early to mid-1900s, the bulk of immigrants to the United States came from Western Europe. Hale (2000) mentions that worsening economic conditions in Mexico and Central America over the past decade are largely

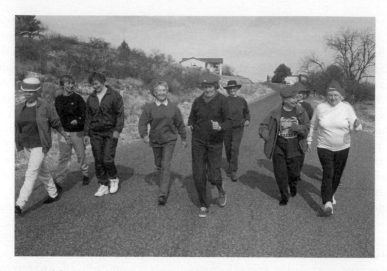

**Figure 10.1** Health promotion for the elderly will be in increasing demand in the next century.

Chad Ehlers/Photolibrary

responsible for the large number of immigrants from those areas. Gheisar and Clark (2000) write that the refugee populations streaming to America from war-ravaged regions of Asia, Africa, and Eastern Europe are presenting new challenges (and opportunities) for the public health community. This wave of new immigration, coupled with the fact that, regardless of country of origin, immigrants have higher rates of fertility than native-born peoples, means that the shifts in culture and the challenges to majority norms alluded to by Clark are likely here to stay.

Statistics from the U.S. Bureau of the Census (2010) indicate that in 2008 the U.S. minority population was 12.3 percent African American, 15.1 percent Hispanic, 4.4 percent Asian or Pacific Islander, and 0.8 percent Native American. **Table 10.1** shows the projected percentage figures for each of these population groups for the years 2010, 2020, 2030, 2040, and 2050 (U.S. Bureau of the Census, 2010).

**Table 10.1**   Projected U.S. population percentages of African Americans, Hispanics, Native Americans, and Asians or Pacific Islanders: 2010, 2020, 2030, 2040, and 2050

| Race | Year | | | | |
| --- | --- | --- | --- | --- | --- |
| | **2010** | **2020** | **2030** | **2040** | **2050** |
| African American | 12.3% | 13.5% | 13.9% | 14.3% | 14.6% |
| Hispanic | 15.1% | 17.8% | 20.1% | 22.3% | 24.4% |
| Native American | 0.9% | 0.8% | 0.8% | 0.8% | 0.7% |
| Asian/Pacific Islander | 5.8% | 6.2% | 6.7% | 7.8% | 8.8% |

(U.S. Census Bureau, 2004)

From Table 10.1 it is readily apparent that the greatest percentage increase over the next thirty years will come from the Hispanic and Asian/Pacific Islander groups. The percentage increase of Hispanics and Asians from 2010 until 2050 is 83 percent and 57 percent, respectively. During this same time period, the percentage of non-Hispanic whites in the population will fall from 65 percent in the year 2010 to about 50 percent in the year 2050, a decrease of about 21 percent.

At least one ramification of these changes, increasing numbers of ethnic minority students in public school, is already being felt in the classrooms of our nation. In 2008, approximately 43 percent of the children in public schools in the United States were minorities. Additionally, in New York City in the next decade, 35 to 40 percent of the residents will be Hispanic, 25 percent African American, and 25 percent white. The escalating minority population makes an already diverse nation even more so and presents health education specialists with an ever widening array of opportunities and challenges as the twenty-first century continues to unfold.

## Aging

Another demographic factor that will impact the practice of health education/promotion in the future is the aging population. The U.S. Bureau of the Census (2010) lists persons age sixty-five or older as representing 12.6 percent of the U.S. population. Between the years 2010 and 2040, the population over sixty-five is expected to grow to equal 20.5 percent of the total. To further illustrate this trend, the estimated median age of the U.S. population in 2010 is 36.7. In the year 2020, it is estimated to be 37.6; and in 2030, it will be approximately 39.

One of the major reasons for the aging trend is that older Americans are living longer than ever before. Other causative factors accentuating changes in age demographics are that married couples in the United States are having fewer children, and the oldest of the baby boomers (those born between 1946 and 1964) are now nearing retirement age. This group's massive size causes it to have a dominant effect on U.S. population statistics.

## Societal Trends

There probably has not been a time when societal change was as rapid as in the latter decades of the twentieth century. For example, since 1960, there have been changes in societal mores and practices, such as more openness to cohabitation, a greater tolerance for premarital sex, more vocal and open gay relationships, a greater number of single-parent households, an increase in child abuse, more violence, an increase in the amount and availability of pornographic materials, massive changes in the number of ethical issues related to medicine, alterations in the way the medical establishment is organized and medical care is delivered, a decreasing respect for authority of any kind, declining support for K–12 public schools and higher education institutions, an infusion of and a reliance on technology, and a distrust of the political establishment in general. All of these factors play a big role in shaping the structure of society in the future. This section discusses several of the major societal trends that experts agree will impact health education/promotion in the new millennium.

## Technology

Certainly, the boom in **technology** has affected, if not transformed, the lives of many people around the globe. Many of the advances in communication, transportation, medicine, engineering, and ease of access to information have created an enhanced quality of life for people worldwide. The increased availability and use of technology also creates myriad opportunities for the prospective health education specialist in the planning, design, implementation, and evaluation of programs and materials.

It is next to impossible to find a campus today that does not feature student computer labs in numerous locations and wireless technology in all buildings. In today's environment, many courses and even entire degree programs are offered using Web-based technologies, enabling the student to participate in class sessions in "real time" no matter where she/he resides. The constantly expanding technological capabilities in the field of education have created a learning environment in which information is readily available and lessons can be easily structured to require a greater degree of critical thinking and be more interactive than was possible only a few years ago. Several journals are published only in electronic form; no printed hard copy is available, and projects are under way to digitize entire collections of books and monographs, making the information contained in those publications not only more readily accessible but content searchable. There is no doubt that the knowledge explosion trend fueled by new innovations in educational technology will continue.

What does this rapid acceleration mean for health education specialists? Gold and Atkinson (2006) offer several intriguing considerations on how the advances in technology can/will revolutionize the delivery of health education/promotion.

- Extending our traditional health education/promotion delivery systems by reaching out across time and space, as well as literacy and language.

- Allowing both synchronous and asynchronous communications in pictures, sounds, movement, and virtual reality.

- Individualizing and personalizing communication and instruction through tailored messages and interventions based on the variables we know are likely to influence interest, ability, readiness, and a host of other relevant variables.

- Extending the way we internalize, understand, individualize, and use massive amounts of data through instant access to even the minutest detail in a large data repository.

- Enhancing opportunities to provide new services and interventions by creating new practices and strategies (p. 46).

Gold and Atkinson also posit potential applications for health education specialists from the list just presented. These include creating tailored content of interest and pertinence delivered to individual desktops daily, using simulation to "improve decision-making skills of the public regarding the use of health information, podcasting relevant information directly to both individuals and groups, utilizing GIS capabilities to map out and investigate problems in a more complete manner" (p. 45).

Clearly technology will greatly shape the face of the delivery of health education/promotion into the future. Students of health education/promotion must become familiar with the methods available to gather and deliver information in order to take maximum advantage of the potential applications in the years ahead.

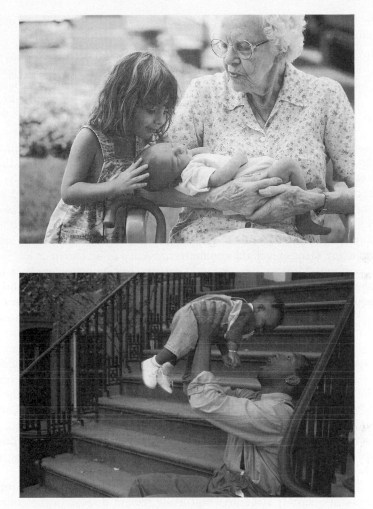

**Figure 10.2** An awareness of different family structures, such as extended families or single parents, is an important consideration when planning prevention messages.

(Sue Ann Miller/Getty; Richard Lord/The Image Works)

## Family Structure

The American family structure has changed dramatically since the 1960s (see **Figure 10.2**). The **traditional family** (two parents and their children) is becoming less and less common because of factors such as high rates of divorce, smaller families, postponed marriage and childbearing, teenage and nonmarital childbearing, stepfamilies, homosexual couples, and dual-earner marriages (Acock & Demo, 1994). These changes have spawned a new sociological family descriptor, the **postmodern family** (Cheal, 1991; Stacy, 1991).

Hale (2000) summarizes the "new paradigm" in family structure in the United States when she states:

> About 30% of Americans live alone or in non-family combinations, such as with house-mates, friends, or partnerships outside legal marriage. Even if we restrict families to the standard definition, 43% are married couples without children younger than 18, and 35% are married couples with children. Another 10% are female-headed families with children, 3% are male-headed families with children, and 10% are other family types. (p. 1)

In 1980, 77 percent of children under the age of eighteen lived with both parents, and 18 percent lived with the mother only. In 2005, 67 percent of those under eighteen lived with both parents, and 23 percent lived with the mother only. Of note is the fact that slightly more than 4 percent of 0–17-year-olds in 2005 lived with grandparents, other relatives, or in the homes of nonrelatives (National Vital Statistics System, 2006).

The impact caused by these new structures is being felt throughout our society. Children are the most affected. Many parents today provide less guidance and support, and many seem to lack the commitment needed to be parents.

Simons-Morton, Greene, and Gottlieb (1995) document other stressful changes in the family. They mention that the high costs of providing for a family today practically require that a family have two incomes. This places a strain even on nuclear families with two parents; affordable daycare services for the children must be obtained. For many low-income and single-parent families, the choice is no care or supervision at all—a situation that puts children at risk. In addition, fewer employers are offering health insurance, particularly in service-oriented positions that often pay minimum wage and are a major source of employment for many low-skilled workers. As a result, nearly 19 percent of children in the United States are living in poverty. This is the highest rate in the industrialized world (*Kids Count* Data Book, 2010). The linkage between these factors may be a predisposing condition leading to an increased rate of child abuse (McKenzie, Kotecki, & Pinger, 2008). Finally, it is no secret that the economic downturn since 2008 has contributed significantly to increasing the number of families and children under economic stress due to job loss or underemployment.

The changes previously noted have significant implications for health education specialists. Family structures will likely remain diverse in the coming years and will probably operate on a new set of norms. In other words, new methods of reaching individuals, families, and communities will need to be created in order to improve the health of all family members in accordance with their needs.

## Political Climate

As was mentioned earlier, there remains little doubt that today there is an increasing frustration with politics and politicians in general. Whether a person is a **conservative**, one who generally distrusts governmental regulations and tax-supported programs for addressing social or economic problems; a **moderate**, one who usually acts in a more situationally specific manner in regard to using tax-supported programs to solve societal problems; or a **liberal**, one who generally desires more government programs to attack social and economic problems, there seems to be no end to the bickering and infighting among members of various political parties. Many of the political issues considered in Congress relate to health. For example, the landmark agreement between the tobacco industry and the states over the sale and marketing of tobacco products to minors, the

**Figure 10.3** An awareness of political issues that affect health will be even more crucial in the future.

(Rachel Epstein/PhotoEdit Inc.)

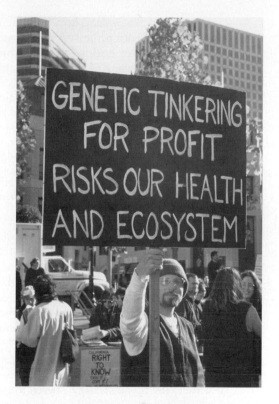

addition of prescription drug benefits to Medicare, the repeal of a motorcycle helmet law in Texas, the development of the Department of Homeland Security after September 11, 2001, the passage of a physician-assisted suicide law in Oregon, the settlement of a lawsuit related to the storage of nuclear waste in Idaho, the funding for the wars in Iraq and Afghanistan, passage of the Affordable Care Act, community health center legislation, and the lack of oversight of distribution of funds following Hurricane Katrina are examples of political issues that directly impact the health of the populace (see **Figure 10.3**).

Politics and health seem to be inextricably linked. Some governmental officials and legislators claim that public health programs infringe on personal autonomy by advocating for seat belt laws, tobacco laws, helmet laws, air bags, healthier options in fast foods, gun control laws, and health insurance for all. Others believe that legislation fostering an environment that enhances the health of the population as a whole is worth the sacrifice of some personal choice and autonomy.

As citizens and professionals, the involvement of health education specialists in the political process is important. O'Rourke (2006) states, "Health education not only seeks to change lifestyles, but to create public understanding of the political issues involved in public health programs" (p. 9). He goes on to challenge all health education specialists to assume a **macrolevel** view of health problems. Using this approach, health education specialists move from a position of assisting behavior change one person at a time to community-based interventions. In implementing the community-based programs, success often depends on the health education specialist's having a working knowledge of the political process and how it impacts every decision. Hunter (2008) supports the fact that public health professionals can no longer be bystanders but must become passionate advocates for healthy change in individuals and communities. He believes that the collective advocacy of all public health practitioners is vital in moving governmental bodies to support and improve health.

There is little doubt that health education specialists must become participants in the political process. O'Rourke (2006) eloquently makes a case for enhancing the effectiveness of health education/promotion through an approach that

> encompasses collective responsibility and community involvement through participation in the political process and service on county health boards, city councils, and school boards. In these capacities, health educators can influence the health of entire communities and not rely on the 'one person at a time' model of improving health through individual responsibility. (p. 8)

To that end, a method for health education specialists to increase their visibility and political clout is advanced by McDermott (2000) when he challenges present and future health education specialists to consider the importance of research in the practice of health education/promotion. For interventions to be effective, health education specialists must use tested best practices when these practices are known. Future gains in the effectiveness and scope of prevention programs probably will be made only when health education specialists insist on pushing the research envelope to determine the factors that affect health and cause health disparities in populations, are components of effective intervention programs, and allow for dissemination of these programs across a variety of settings. Including community partners and legislators in these research efforts is a strategy proven to gain trust and allies more welcoming to the benefit of macrolevel initiatives.

## Medical Care Establishment and the Affordable Care Act

The health care system in the United States continues to be in need of an overhaul. Passage of the Affordable Care Act in early 2010 is a start in the right direction, but the exact impact of that legislation is far from certain as many of the provisions in the plan are set to be enacted three to six years from now. Meanwhile, the cost of care continues to escalate, and the system seems stuck in an unsustainable model of reimbursement for procedures instead of reimbursement for helping people stay well. Citizens increasingly desire to be participants in their own care and to be provided with options. Enhancing the quality of life as opposed to simply increasing longevity is becoming a prevalent goal of U.S. health care consumers.

There are several reasons for this trend. Although few would deny that our medical care system has been responsible for saving countless lives, clearly health is largely a reflection of the nature of the environments in which a person resides, personal lifestyle choices, and standards of living, and not the medical care system. Medical care tends to concentrate on secondary and tertiary care and to ignore the value of primary prevention.

These points are substantiated by Williams, McClellan, and Rivlin (2010) and Goodartz et al. (2010) when they state that healthier lives are best fostered in a climate of a culture of health. What seems to be most important in creating and maintaining health are the actions taken by individuals and communities to select and support habits like choosing what food we eat, having healthy relationships, staying physically active, and investing in safe and environmentally friendly neighborhoods. Much of health is tied not to medical intervention, but to primary prevention.

The Affordable Care Act has increased the opportunities for health education specialists. Koh and Sebelius (2010) document that this law "promotes wellness in the workplace, providing new health promotion opportunities for employers and employees" (p. 4). In addition, the act strengthens the community role in promoting prevention and serves to enhance partnerships between state and local government and community groups and nonprofits.

Another example of how health education/promotion has a place in the medical care arena can be demonstrated by examining the mission of the Boise, Idaho–based nonprofit corporation, Healthwise. Healthwise is the provider of the Web-based health information found in WebMD and also is responsible for much of the health education/promotion content disseminated by major insurance companies and hospitals around the country. Chairman and CEO Don Kemper (2007) has authored a white paper entitled "The Healthwise Ix Solution" in which he states that a health care transformation is possible if consumers are able to: "1) gain access to information that helps them do as much for themselves as possible, 2) gain tools necessary to ask for the care they need, and 3) help them say no to the care they don't need providing them with a sense of autonomy" (p. 4).

Kemper's approach bodes well for enhanced opportunities for health education specialists who desire to practice in a health care setting in large part because of the set of situations, policies, and approaches that seem to have no end solution: managed care, the fact that almost 47 million Americans have no health insurance (although, we hope, the Affordable Care Act will decrease this number), the continuous federal tinkering with both the Medicare and Medicaid systems, lack of oversight for universal quality of care standards, huge disparities in the cost-quality sphere (Abelson, 2007), the growing influence of insurers, lack of affordability of private pay insurance with a set of benefits equal to most employer-provided or public insurance plans, poor chronic disease management protocols, and frustration with a lack of emphasis on prevention. Given these circumstances, health education specialists can facilitate patient choice by helping patients understand their options regarding physician choice, health care insurance plan, type of care, and intensity of services. In addition, they can assist medical organizations by increasing patient satisfaction through contributing to more one-on-one contact, improving patterns of communication between patient and provider, and enhancing patient compliance with treatment regimens (T. Epperly, personal communication, Family Medicine Residency of Idaho, Boise, May 2009; C. Spear, personal communication, Boise State University, Boise, August 2010).

# Professional Preparation and Credentialing

Although the issues of professional preparation and credentialing were extensively covered in Chapter 6, both have implications for the future practice of health education/promotion. Thus, the reasons why health education/promotion practice might be affected by these issues are of some importance.

## Professional Preparation

In this discussion, it is not our intent to provide a list of courses that must be taken to become a "better" health education specialist. Coursework is by nature specific to the institution you are attending. Course titles and descriptions vary widely from one program to another. As you are aware, the coursework you will take in your degree program is interdisciplinary. We attempt to provide some ideas, concepts, and objectives for you to consider as you enter your preparation program.

The social changes previously discussed in this chapter are the challenges driving health education specialists of the future to be proactive in meeting the demands placed on them. What tasks will a health education specialist need to be able to perform to be effective in the decades ahead? Clark (1994) helps answer this question by making several salient points about health education/promotion in the future:

1. The mission will be less providing factual information and more helping people become more analytical thinkers—thus enabling them to deal better with complex issues and uncertainty.

2. There will be newer, stronger partnerships with the medical establishment. This collaboration will give a new power to health education/promotion and will capitalize on the idea that health education/promotion makes a difference in disease management.

3. Health education specialists will need to analyze situations and examine past and future trends to see the threats to quality of life. Long-term, not short-term, thinking will be a must.

4. A greater emphasis will be placed on values clarification. Health education specialists must learn to account for the effects of culture and then find processes that reach people with different values.

5. Mechanisms need to be perfected for designing and delivering multilevel approaches to optimize health education/promotion in addressing priority health problems. Education at the community level will be the focus of most health interventions.

6. There will be an enhanced need for quality research, so that the effectiveness of health education/promotion methodologies can be ascertained. The need for cost-effective, efficient strategies will remain.

7. Health education specialists must determine how to use technology to help people learn.

8. The need to integrate education, health, and social services within the schools will become more recognized. The gap between school and community services will close.

9. Environmental activism will continue to emerge, and health education specialists can play an important role in facilitating multidimensional programs that cross all socioeconomic and political boundaries.

10. In the final analysis, people will judge the success of health education/promotion by whether or not their quality of life has improved.

Several of Clark's thoughts echo those of O'Rourke (2006), who challenges health education specialists to be more macrolevel-oriented. In other words, there is an ever growing need to facilitate health education/promotion interventions at the community level (as opposed to the individual level, or **microlevel**). Inherent in this charge is that those who reside in the community where the intervention occurs will be totally involved in the planning from the outset. English and Videto (1997) affirm these observations when they state, "Regardless of our place of practice, our ability to identify and meet the needs of our local communities and neighborhoods is likely to be the measure that will determine our success as health educators . . . successful programs use community involvement" (p. 4).

Three additional documents that provide information about the competencies health education specialists must possess into the future are described below. The first two can be found using the Weblinks at the end of this chapter. The first document features the deliberations by members of the Committee on Educating Public Health Professionals for the 21st Century. The workshop participants who wrote the article "Who Will Keep the Public Healthy? Workshop Summary" (Weblinks #3) identify eight new content areas that should be added to the curricula of individuals studying to practice public health: informatics, genomics, communication, community-based participatory research, global health, health policy, health law, and public health ethics. Although the report is largely directed at universities offering graduate programs, even a cursory glance finds several suggested content areas that are relevant to the practice of health education/promotion. The list also shows the rapidly expanding knowledge base the future health education specialist will need to have in order to successfully interact with health professionals from a variety of other fields. The more understanding a health education specialist has about the vocabulary and nature of the work of other health providers, the more likely she or he is to be an accepted and valued member of the health care community.

The second document presents the results of a study titled "Health Educator Job Analysis 2010." The study was commissioned by the American Association for Health Education (AAHE), the Society for Public Health Education (SOPHE), and the National Commission for Health Education Credentialing (NCHEC). In short, the study describes current health education/promotion practice in the United States and helps set the stage for revisiting competencies for entry level and advanced practitioners

The third document, a cogent paper written by McKenzie (2004), cautions that those in charge of health education preparation programs must not assume that it is possible or even advisable to prepare "generic" health education specialists. The four practice settings to which he refers in the quote that follows are discussed later in this chapter. McKenzie states, ". . . even though the responsibilities and competencies of health educators are similar regardless of the settings, the work is indeed different and the preparation cannot be the same . . ." (p. 48).

It is apparent that tomorrow's health education specialists must be able to respond rapidly to changes in all avenues of society. When planning, implementing, and evaluating programs and working in multidimensional settings, they must enter into collaborative relationships with health care professionals from other disciplines in a spirit of cooperation. Health education specialists who are not afraid to be innovative, who respect but do not fear change, who are not just purveyors of information but community builders and facilitators of learning, who continue to be curious and learn themselves, who have a sense of adventure, and who seek the truth through thoughtful research, study, and dialogue are the individuals who will lead our profession into the next several decades.

## Credentialing

The history of and reasons for credentialing were thoroughly covered in Chapter 6. There are, however, several facets of credentialing that need reemphasis because they have profound implications for the future practice of health education/promotion.

The credentialing process as it now stands begins with the candidate's submitting a transcript of coursework in health education to the National Commission for Health

Education Credentialing (NCHEC). Upon verification by NCHEC that the candidate has completed coursework leading to a degree in health education and the coursework has focused on the responsibilities and competencies of an entry-level health education specialist, the applicant is permitted to sit for the certification exam. Exam questions are based on the seven responsibilities and competencies for entry-level health education specialists, Individuals who pass the exam are awarded a Certified Health Education Specialist (CHES) credential. Those individuals must then complete continuing education units to maintain their credential.

This process is not without its detractors. The major reason for this is that all individuals who seek a CHES certification must complete the same process. This tends to skew the credential in favor of creating a generic health education specialist (see McKenzie, 2004). Many practicing health education specialists argue that the skills needed to teach health in a school setting differ from those needed to conduct a community program at a local American Cancer Society office or to direct health promotion programs at a worksite. For example, school health education specialists often see the need to be content specialists, whereas community health education specialists are more process and skills oriented.

Simons-Morton, Greene, and Gottlieb (1995) accurately mention that health education is a diverse profession. Health education specialists practice in a variety of settings (e.g., school, worksite, community, health care); they may work with different populations (e.g., adults, the aged, children, minorities); they may be process specialists (e.g., program planners, program implementers, program evaluators); or they may be content specialists (e.g., specialists in HIV/AIDS, chronic diseases, injury or violence prevention, nutrition). Should there be a generic credential? Perhaps in the future there will be "practice-specific" credentials. A potential important consequence of having a CHES credential is that of eligibility for reimbursement for services rendered. As different care models are advanced with prevention as a focus (thanks to the Affordable Care Act), insurers are increasingly limiting the types of providers eligible for reimbursement. Without some external credential or license, it is highly unlikely that any health education services rendered in a medical care setting will be reimbursed (Idaho Blue Shield Human Resources Department, 2008).

Though discussions related to this issue doubtless will continue, the credentialing process is here to stay. The bottom line is that this certification program does "establish a national standard for individual health education specialists. It differs from state and local certifications and registries in that the requirements do not vary from one locale to another" (NCHEC, 2010). The CHES process as currently configured seems to work well and is increasingly endorsed by prevention specialists and organizations nationwide. Potential changes to the credentialing process and necessary competencies that emanate from the study, "Health Educator Job Analysis 2010," referenced in the previous section of this chapter will most likely occur. Students should stay abreast of developments in credentialing by visiting the AAHE, NCHEC, and SOPHE Web sites on a regular basis.

Caile Spear, President-Elect of the American Association for Health Education (AAHE), posits that the public health professions that focus on prevention need to unify (perhaps under a common credential) to make their voice more clearly heard and their message more uniform. She goes on to say that unification of these professions would mimic what funding agencies are doing in that they would be soliciting projects that encompass holistic approaches to addressing health issues. Funding agencies are moving away from providing funds for specific health problems (e.g., substance abuse, child abuse, lack of physical activity, etc.) to funding more global strategies. Similarly, a united group of prevention professionals (including health education specialists), regardless of practice setting, would be more powerful in making a local and national case for the role of prevention in overall health than the current model in which prevention professionals often are members of several different professional organizations (personal communication, August 2010).

As the profession of health education/promotion continues to evolve and health education specialists become more visible partners in the delivery of health services, students considering careers in this field should seriously consider obtaining CHES certification. To that end, Spear also encourages all health educators to become health education specialists by seeking CHES certification. The CHES credential assists employers in identifying practitioners who have met national standards, and it assures the consumers of health education/promotion services that the health educators with whom they work are competent professionals (personal communication, August 2010).

# Implications for Practice Settings

Chapter 7 detailed the variety of settings in which health education specialists can practice: the worksite, school, health care, or public health. Each setting has unique characteristics. The content areas covered, the population characteristics, and the competencies required differ according to the organization's mission and structure (Simons-Morton, Greene, & Gottlieb, 1995, p. 425). However, the settings also are similar in that the goal of health education/promotion is to create a climate that facilitates the improvement of health status for every member of the population served by the setting. The first part of this chapter described various influences destined to impact the health of the populace into the next century. This section briefly summarizes the future role of the health education specialist in each setting.

## School Setting

"Children don't learn as well when they are not healthy" (Seffrin, 1994, p. 397). "Schools are an integral part of the community, and, if we don't have high quality school health education we will pay the price later in higher costs to all of us. Health education specialists regardless of practice setting should support and be champions for well-funded, vigorous and vital school health programs" (Spear, personal communication, August 2010). These statements characterize the goal and importance of school health education and provide direction for school health education specialists (see **Figure 10.4**). If children's well-being is to be maintained or enhanced, a comprehensive approach (sometimes called a coordinated approach) to providing health education is needed (Allensworth & Kolbe, 1987). The coordinated approach consists of eight components integrated to meet all of the health needs of the children and adolescents attending the school: (1) classroom school health education lessons, (2) the school lunch program, (3) health screenings, (4) physical education, (5) a healthy and safe school environment, (6) the availability of trained school counselors, (7) faculty and staff health promotion, and (8) family and community support for education and health. Actually implementing this model is a tall order. In their discussion summarizing a study on school health policies and programs, Kolbe and colleagues (1995) note:

> School health policies and programs, particularly at the school level, may not adequately address several of the most serious public health problems today such as

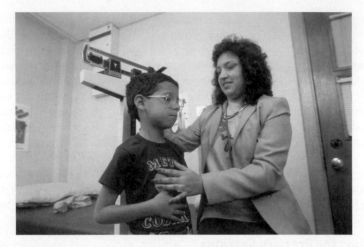

**Figure 10.4** Schools can serve as sites for offering preventive health services and education.

(Bob Daemmrich/The Image Works)

violence, unintentional injuries such as motor vehicle crashes, and unintended pregnancies. School health services that do not respond to these problems, classroom instruction that is inadequate in scope and depth, and school health policies that only include punitive rather than remedial responses to violations must be replaced with more responsive programs. (p. 343)

Should you choose to practice health education/promotion in a school setting, what skills and abilities must you possess if schools are to incorporate a coordinated health education/promotion program to address the health needs of children and adolescents, both now and in the future? In light of the information on influences on health in this chapter and that on settings for health education/promotion from Chapter 7, we think that the following skills are imperative. You must be able to:

1. Read and interpret the findings of health research on effective health programs and practices.

2. Create a logical scope and sequence to health content units that incorporate age-appropriate information.

3. Prepare and deliver lessons that are participatory in nature, stress skill development, and foster attitudes necessary for problem solving and informed decision making.

4. Use both qualitative and quantitative strategies to evaluate your lessons, your units, and the district health education/promotion program.

5. Assess the health needs of the students, faculty, and staff.

6. Ensure that health and counseling services are provided for students.

7. Create or coordinate a parent/community health education/promotion advisory council.

8. Actively participate in local, state, regional, and national professional organizations.

9. Use technology to assist in both updating your own skills and delivering health education/promotion messages to your school and community.

10. Learn about the influence of culture on health, cultivate sensitivity toward it, and instill an awareness of it in your teaching.

11. Assist teachers at all grade levels in obtaining age-appropriate health education materials and help coordinate a classroom scope and sequence for all grade levels in your district.

12. Serve as resource person and liaison between the school health setting and other settings in which health education might occur.

13. Acquire sound oral and written communication techniques.

14. Work both independently and as a member of a team.

15. Apply behavior-change strategies and what is known about environmental influences on behavior to the classroom setting.

16. Collaborate with health education specialists practicing in the community, worksite, or health care setting to coordinate the delivery of disease prevention and health promotion messages and programs.

17. Teach and promote the enhancement of strategies to increase health literacy among the population served to reduce health disparities (Hasnain-Wynia & Wolf, 2010).

School health educators who possess these skills will be well prepared to lead programs that enhance the health of the students and teachers in their schools.

## Worksite Setting

The workplace of today bears little resemblance to that of only twenty years ago. Because many employers want to attract the best employees and they realize that employee satisfaction is key in productivity and retention, worksites have introduced programs for employees and their families that provide continuing education, recreational opportunities, health promotion, and financial planning. In particular, worksites have become an increasingly important setting for health education/promotion programs. Typically, the health education/promotion programs in these settings address injury prevention, exercise, the control of smoking, stress management, and alcohol and other drug abuse (Simons-Morton, Greene, & Gottlieb, 1995). As noted earlier in this chapter, the Affordable Care Act also signals the advent of a renewed emphasis on worksite health promotion (Koh & Sebelius, 2010).

The influence of changing demographic patterns on health education/promotion in general was discussed previously. However, another factor must be taken into account when specifically anticipating the future direction of worksite health promotion. The greatest percentage of persons joining the workforce in the decade between 2010 and 2020 will be women and minorities.

The expansion of worksite health promotion programs bodes well for the future of health education/promotion and the concurrent need for an increasing number of trained health education specialists. This truth has broad implications for the future practice of worksite health education/promotion. Together with the information presented both earlier in this chapter and in Chapter 7, the following competencies represent a baseline for the future practice of health education/promotion in worksite settings:

1. Recognize the importance of cultural and demographic influences on individual and group health behavioral choices.

2. Coordinate needs assessments of worksite populace and conduct evaluations of program components.

3. Identify and work with aspects of the corporate organizational climate that facilitate or impede participation.

4. Become familiar with the culture inherent in a business setting.

5. Prepare and conduct prevention presentations to worksite subgroups.

6. Conduct fitness assessments and participate in health screenings.

7. Use up-to-date technology to market programs to worksite supervisors, employees, and their families through newsletters, brochures, Internet chat groups, and other media.

8. Plan and manage a budget.

9. Coordinate employee coalitions/steering committees to maximize employee input into program components.

10. Function as a resource person for health information for employees and their families.

11. Be able to apply behavior-change strategies and what is known about environmental influences on behavior to the worksite setting.

12. Implement programs in a manner consistent with management philosophy.

13. Attain a working knowledge of epidemiological and statistical principles and applications.

14. Acquire sound oral and written communication techniques.

15. Work both independently and as a member of a team.

16. Design and employ evaluation strategies that are outcomes-based to assess program effectiveness.

17. Gain a thorough understanding of current, relevant literature and well-designed research studies that influence practice in the worksite setting.

18. Teach and promote the enhancement of strategies to increase health literacy among the population served to reduce health disparities (Hasnain-Wynia & Wolf, 2010).

Incorporating competencies such as those listed previously into the professional preparation program will help ensure that you are ready to begin practice as a worksite health education specialist.

## Public Health Setting

The community setting (called the "public health setting" in this text) has the greatest variety of options for the practice of health education/promotion. For example, health education specialists are employed in many local, city, state, and federal health departments; in many federal agencies; in county extension agencies; in volunteer health organizations (e.g., American Cancer Society, American Heart Association, American

Red Cross); in churches; in homeless shelters; in grassroots community organizations; and in prisons. One reason for the diversity of opportunities is that the mission, goals, and objectives of one community agency may differ dramatically from those of another. Some agencies might have a health education specialist serving as a coordinator of services or as a fund-raiser, while in another agency the educator might plan, conduct, and evaluate programs. Another, more obvious reason for increased employment opportunities is that almost every locale in the United States has one of the aforementioned groups.

The purpose of community health organizations is to both monitor and improve the health of the public they serve. Goodman (2000) notes that when health education specialists combine forces with people from other professional disciplines (e.g., ecologists, economists, anthropologists, communication specialists), the probability of reducing the health risks of populations is heightened. Consequently, collaboration with community organizations and with other professionals to address population health is a skill that all health education specialists must develop. In this era of using health education/promotion to help reduce health care costs, and with an increasing need for community-level programs, public health education specialists are well positioned to participate in improving the health of citizens from all regions of the United States.

With employment opportunities for public health education specialists on the rise, what skills will the public health education specialists of the future need in order to function effectively? Following is a list of competencies or attributes that will be critical to the effective practice of public health education. They are not in any specific order of importance.

1. Recognize the importance of cultural and demographic influences on individual and group health behavioral choices.

2. Maintain competence in the use of technology to access and deliver health-related information.

3. Learn and use strategies to seek information, guidance, and support from community members regarding their health needs.

4. Assess strengths of communities in building a plan to assist them in meeting their health needs.

5. Be able to apply behavior-change strategies and what is known about environmental influences on behavior to the public health setting.

6. Learn coalition-building strategies.

7. Actively participate in local, state, regional, and national professional organizations.

8. Study and apply the fundamentals of obtaining extramural funding.

9. Use a variety of marketing strategies to reach diverse community constituencies.

10. Learn to be flexible, as the job probably will involve changing and varied responsibilities.

11. Learn another language.

12. Advocate policies that enhance the role of prevention and provide for universal access to health services when needed.

13. Foster the ability to work in a multidisciplinary environment.

14. Attain a working knowledge of epidemiological and statistical principles and applications.

15. Acquire excellent oral and written communication techniques.

16. Work independently and as a member of a team.

17. Design and employ evaluation strategies that are outcomes based to assess program effectiveness.

18. Gain a thorough understanding of current, relevant literature and well-designed research studies that influence practice in the community setting (i.e., community-based participatory research).

19. Teach and promote the enhancement of strategies to increase health literacy among the population served to reduce health disparities (Hasnain-Wynia & Wolf, 2010).

A well-trained community health education specialist will undoubtedly make an increased contribution to the health of populations. With the increasing health awareness of U.S. citizens and the multitude of cultural changes in society, community health education specialists have a bright and exciting future.

## Health Care Setting

Health care settings employ health education specialists in a variety of institutions and a multitude of ways. Health education specialists can be employed in for-profit and public hospitals, health maintenance organizations (HMOs), medical care clinics, and home health agencies. They might be involved in conducting one-on-one patient education; planning and implementing education programs for enrollees or other medical providers; coordinating community education programs on a variety of health topics; conducting program evaluations; marketing the health services available through the hospital, clinic, or HMO; conducting health education/promotion activities for the employees; or serving as a member of a community health promotion team.

Epperly (personal communication, May 2009.) feels that health care providers, insurance companies, and the public in general are becoming more receptive to the notion that accurate and timely health information is an important part of any treatment regimen. Lack of adequate health education/promotion can negate potential positive contributions in the prevention and management of disease. With no end in sight to the skyrocketing costs of health care, the word "prevention" is being incorporated into more care plans than ever before.

Yarnall et al. (2003) notes that the evidence of preventive services is well established but the rate of the delivery of preventive services by medical providers is severely lacking. Their study of time burdens required to deliver preventive care concluded that the major reason for the lack of delivery is that, in order to fulfill the U.S. Preventive Health Services Task Force recommendations, a primary care physician with a "normal" practice would have to dedicate nearly 7.5 hours per day solely to the delivery of preventive services. Obviously, this time allocation is impossible because physicians need to spend most their time diagnosing and treating disease. Yarnall's study concludes with the following statement: "Our current system of preventive care delivery—provided by physicians . . . no longer meets national needs. New methods of preventive care delivery are required, as well as a clearer focus on which services can be best provided, and by whom" (p. 640).

The shift in practice norms by most clinical health care professionals requires trained personnel to ensure that education in the health care setting meets the needs of both the patient and the provider and motivates the patient to both adopt a healthier lifestyle and comply with any treatment regimen. Given the medical community's acceptance of the value of health education/promotion in patient care, the outlook is positive for more employment opportunities for health education specialists in health care settings. What skills, competencies, and attributes will be absolutely necessary for the health education specialist of the future who seeks employment in a health care setting? Following is a list (in no particular order):

1. Obtain a working knowledge of epidemiological and statistical principles and applications.

2. Maintain competence in the use of technology to access and deliver health-related information.

3. Be able to apply behavior-change strategies and what is known about environmental influences on behavior to the health care setting.

4. Recognize the importance of cultural and demographic influences on individual and group health behavioral choices.

5. Become familiar with technological innovations to provide better outreach to patients, employees, and their families through a variety of electronic and hard copy newsletters, brochures, Internet chat groups, Web sites, and other media outlets.

6. Provide training in health education/promotion theory to other members of the health care team.

7. Become familiar with the clinical disease process.

8. Advocate policies that enhance the role of prevention and provide for universal access to health services when needed.

9. Prepare and deliver lessons that are participatory in nature and research-based, that stress skill development, and that foster attitudes necessary for problem solving and informed decision making.

10. Coordinate interdisciplinary teams/steering committees to maximize input into program components.

11. Learn to be flexible, as the job probably will involve changing and varied responsibilities.

12. Serve as a liaison between the health care setting and other settings in which health education might occur.

13. Function as a resource person for health information for patients and their families.

14. Learn another language.

15. Acquire sound oral and written communication techniques.

16. Work independently and as a member of a team.

17. Obtain a working knowledge of the role of informatics in assisting in prevention at all vulnerable points in the causal chains leading to disease, injury, or disability (Davies, Smith, & Gustafson, 2001).

18. Teach and promote the enhancement of strategies to increase health literacy among the population served to reduce health disparities (Hasnain-Wynia & Wolf, 2010).

With rapid changes occurring in medical care delivery today, there is much reason for health education specialists to be optimistic about employment opportunities. As the public demands health education/promotion and disease prevention as a part of their medical care treatment plan, health education specialists will increasingly be identified as the best prepared to assist individuals in adopting healthy lifestyles.

## Alternative Settings

Besides the four traditional practice settings previously discussed, there are several other viable alternatives for the practice of health education/promotion into the next century. In this section, we very briefly introduce these choices so that individuals who are interested can research them further.

The first alternative is to teach health education/promotion in a **postsecondary institution**, usually defined as an institution that educates people after they graduate from high school. There will continue to be a need for qualified instructors. Minimum standards for obtaining one of these positions is usually a master's degree in health education and two to five years of experience for a community college or vocational school position, and a doctorate and two to five years of experience for a college or university position.

Students who are interested in combining the fields of health education/promotion and journalism can find positions in both the print and TV media as health reporters for newspapers, magazines, and TV stations. A broad-based knowledge of health issues and a passion for writing and/or speaking are necessary qualifications.

Because of the increasing interdependence among nations and because there are many areas of the world in which health assistance is badly needed, health education specialist positions will continue to be available in foreign countries. Examples include positions with organizations such as the Peace Corps, Project Hope, the United Nations, the Pan American Health Organization, and the World Health Organization. Many national church organizations also send interdisciplinary health teams to international locations to improve the health of the populace. Often, the health education specialist must have a college degree, some experience, and ability to speak a foreign language.

Medical supply companies, pharmaceutical companies, sports equipment manufacturers, health food stores, and textbook publishers often employ health education specialists in sales positions. A college degree is required. In addition, a willingness to travel, excellent oral and written communication skills, and an ability to work with all types of people are necessary prerequisites.

Because of the aging of the U.S. population, demand for health education specialists in long-term care institutions and retirement communities is escalating. Usually, a college degree is required. Excellent oral and written communication skills are essential, as is a desire to listen and learn from the wisdom of individuals residing in these communities.

There continues to be an increasing number of opportunities for health education specialists in entrepreneurial and consultant roles. As self-employed persons, these individuals are free to set up their own practice, hiring out as consultants to organizations that temporarily need someone with expertise in grant writing, program planning and evaluation, software development, professional speaking, or technical writing. Other possibilities include contracting with several small businesses to conduct worksite health promotion, freelancing with HMOs and other insurance providers to offer health education/promotion services (reimbursement will be an issue), serving as a content specialist (e.g., stress management, eating disorders, substance abuse) to businesses and corporations, becoming a certified personal trainer, and teaching part-time in colleges, community colleges, or evening community education/promotion programs.

Now that we have explored the differences in the various practice settings, we reemphasize the fact that there are common tasks for health education specialists that transcend the individual practice settings. Dr. John Seffrin, director of the American Cancer Society, eloquently reminds us of the direction health education/promotion must take, no matter what the practice setting, if it is to realize its potential. His scholar's address (Seffrin, 1997), given to members of the American Association for Health Education (AAHE), describes four actions for present and future health education specialists that still ring true today:

1. Look at ourselves as major players in keeping Americans healthy; to that end, work with policy makers to affect legislation that truly promotes health.

2. Collaborate with other health professionals in both the for-profit and the not-for-profit sectors.

3. Strive to exhibit greater professional solidarity; be an advocate for the profession of health education/promotion and the role that trained health education specialists can play as part of the health care team.

4. Advocate for those who do not have a voice; be a spokesperson in the political arena, and work to ensure that health services and health education/promotion are available for all.

## SUMMARY

This chapter began with the notion of change as a constant. Although no one can actually "see" into the future, it is obvious that flexibility is imperative in order to adapt to ongoing change. This is an exciting time to become a health education specialist. Opportunities have never been greater, and the future has never looked brighter. There is little doubt that health education/promotion will continue to expand in all of the more traditional as well as some of the nontraditional settings. Health education specialists have the training and expertise to make a positive difference in enhancing the quality of life for all people. We wish you success as you begin your journey.

## REVIEW QUESTIONS

1. Identify three worksite settings in which health education specialists will practice to a greater degree than they currently do.

2. How will each of the societal changes discussed in the chapter impact the practice of health education/promotion in the worksite setting? The medical care setting? The school setting? The public health setting?

3. What are the implications for health education/promotion graduates who choose not to become credentialed (CHES)?

4. How will changing demographic patterns affect the practice of health education/promotion in nontraditional settings?

5. What is meant by the statement "Health education specialists need to become enhanced advocates for the profession"?

6. How will the passage of the Affordable Care Act impact the practice of health education/promotion?

## CASE STUDY

One day, while leaving the health education/promotion office on your campus, you notice an announcement posted on the message board that the health education/promotion program in which you are enrolled is seeking national accreditation. The announcement includes information from the department chair on the reasons for accreditation along with a request for student assistance in working with faculty to prepare the necessary self-study documentation prior to the visit from an outside review team. Because you are entering the second semester of your junior year, you decide that a great way to learn more about the health education/promotion program and the field of health education/ promotion in general would be to volunteer.

You notify the department chair of your willingness to help, and she appoints you to one of the program study committees, specifically the committee dealing with the use of Web-based teaching in delivering the health education/promotion curriculum. You are excited about that committee because you have some opinions on the value of Web-based courses. Although you have never enrolled in a Web-based course yourself, you know people who have, and they seem to have mixed feelings about the courses they have taken. The ambivalence of your classmates has led you to believe that Web-based courses are not as rigorous as courses offered by more traditional methods.

At the first meeting of the study committee, the committee chair outlines tasks that will need to be accomplished and suggests a timeline for completion. One of the major tasks is to determine whether the Web-based courses offered by the department are meeting the goals for which they are designed. How might that task be accomplished? What questions would you need to ask to obtain that information? What methods would you use to collect the necessary data? How might the findings be used by health education/promotion programs in planning for the future?

## CRITICAL THINKING QUESTIONS

1. What major demographic trend will most impact the delivery of health education/promotion in the next several decades? Given your answer, describe the health education specialist in the year 2020.

2. Compare and contrast the lists of competencies noted in the chapter for the four major practice settings in which a health education specialist might practice. Use your findings to support or refute the claim made by some professionals that health education specialists will be much more effective if their preparation programs include coursework specific to the settings in which they will practice.

3. Suppose that the year is 2015. If you had the power to decide how our health care system utilizes health education specialists, what duties might you assign to them in the clinical setting? How might your choices influence the goal of eliminating health disparities in the United States within the next ten years?

4. Assume that it is the year 2030 and you are retiring after many years as a practicing health education specialist. At your retirement banquet, you have been asked to spend five minutes summarizing the accomplishments of your profession. What will you say?

5. What are some ways in which the health education/health promotion community can make the message of prevention more palatable to the public? How might you implement your ideas?

## ACTIVITIES

1. Make a list of your five strongest attributes. Make a second list of the five tasks you most like to do. Using these lists and what you know about health education/promotion, write a paragraph describing the "perfect" health education/promotion job for you.

2. Construct and administer a short survey to the health education/promotion faculty at your institution on what they see as major influences on the future practice of health education/promotion. Compile your results and share them with the class.

3. Interview two graduates from your school's health education/promotion program who are now practicing in the field as certified health education specialists. Make certain they are from different settings—for instance, one in a school and one in public health. Try to ascertain their feelings about their jobs and the influences they see impacting the way they practice, both now and in the future.

4. Assume that the year is 2015. You are responsible for writing a job description that will be used to advertise for a new public health education specialist position. Write out the description, making sure to include the qualifications and duties the applicant will have to possess.

## WEBLINKS

1. **http://www.healthypeople.gov**

   Healthy People 2020

   Web site of the national Healthy People 2020 documents that describe U.S. goals and objectives for creating a healthier population by 2020.

2. **http://www.kingcounty.gov/healthservices/health.aspx**

   Seattle and King County Public Health Section

   This outstanding Web site was launched by the Seattle King County Health Department to help health education specialists and the public obtain current information on a variety of pertinent public health topics such as bioterrorism preparedness, family planning and reproductive health, diabetes, HIV/AIDS, and others.

3. **http://www8.nationalacademies.org/onpinews/newsitem.aspx?RecordID=10542**

   "Who Will Keep the Public Healthy"

   Link to a 2003 report from the Institute of Medicine of the National Academies that suggests specific ways to improve public health professionals' capabilities to address new and complex challenges. The report emphasizes that public health professionals in government health departments, other health services, community agencies, and universities have a shared responsibility to prevent illness and injury and keep communities healthy.

4. http://www.cnheo.org/

   Coalition of National Health Education Organizations Web site

   Provides a link to the study on Health Educator Job Analysis 2010 that was referenced in the chapter.

5. http://www.kaiseredu.org

   The Henry J. Kaiser Family Foundation

   The Kaiser Family Foundation Web site highlights health policy issues and enables the user to access background information on several current health policy topics. Modules and slide tutorials explaining the policy issues are also included.

6. http://www.rwjf.org/

   Web site of the Robert Wood Johnson Foundation featuring papers on health policy, health issues analyses, grant opportunities, and research and commentaries on health care reform.

7. http://www.aahe4me.org/

   AAHE4Me is a health education student Web site sponsored by the American Association for Health Education (AAHE). It is designed to provide undergraduate and graduate students a mechanism to become active participants within the profession and to interact with one another and, from time to time, with more experienced professionals.

## REFERENCES

Abelson, R. (2007). *In health care, cost isn't proof of high quality.* Retrieved on December 21, 2010, from http://www.nytimes.com/2007/06/14/health/14insure.html

Acock, A. C., & Demo, D. H. (1994). *Family diversity and well-being.* Thousand Oaks, CA: Sage.

Allensworth, D. D., & Kolbe, L. J. (1987). The comprehensive school health program: Exploring an expanded concept. *Journal of School Health, 57* (10), 409–412.

Cheal, D. (1991). *The family and the state of theory.* Toronto: University of Toronto Press.

Clark, N. M. (1994). Health educators and the future: Lead, follow, or get out of the way. *Journal of Health Education, 25* (3), 136–141.

Davies, J., Smith, G., & Gustafson, D. (2001). Public health informatics transforms the notifiable condition system. *Northwest Public Health, Spring/Summer,* 14–17.

English, G. M., & Videto, D. M. (1997). The future of health education: The knowledge to practice paradox. *Journal of Health Education, 28* (1), 4–8.

Gheisar, R. E., & Clark, C. J. (2000). New immigrant and refugee communities mean new challenges for public health. *Washington Public Health, Fall,* University of Washington, 2.

Gold, R. S., & Atkinson, N. L. (2006). Imagine this, imagine that. A look into the future of technology for health educators. *The Health Education Monograph Series, 23* (1), 44–48.

Goodartz, D., et al. (2010). The promise of prevention: The effects of four preventable factors on national life expectancy and life expectancy disparities by race and county in the United States. *PLoS Medicine, 7* (3), 1–13.

Goodman, R. M. (2000). On contemplation at 50: SOPHE Presidential Address. *Health Education and Behavior, 27* (4), 423–429.

Hale, C. (2000). Demographic trends influencing public health practice. *Washington Public Health, Fall,* University of Washington, 1–3.

Hasnain-Wynia, R., & Wolf, M. (2010). Promoting health care equity: Is health literacy a missing link? *Health Services Research, 45* (4), 897–903.

Hunter, D. J. (2008). Health needs more than healthcare: The need for the new paradigm. *European Journal of Public Health, 18* (3), 217–219.

Idaho Blue Shield Human Resources Department. (May 2008). Personal communication.

Kemper, D. W. (2007). The Healthwise Ix Solution. Retrieved on December 14, 2010, from https://www.physiciansacademy.com/events/HR09000/pdf/thoughtleadership/The%20Healthwise%20Ix%20Solution.pdf

*Kids Count* Data Book. (2010). New York: Annie E. Casey Foundation. Retrieved on September 9, 2010, from http://www.aecf.org/MajorInitiatives/KIDSCOUNT.aspx

Koh, H. K., & Sebelius, K. G. (2010). Promoting prevention through the Affordable Care Act. *The New England Journal of Medicine,* 1–5. Retrieved on September 9, 2010, from http://healthpolicyandreform.nejm.org/?p=12171

Kolbe, L. J., et al. (1995). The School Health Policies and Programs Study (SHPPS): Context, methods, general findings, and future efforts. *Journal of School Health, 65* (8), 339–343.

McDermott, R. J. (2000). Health education research: Evolution or revolution (or maybe both)? *Journal of Health Education, 31* (5), 264–271.

McKenzie, J. F. (2004). Professional preparation: Is a generic health educator really possible? *American Journal of Health Education, 35* (1), 46–48.

McKenzie, J. F., Kotecki, J. E., & Pinger, R. R. (2008). An introduction to community health. Boston, MA: Jones and Bartlett.

National Commission for Health Education Credentialing. (2010). *CHES requirements.* Retrieved on December 23, 2010, from http://www.nchec.org/

National Vital Statistics System. (2006). Retrieved on June 14, 2007, from http://www.childstats/gov/americaschildren/pop/asp

O'Rourke, T. (2006). Philosophical reflections on health education and health promotion: Shifting sands and ebbing tides. *The Health Education Monograph Series, 23* (1), 7–10.

Seffrin, J. R. (1994). America's interest in comprehensive school health education. *Journal of School Health, 64* (10), 397–399.

Seffrin, J. R. (March 1997). *AAHE scholar's address.* St. Louis: American Alliance for Health, Physical Education, Recreation, and Dance Convention.

Simons-Morton, B. G., Greene, W. H., & Gottlieb, N. H. (1995). *Introduction to health education and health promotion* (2nd ed.). Prospect Heights, IL: Waveland Press.

Stacy, J. (1991). *Brave new families.* New York: Basic Books.

U.S. Census Bureau. (2010). American Factfinder. Retrieved September 9, 2010, from http://factfinder.census.gov

Williams, D. R., McClellan, M. B., & Rivlin, A. M. (2010). Beyond the Affordable Care Act: Achieving real improvements in American's health. *Health Affairs, 29* (8), 1481–1488.

Yarnall, K.S. H., et al. (2003). Primary care: Is there enough time for prevention? *American Journal of Public Health, 93* (4), 635–641.

# Development of a Unified Code of Ethics for the Health Education Profession[1]

The earliest code of ethics for health educators appears to be the 1976 SOPHE Code of Ethics, developed to guide professional behaviors toward the highest standards of practice for the profession. Following member input, Ethics Committee Chair Elizabeth Bernheimer and Paul Mico refined the Code in 1978. Between 1980 and 1983 renewed attention to the code of ethics resulted in a revision that was to be reviewed by SOPHE Chapters and, if accepted, then submitted to other health education professional associations to serve as a guide for the profession (Bloom, 1999). The 1983 SOPHE Code of Ethics was a combination of standards and principles but no specific rules of conduct at that time (Taub et al., 1987).

Following the earlier recommendation of SOPHE President, Lawrence Green, that SOPHE, AAHE, and the Public Health Education section of APHA consider appointing joint committees, a SOPHE–AAHE Joint Committee was appointed by then AAHE president Peter Cortese and then SOPHE president Ruth Richards in 1984. This committee was charged with developing a profession-wide code of ethics (Bloom, 1999). Between August 1984 and November 1985 the Committee, chaired by Alyson Taub, carried out its charge to (1) identify and use all existing health education ethics statements, (2) determine the appropriate relationship between the code of ethics and the Role Delineation guidelines, including recommendations for enforcement, and (3) to prepare an ethics document for approval as a profession-wide code of ethics. The Joint Committee found that the only health education organization to work on ethics, other than SOPHE, was the American College Health Association, which included a section on ethics in their *Recommended Standards and Practices for a College Health Education Program*. The committee concluded that it was premature to describe how the Code might relate to the Role Delineation guidelines and further recommended that individual responsibility for adhering to the Code of Ethics be the method of enforcement. Finally, the Joint Committee recommended that, in the absence of resources to retain expert consultation in development of ethical codes of conduct, the 1983 SOPHE Code of Ethics be adopted profession-wide and serve as a basis for the next step involving development of rules of conduct (Taub et al., 1987). While SOPHE accepted the Joint Committee's recommendation, there was no similar action by AAHE (Bloom, 1999). The AAHE Board chose not to accept the suggestion of adopting the SOPHE Code on behalf of the profession because they realized that the membership of AAHE needed to be more completely involved in discussing and formulating a Code of Ethics before the AAHE Board could adequately

---

[1]This introduction was prepared through the joint efforts of Ellen Capwell (SOPHE), Becky Smith (AAHE), Janet Shirreffs (AAHE), and Larry K. Olsen (ASHA). Prepared 11/14/99.

represent the interests and needs of AAHE members in collaborative work on ethics with other professional societies.

In September of 1991, an ad hoc AAHE Ethics Committee, chaired by Janet Shirreffs, was charged by President Thomas O'Rourke to develop a code of ethics that represented the professional needs of the variety of health education professionals in the membership of AAHE. They were to review the literature, including other professional codes of ethics, and conduct in-depth surveys of AAHE members. For the next two years, the AAHE Ethics Committee executed its charge through a variety of venues, including correspondence, surveys, face-to-face meetings, presentations and discussion sessions at the national conventions of AAHE, ASHA, and APHA, and through conducting focus group sessions at strategic locations around the country. Based upon the work of this committee, an AAHE Code of Ethics was adopted by the AAHE Board of Directors in April 1993 (AAHE, 1994). Subsequently, both AAHE and SOPHE continued to focus on ethical issues. SOPHE has promoted programming in ethics through its annual and midyear meetings. In December 1992 a summary of the 1983 SOPHE Code of Ethics was prepared by Sarah Olson and distributed as a promotional piece. The SOPHE Board of Trustees supported the summary Code of Ethics in 1994. Since 1993 AAHE has had a standing committee on ethics that recently proposed convention programming and publications in the area of ethics. Recognizing the need to work with other organizations toward a profession-wide Code of Ethics, the SOPHE Board requested that the Coalition of National Health Education Organizations (CNHEO) propose a strategy for accomplishing this goal. In July 1994 the Board adopted a motion that SOPHE support a profession-wide Code of Ethics based on ethical principles and that AAHE should be contacted for support in the effort (Bloom, 1999).

In 1995, the National Commission for Health Education Credentialing, Inc. (NCHEC) and CNHEO co-sponsored a conference, The Health Education Profession in the Twenty-First Century: Setting the Stage (Brown et al., 1996). During that conference, it was recommended that efforts be expanded to develop a profession-wide Code of Ethics.

Shortly thereafter, delegates to the Coalition of National Health Education Organizations pledged to work toward development of a profession-wide Code of Ethics using the existing SOPHE and AAHE Codes as a starting point (Bloom, 1999). A National Ethics Task Force was subsequently developed, with representatives from the various organizations represented on the coalition. It was decided that the coalition delegates would not be the Task Force. As a result, the various member organizations of the coalition were asked to recommend individuals for inclusion on this important Task Force.

During the November 1996 APHA meeting, Larry Olsen, who was the coordinator of the Coalition of National Health Education Organizations and delegate to the coalition from ASHA, William Livingood (SOPHE), and Beverly Mahoney (AAHE) led a session on ethics sponsored by the CNHEO. At that meeting, the basic conceptual plan that had been developed by the coalition's Ethics Task Force was presented. Those attending the session were asked to provide input, both for the process and the content of the "new" Code of Ethics. Those in attendance were strong in their support for the importance of having a Code of Ethics for the profession that would provide an ethical framework for health educators, regardless of the setting in which health education was practiced.

The Ethics Task Force of the Coalition reviewed the two existing codes (SOPHE and AAHE) along with the supporting documents for both, and decided that they would enlist the support of a consultant to assist in the unification process. Claire Stiles of Eckerd College was subsequently retained to offer comments about the proposals of the Task Force, as well as the various drafts that would be developed.

A presentation on behalf of the Ethics Task Force was made in November 1997 at the national APHA meeting in Indianapolis, and the first draft of the "Unified Code of Ethics" was presented. Attendees were asked to comment about the draft document and were asked to take copies of the draft document to distribute among their constituencies. Comments from professionals in the field were returned to and considered by the Task Force.

A second (revised) draft of the Unified Code was presented during the March 1998 AAHE meeting in Reno. Comments received from the APHA Indianapolis meeting and field distribution had been incorporated into the document. In addition, the AAHE Ethics Committee had the opportunity to comment about the "new" document. During the presentation in Reno, participants were put into small groups to discuss and comment on each of the articles included in the draft document. These comments were subsequently incorporated into the document and the stage was set for a series of meetings designed to elicit commentary from professionals in the field, as well as those who attended the meetings of national professional health education organizations.

Following yet another revision of the emerging code, presentations on behalf of the Task Force were made in San Antonio in May 1998 at the joint SOPHE/ASTDHPPHE meeting; in San Diego in June 1998 at the national meeting of ACHA; and in Colorado Springs in October 1998 at the national meeting of ASHA. Throughout this process, comments and suggestions about the code were received and examined by the Task Force. Throughout this process of revision and refinement, care was taken to retain the context and concepts present in the "parent" SOPHE and AAHE documents.

The "first final draft" of the Unified Code of Ethics was presented in Washington, DC, at the November 1998 meeting of the APHA. The coalition also met in conjunction with APHA and it was decided that the final draft of the Unified Code would be prepared for presentation to the field in 1999.

In April 1999 the Unified Code of Ethics was presented in Boston at the national AAHE meeting. During that meeting the coalition also met and it was decided that all delegates to the coalition, as well as the Ethics Task Force members, would examine closely the work that had been done and offer comments and suggestions. It was further decided that coalition delegates would be sent a copy of the entire document (both the long and short forms), so that the documents could be discussed during the coalition's May 1999 conference call. During that conference call, the delegates voted to present the Code of Ethics to their respective organizations, for ratification during the remainder of 1999.

On November 8, 1999, the coalition delegates met in Chicago in conjunction with the American Public Health Association's annual meeting. At that meeting, the Code of Ethics was a topic of discussion. Letters had been received from all the delegate organizations indicating that they had approved the document. It was moved and seconded that the Code of Ethics be approved and distributed to the profession. There being no further comments by the CNHEO delegates, the Code of Ethics was approved, unanimously, as a Code of Ethics for the profession of Health Education.

The Code of Ethics that has evolved from this long and arduous process is not seen as a completed project. Rather, it is envisioned as a living document that will continue to evolve as the practice of Health Education changes to meet the challenges of the new millennium.

### References

Association for the Advancement of Health Education. (1994). Code of ethics for health educators. *Journal of Health Education, 25* (4), 197–200.

Bloom, F. K. (1999). The Society for Public Health Education: Its development and contributions: 1976–1996. Unpublished doctoral dissertation, Columbia University.

Brown, K. M., Cissell, W., DuShaw, M., Goodhart, F., McDermott, R., Middleton, K., Tappe, M., & Welsh, V. (1996). The health education profession in the twenty-first century: Setting the stage. *Journal of Health Education, 27* (6), 357–364.

Taub, A., Kreuter, M., Parcel, G., & Vitello, E. (1987). Report from the AAHE/SOPHE Joint Committee on Ethics. *Health Education Quarterly, 14* (1), 79–90.

*Members of the Ethics Task Force*

Mal Goldsmith (ASHA)

Alyson Taub (SHES Section, APHA)

June Gorski (SOPHE)

Ken McLeroy (PHEHP Section, APHA)

Larry K. Olsen (ASHA), Committee Chair

Wanda Jubb (SSDHPER)

# Code of Ethics for the Health Education Profession

## Long Version[2]

### *Preamble*

The health education profession is dedicated to excellence in the practice of promoting individual, family, organizational, and community health. Guided by common ideals, health educators are responsible for upholding the integrity and ethics of the profession as they face the daily challenges of making decisions. By acknowledging the value of diversity in society and embracing a cross-cultural approach, health educators support the worth, dignity, potential, and uniqueness of all people.

The Code of Ethics provides a framework of shared values within which health education is practiced. The Code of Ethics is grounded in fundamental ethical principles that underlie all health care services: respect for autonomy, promotion of social justice, active promotion of good, and avoidance of harm. The responsibility of each health educator is to aspire to the highest possible standards of conduct and to encourage the ethical behavior of all those with whom they work.

Regardless of job title, professional affiliation, work setting, or population served, health educators abide by these guidelines when making professional decisions.

### *Article I: Responsibility to the Public*

A health educator's ultimate responsibility is to educate people for the purpose of promoting, maintaining, and improving individual, family, and community health. When a conflict of issues arises among individuals, groups, organizations, agencies, or institutions, health educators must consider all issues and give priority to those that promote wellness and quality of living through principles of self-determination and freedom of choice for the individual.

*Section 1* Health educators support the right of individuals to make informed decisions regarding health, as long as such decisions pose no threat to the health of others.

*Section 2* Health educators encourage actions and social policies that support and facilitate the best balance of benefits over harm for all affected parties.

*Section 3* Health educators accurately communicate the potential benefits and consequences of the services and programs with which they are associated.

*Section 4* Health educators accept the responsibility to act on issues that can adversely affect the health of individuals, families, and communities.

*Section 5* Health educators are truthful about their qualifications and the limitations of their expertise and provide services consistent with their competencies.

*Section 6* Health educators protect the privacy and dignity of individuals.

---

[2]Used with the permission of the Coalition of National Health Education Organizations.

**Section 7** Health educators actively involve individuals, groups, and communities in the entire educational process so that all aspects of the process are clearly understood by those who may be affected.

**Section 8** Health educators respect and acknowledge the rights of others to hold diverse values, attitudes, and opinions.

**Section 9** Health educators provide services equitably to all people.

## Article II: Responsibility to the Profession

Health educators are responsible for their professional behavior, for the reputation of their profession, and for promoting ethical conduct among their colleagues.

**Section 1** Health educators maintain, improve, and expand their professional competence through continued study and education; membership, participation, and leadership in professional organizations; and involvement in issues related to the health of the public.

**Section 2** Health educators model and encourage nondiscriminatory standards of behavior in their interactions with others.

**Section 3** Health educators encourage and accept responsible critical discourse to protect and enhance the profession.

**Section 4** Health educators contribute to the development of the profession by sharing the processes and outcomes of their work.

**Section 5** Health educators are aware of possible professional conflicts of interest, exercise integrity in conflict situations, and do not manipulate or violate the rights of others.

**Section 6** Health educators give appropriate recognition to others for their professional contributions and achievements.

## Article III: Responsibility to Employers

Health educators recognize the boundaries of their professional competence and are accountable for their professional activities and actions.

**Section 1** Health educators accurately represent their qualifications and the qualifications of others whom they recommend.

**Section 2** Health educators use appropriate standards, theories, and guidelines as criteria when carrying out their professional responsibilities.

**Section 3** Health educators accurately represent potential service and program outcomes to employers.

**Section 4** Health educators anticipate and disclose competing commitments, conflicts of interest, and endorsement of products.

**Section 5** Health educators openly communicate to employers expectations of job-related assignments that conflict with their professional ethics.

**Section 6** Health educators maintain competence in their areas of professional practice.

## Article IV: Responsibility in the Delivery of Health Education

Health educators promote integrity in the delivery of health education. They respect the rights, dignity, confidentiality, and worth of all people by adapting strategies and methods to meet the needs of diverse populations and communities.

**Section 1** Health educators are sensitive to social and cultural diversity and are in accord with the law when planning and implementing programs.

**Section 2** Health educators are informed of the latest advances in theory, research, and practice, and use strategies and methods that are grounded in and contribute to development of professional standards, theories, guidelines, statistics, and experience.

**Section 3** Health educators are committed to rigorous evaluation of both program effectiveness and the methods used to achieve results.

**Section 4** Health educators empower individuals to adopt healthy lifestyles through informed choice rather than by coercion or intimidation.

*Section 5* Health educators communicate the potential outcomes of proposed services, strategies, and pending decisions to all individuals who will be affected.

## Article V: Responsibility in Research and Evaluation

Health educators contribute to the health of the population and to the profession through research and evaluation activities. When planning and conducting research or evaluation, health educators do so in accordance with federal and state laws and regulations, organizational and institutional policies, and professional standards.

*Section 1* Health educators support principles and practices of research and evaluation that do no harm to individuals, groups, society, or the environment.

*Section 2* Health educators ensure that participation in research is voluntary and is based upon the informed consent of the participants.

*Section 3* Health educators respect the privacy, rights, and dignity of research participants, and honor commitments made to those participants.

*Section 4* Health educators treat all information obtained from participants as confidential unless otherwise required by law.

*Section 5* Health educators take credit, including authorship, only for work they have actually performed and give credit to the contributions of others.

*Section 6* Health educators who serve as research or evaluation consultants discuss their results only with those to whom they are providing service, unless maintaining such confidentiality would jeopardize the health or safety of others.

*Section 7* Health educators report the results of their research and evaluation objectively, accurately, and in a timely fashion.

## Article VI: Responsibility in Professional Preparation

Those involved in the preparation and training of health educators have an obligation to accord learners the same respect and treatment given other groups by providing quality education that benefits the profession and the public.

*Section 1* Health educators select students for professional preparation programs based upon equal opportunity for all, and the individual's academic performance, abilities, and potential contribution to the profession and the public's health.

*Section 2* Health educators strive to make the educational environment and culture conducive to the health of all involved, and free from sexual harassment and all forms of discrimination.

*Section 3* Health educators involved in professional preparation and professional development engage in careful preparation; present material that is accurate, up-to-date, and timely; provide reasonable and timely feedback; state clear and reasonable expectations; and conduct fair assessments and evaluations of learners.

*Section 4* Health educators provide objective and accurate counseling to learners about career opportunities, development, and advancement, and assist learners to secure professional employment.

*Section 5* Health educators provide adequate supervision and meaningful opportunities for the professional development of learners.

## Code of Ethics for the Health Education Profession

### Short Version[2]

#### Preamble

The health education profession is dedicated to excellence in the practice of promoting individual, family, organizational, and community

[2]Used with the permission of the Coalition of National Health Education Organizations.

health. The Code of Ethics provides a framework of shared values within which health education is practiced. The responsibility of each health educator is to aspire to the highest possible standards of conduct and to encourage the ethical behavior of all those with whom they work.

### Article I: Responsibility to the Public

A health educator's ultimate responsibility is to educate people for the purpose of promoting, maintaining, and improving individual, family, and community health. When a conflict of issues arises among individuals, groups, organizations, agencies, or institutions, health educators must consider all issues and give priority to those that promote wellness and quality of living through principles of self-determination and freedom of choice for the individual.

### Article II: Responsibility to the Profession

Health educators are responsible for their professional behavior, for the reputation of their profession, and for promoting ethical conduct among their colleagues.

### Article III: Responsibility to Employers

Health educators recognize the boundaries of their professional competence and are accountable for their professional activities and actions.

### Article IV: Responsibility in the Delivery of Health Education

Health educators promote integrity in the delivery of health education. They respect the rights, dignity, confidentiality, and worth of all people by adapting strategies and methods to meet the needs of diverse populations and communities.

### Article V: Responsibility in Research and Evaluation

Health educators contribute to the health of the population and to the profession through research and evaluation activities. When planning and conducting research or evaluation, health educators do so in accordance with federal and state laws and regulations, organizational and institutional policies, and professional standards.

### Article VI: Responsibility in Professional Preparation

Those involved in the preparation and training of health educators have an obligation to accord learners the same respect and treatment given other groups by providing quality education that benefits the profession and the public.

# Health Education Job Analysis 2010 New Competencies

The Seven Areas of Responsibility are a comprehensive set of Competencies and Sub-competencies defining the role of the health education specialist. These Responsibilities were verified through the 2010 Health Educator Job Analysis Project and serve as the basis of the CHES exam beginning in April 2011 and the MCHES exam in October 2011. The Sub-competencies shaded are advanced-level only and will not be included in the entry-level, CHES examination. However the advanced-level Sub-competences will be included in the October 2011 MCHES examination.

### Area of Responsibility I

ASSESS NEEDS, ASSETS AND CAPACITY FOR HEALTH EDUCATION

*COMPETENCY 1.1:    Plan Assessment Process*

1.1.1  Identify existing and needed resources to conduct assessments

1.1.2  Identify stakeholders to participate in the assessment process

1.1.3  Apply theories and models to develop assessment strategies

1.1.4  Develop plans for data collection, analysis, and interpretation

1.1.5  Engage stakeholders to participate in the assessment process

1.1.6  Integrate research designs, methods, and instruments into assessment plan

*COMPETENCY 1.2:    Access Existing Information and Data Related to Health*

1.2.1  Identify sources of data related to health

1.2.2  Critique sources of health information using theory and evidence from the literature

1.2.3  Select valid sources of information about health

1.2.4  Identify gaps in data using theories and assessment models

1.2.5  Establish collaborative relationships and agreements that facilitate access to data

1.2.6  Conduct searches of existing databases for specific health-related data

*COMPETENCY 1.3:    Collect Quantitative and/or Qualitative Data Related to Health*

1.3.1  Collect primary and/or secondary data

1.3.2  Integrate primary data with secondary data

1.3.3  Identify data collection instruments and methods

1.3.4  Develop data collection instruments and methods

1.3.5  Train personnel and stakeholders regarding data collection

1.3.6  Use data collection instruments and methods

1.3.7 Employ ethical standards when collecting data

COMPETENCY 1.4: *Examine Relationships Among Behavioral, Environmental and Genetic Factors That Enhance or Compromise Health*

1.4.1 Identify factors that influence health behaviors

1.4.2 Analyze factors that influence health behaviors

1.4.3 Identify factors that enhance or compromise health

1.4.4 Analyze factors that enhance or compromise health

COMPETENCY 1.5: *Examine Factors That Influence the Learning Process*

1.5.1 Identify factors that foster or hinder the learning process

1.5.2 Analyze factors that foster or hinder the learning process

1.5.3 Identify factors that foster or hinder attitudes and belief

1.5.4 Analyze factors that foster or hinder attitudes and beliefs

1.5.5 Identify factors that foster or hinder skill building

1.5.6 Analyze factors that foster or hinder skill building

COMPETENCY 1.6: *Examine Factors That Enhance or Compromise the Process of Health Education*

1.6.1 Determine the extent of available health education programs, interventions, and policies

1.6.2 Assess the quality of available health education programs, interventions, and policies

1.6.3 Identify existing and potential partners for the provision of health education

1.6.4 Assess social, environmental, and political conditions that may impact health education

1.6.5 Analyze the capacity for developing needed health education

1.6.6 Assess the need for resources to foster health education

COMPETENCY 1.7: *Infer Needs for Health Education Based on Assessment Findings*

1.7.1 Analyze assessment findings

1.7.2 Synthesize assessment findings

1.7.3 Prioritize health education needs

1.7.4 Identify emerging health education needs

1.7.5 Report assessment findings

## Area of Responsibility II

### PLAN HEALTH EDUCATION

COMPETENCY 2.1: *Involve Priority Populations and Other Stakeholders in the Planning Process*

2.1.1 Incorporate principles of community organization

2.1.2 Identify priority populations and other stakeholders

2.1.3 Communicate need for health education to priority populations and other stakeholders

2.1.4 Develop collaborative efforts among priority populations and other stakeholders

2.1.5 Elicit input from priority populations and other stakeholders

2.1.6 Obtain commitments from priority populations and other stakeholders

COMPETENCY 2.2: *Develop Goals and Objectives*

2.2.1 Use assessment results to inform the planning process

2.2.2 Identify desired outcomes utilizing the needs assessment results

2.2.3  Select planning model(s) for health education

2.2.4  Develop goal statements

2.2.5  Formulate specific, measurable, attainable, realistic, and time-sensitive objectives

2.2.6  Assess resources needed to achieve objectives

*COMPETENCY 2.3:    Select or Design Strategies and Interventions*

2.3.1  Assess efficacy of various strategies to ensure consistency with objectives

2.3.2  Design theory-based strategies and interventions to achieve stated objectives

2.3.3  Select a variety of strategies and interventions to achieve stated objectives

2.3.4  Comply with legal and ethical principles in designing strategies and interventions

2.3.5  Apply principles of cultural competence in selecting and designing strategies and interventions

2.3.6  Pilot test strategies and interventions

*COMPETENCY 2.4:    Develop a Scope and Sequence for the Delivery of Health Education*

2.4.1  Determine the range of health education needed to achieve goals and objectives

2.4.2  Select resources required to implement health education

2.4.3  Use logic models to guide the planning process

2.4.4  Organize health education into a logical sequence

2.4.5  Develop a timeline for the delivery of health education

2.4.6  Analyze the opportunity for integrating health education into other programs

2.4.7  Develop a process for integrating health education into other programs

*COMPETENCY 2.5:    Address Factors That Affect Implementation*

2.5.1  Identify factors that foster or hinder implementation

2.5.2  Analyze factors that foster or hinder implementation

2.5.3  Use findings of pilot to refine implementation plans as needed

2.5.4  Develop a conducive learning environment

### Area of Responsibility III

IMPLEMENT HEALTH EDUCATION

*COMPETENCY 3.1:    Implement a Plan of Action*

3.1.1  Assess readiness for implementation

3.1.2  Collect baseline data

3.1.3  Use strategies to ensure cultural competence in implementing health education plans

3.1.4  Use a variety of strategies to deliver a plan of action

3.1.5  Promote plan of action

3.1.6  Apply theories and models of implementation

3.1.7  Launch plan of action

*COMPETENCY 3.2:    Monitor Implementation of Health Education*

3.2.1  Monitor progress in accordance with timeline

3.2.2  Assess progress in achieving objectives

3.2.3  Modify plan of action as needed

3.2.4  Monitor use of resources

3.2.5  Monitor compliance with legal and ethical principles

*COMPETENCY 3.3:    Train Individuals Involved in Implementation of Health Education*

3.3.1  Select training participants needed for implementation

3.3.2 Identify training needs

3.3.3 Develop training objectives

3.3.4 Create training using best practices

3.3.5 Demonstrate a wide range of training strategies

3.3.6 Deliver training

3.3.7 Evaluate training

3.3.8 Use evaluation findings to plan future training

### Area of Responsibility IV

### CONDUCT EVALUATION AND RESEARCH RELATED TO HEALTH EDUCATION

COMPETENCY 4.1: *Develop Evaluation/Research Plan*

4.1.1 Create purpose statement

4.1.2 Develop evaluation/research questions

4.1.3 Assess feasibility of conducting evaluation/research

4.1.4 Critique evaluation and research methods and findings found in the related literature

4.1.5 Synthesize information found in the literature

4.1.6 Assess the merits and limitations of qualitative and quantitative data collection for evaluation

4.1.7 Assess the merits and limitations of qualitative and quantitative data collection for research

4.1.8 Identify existing data collection instruments

4.1.9 Critique existing data collection instruments for evaluation

4.1.10 Critique existing data collection instruments for research

4.1.11 Create a logic model to guide the evaluation process

4.1.12 Develop data analysis plan for evaluation

4.1.13 Develop data analysis plan for research

4.1.14 Apply ethical standards in developing the evaluation/research plan

COMPETENCY 4.2: *Design Instruments to Collect*

4.2.1 Identify useable questions from existing instruments

4.2.2 Write new items to be used in data collection for evaluation

4.2.3 Write new items to be used in data collection for research

4.2.4 Establish validity of data collection instruments

4.2.5 Establish reliability of data collection instruments

COMPETENCY 4.3: *Collect and Analyze Evaluation/ Research Data*

4.3.1 Collect data based on the evaluation/research plan

4.3.2 Monitor data collection and management

4.3.3 Analyze data using descriptive statistics

4.3.4 Analyze data using inferential and/or other advanced statistical methods

4.3.5 Analyze data using qualitative methods

4.3.6 Apply ethical standards in collecting and analyzing data

COMPETENCY 4.4: *Interpret Results of the Evaluation/ Research*

4.4.1 Compare results to evaluation/ research questions

4.4.2 Compare results to other findings

4.4.3 Propose possible explanations of findings

4.4.4 Identify possible limitations of findings

4.4.5 Develop recommendations based on results

COMPETENCY 4.5: *Apply Findings From Evaluation/ Research*

4.5.1 Communicate findings to stakeholders

4.5.2 Evaluate feasibility of implementing recommendations from evaluation

4.5.3 Apply evaluation findings in policy analysis and program development

4.5.4 Disseminate research findings through professional conference presentations

### Area of Responsibility V

#### ADMINISTER AND MANAGE HEALTH EDUCATION

COMPETENCY 5.1: *Manage Fiscal Resources*

5.1.1 Identify fiscal and other resources

5.1.2 Prepare requests/proposals to obtain fiscal resources

5.1.3 Develop budgets to support health education efforts

5.1.4 Manage program budgets

5.1.5 Prepare budget reports

5.1.6 Demonstrate ethical behavior in managing fiscal resources

COMPETENCY 5.2: *Obtain Acceptance and Support for Programs*

5.2.1 Use communication strategies to obtain program support

5.2.2 Facilitate cooperation among stakeholders responsible for health education

5.2.3 Prepare reports to obtain and/or maintain program support

5.2.4 Synthesize data for purposes of reporting

5.2.5 Provide support for individuals who deliver professional development opportunities

5.2.6 Explain how program goals align with organizational structure, mission, and goals

COMPETENCY 5.3: *Demonstrate Leadership*

5.3.1 Conduct strategic planning

5.3.2 Analyze an organization's culture in relationship to health education goals

5.3.3 Promote collaboration among stakeholders

5.3.4 Develop strategies to reinforce or change organizational culture to achieve health education goals

5.3.5 Comply with existing laws and regulations

5.3.6 Adhere to ethical standards of the profession

5.3.7 Facilitate efforts to achieve organizational mission

5.3.8 Analyze the need for a systems approach to change

5.3.9 Facilitate needed changes to organizational cultures

COMPETENCY 5.4: *Manage Human Resources*

5.4.1 Develop volunteer opportunities

5.4.2 Demonstrate leadership skills in managing human resources

5.4.3 Apply human resource policies consistent with relevant laws and regulations

5.4.4 Evaluate qualifications of staff and volunteers needed for programs

5.4.5 Recruit volunteers and staff

5.4.6 Employ conflict resolution strategies

5.4.7 Apply appropriate methods for team development

5.4.8 Model professional practices and ethical behavior

5.4.9 Develop strategies to enhance staff and volunteers' career development

5.4.10 Implement strategies to enhance staff and volunteers' career development

5.4.11 Evaluate performance of staff and volunteers

COMPETENCY 5.5: *Facilitate Partnerships in Support of Health Education*

5.5.1 Identify potential partner(s)

5.5.2 Assess capacity of potential partner(s) to meet program goals

5.5.3 Facilitate partner relationship(s)

5.5.4 Elicit feedback from partner(s)

5.5.5 Evaluate feasibility of continuing partnership

## Area of Responsibility VI

### SERVE AS A HEALTH EDUCATION RESOURCE PERSON

COMPETENCY 6.1: *Obtain and Disseminate Health-Related Information*

6.1.1 Assess information needs

6.1.2 Identify valid information resources

6.1.3 Critique resource materials for accuracy, relevance, and timeliness

6.1.4 Convey health-related information to priority populations

6.1.5 Convey health-related information to key stakeholders

COMPETENCY 6.2: *Provide Training*

6.2.1 Analyze requests for training

6.2.2 Prioritize requests for training

6.2.3 Identify priority populations

6.2.4 Assess needs for training

6.2.5 Identify existing resources that meet training needs

6.2.6 Use learning theory to develop or adapt training programs

6.2.7 Develop training plan

6.2.8 Implement training sessions and programs

6.2.9 Use a variety of resources and strategies

6.2.10 Evaluate impact of training programs

COMPETENCY 6.3: *Serve as a Health Education Consultant*

6.3.1 Assess needs for assistance

6.3.2 Prioritize requests for assistance

6.3.3 Define parameters of effective consultative relationships

6.3.4 Establish consultative relationships

6.3.5 Provide expert assistance

6.3.6 Facilitate collaborative efforts to achieve program goals

6.3.7 Evaluate the effectiveness of the expert assistance provided

6.3.8 Apply ethical principles in consultative relationships

## Area of Responsibility VII

### COMMUNICATE AND ADVOCATE FOR HEALTH AND HEALTH EDUCATION

COMPETENCY 7.1: *Assess and Prioritize Health Information and Advocacy Needs*

7.1.1 Identify current and emerging issues that may influence health and health education

7.1.2 Access accurate resources related to identified issues

7.1.3 Analyze the impact of existing and proposed policies on health

7.1.4 Analyze factors that influence decision-makers

COMPETENCY 7.2: *Identify and Develop a Variety of Communication Strategies, Methods, and Techniques*

7.2.1 Create messages using communication theories and models

7.2.2 Tailor messages to priority populations

7.2.3 Incorporate images to enhance messages

7.2.4 Select effective methods or channels for communicating to priority populations

7.2.5 Pilot test messages and delivery methods with priority populations

7.2.6 Revise messages based on pilot feedback.

COMPETENCY 7.3: *Deliver Messages Using a Variety of Strategies, Methods and Techniques*

7.3.1 Use techniques that empower individuals and communities to improve their health

7.3.2   Employ technology to communicate to priority populations

7.3.3   Evaluate the delivery of communication strategies, methods, and techniques

### COMPETENCY 7.4:   *Engage in Health Education Advocacy*

7.4.1   Engage stakeholders in advocacy

7.4.2   Develop an advocacy plan in compliance with local, state, and/or federal policies and procedures

7.4.3   Comply with organizational policies related to participating in advocacy

7.4.4   Communicate the impact of health and health education on organizational and socio-ecological factors

7.4.5   Use data to support advocacy messages

7.4.6   Implement advocacy plans

7.4.7   Incorporate media and technology in advocacy

7.4.8   Participate in advocacy initiatives

7.4.9   Lead advocacy initiatives

7.4.10  Evaluate advocacy efforts

### COMPETENCY 7.5:   *Influence Policy to Promote Health*

7.5.1   Use evaluation and research findings in policy analysis

7.5.2   Identify the significance and implications of health policy for individuals, groups, and communities

7.5.3   Advocate for health-related policies, regulations, laws, or rules

7.5.4   Use evidence-based research to develop policies to promote health

7.5.5   Employ policy and media advocacy techniques to influence decision-makers

### COMPETENCY 7.6:   *Promote the Health Education Profession*

7.6.1   Develop a personal plan for professional growth and service

7.6.2   Describe state-of-the-art health education practice

7.6.3   Explain the major responsibilities of the health education specialist in the practice of health education

7.6.4   Explain the role of health education associations in advancing the profession

7.6.5   Explain the benefits of participating in professional organizations

7.6.6   Facilitate professional growth of self and others

7.6.7   Explain the history of the health education profession and its current and future implications for professional practice

7.6.8   Explain the role of credentialing in the promotion of the health education profession

7.6.9   Engage in professional development activities

7.6.10  Serve as a mentor to others

7.6.11  Develop materials that contribute to the professional literature

7.6.12  Engage in service to advance the health education profession

---

*Source:* From The National Commission for Health Education Credentialing, Inc. http://www.nchec.org. Used by permission of NCHEC.

# Eta Sigma Gamma Chapters: Locations and Dates of Installation

| Chapter | Location | Date of Installation |
|---|---|---|
| Alpha | Ball State University, Muncie, IN | 1968 |
| Beta | Eastern Kentucky University, Richmond, KY | 1969 |
| Gamma | California State University, Long Beach, CA | 1970 |
| Delta* | California State University, San Diego, CA | 1970 |
| Epsilon | University of Maryland, College Park, MD | 1970 |
| Zeta* | Trenton State College, Trenton, NJ | 1970 |
| Eta | Central Michigan University, Mt. Pleasant, MI | 1970 |
| Theta* | University of Nebraska, Lincoln, NE | 1972 |
| Iota | University of Toledo, Toledo, OH | 1973 |
| Kappa | SUNY College of Cortland, Cortland, NY | 1973 |
| Lambda | Indiana State University, Terre Haute, IN | 1974 |
| Mu* | Western Kentucky University, Bowling Green, KY | 1974 |
| Nu | Indiana University, Bloomington, IN | 1974 |
| Xi* | Purdue University, West Lafayette, IN | 1974 |
| Omicron* | Slippery Rock University, Slippery Rock, PA | 1974 |
| Pi | Western Illinois University, Macomb, IL | 1974 |
| Rho | Kent State University, Kent, OH | 1974 |
| Sigma | James Madison University, Harrisonburg, VA | 1974 |
| Tau* | University of Illinois, Champaign-Urbana, IL | 1975 |
| Upsilon* | Russell Sage College, Albany, NY | 1975 |
| Phi | University of Northern Colorado, Greeley, CO | 1976 |
| Chi | University of Utah, Salt Lake City, UT | 1976 |
| Psi* | Brigham Young University, Provo, UT | 1976 |
| Omega | Illinois State University, Normal, IL | 1976 |
| Alpha Alpha | Southern Illinois University, Carbondale, IL | 1976 |
| Alpha Beta* | Kansas State University, Manhattan, KS | 1976 |
| Alpha Gamma | University of North Florida, Jacksonville, FL | 1976 |
| Alpha Delta | Florida State University, Tallahassee, FL | 1976 |
| Alpha Epsilon* | University of New Mexico, Albuquerque, NM | 1977 |
| Alpha Zeta | California State University, Northridge, CA | 1977 |
| Alpha Eta* | Texas Tech University, Lubbock, TX | 1977 |
| Alpha Theta | Adelphi University, Garden City, NY | 1977 |

| | | |
|---|---|---|
| Alpha Iota | University of Southern Mississippi, Hattiesburg, MS | 1977 |
| Alpha Kappa* | University of Central Arkansas, Conway, AK | 1977 |
| Alpha Lambda | University of Florida, Gainesville, FL | 1977 |
| Alpha Mu* | University of Tennessee, Knoxville, TN | 1978 |
| Alpha Nu | University of North Carolina, Greensboro, NC | 1978 |
| Alpha Xi* | Penn State University, University Park, PA | 1978 |
| Alpha Omicron | Temple University, Philadelphia, PA | 1978 |
| Alpha Pi | Texas A & M University, College Station, TX | 1978 |
| Alpha Rho* | Montclair State University, Montclair, NJ | 1978 |
| Alpha Sigma* | Arizona State University, Tempe, AZ | 1978 |
| Alpha Tau* | Oregon State University, Corvallis, OR | 1979 |
| Alpha Upsilon | Central Washington University, Ellensburg, WA | 1979 |
| Alpha Phi | Texas Women's University, Denton, TX | 1979 |
| Alpha Chi | St. Francis College, Brooklyn, NY | 1979 |
| Alpha Psi* | The Ohio State University, Columbus, OH | 1980 |
| Alpha Omega | University of Nebraska, Omaha, NE | 1980 |
| Beta Alpha | University of Minnesota, Duluth, MN | 1980 |
| Beta Beta* | University of South Carolina, Columbia, SC | 1980 |
| Beta Gamma* | Bowling Green State University, Bowling Green, OH | 1980 |
| Beta Delta | Eastern Michigan University, Ypsilanti, MI | 1980 |
| Beta Epsilon | University of Maine, Farmington, ME | 1980 |
| Beta Zeta | Towson State University, Towson, MD | 1980 |
| Beta Eta | Sam Houston State University, Huntsville, TX | 1980 |
| Beta Theta | East Carolina University, Greenville, NC | 1980 |
| Beta Iota* | Eastern Tennessee State University, Johnson City, TN | 1980 |
| Beta Kappa | Minnesota State University, Mankato, Mankato, MN | 1981 |
| Beta Lambda* | University of Oregon, Eugene, OR | 1981 |
| Beta Mu* | Northeastern University, Boston, MA | 1981 |
| Beta Nu | Eastern Illinois University, Charleston, IL | 1982 |
| Beta Xi* | West Chester University, West Chester, PA | 1982 |
| Beta Omicron | Worcester State College, Worcester, MA | 1982 |
| Beta Pi* | University of Georgia, Athens, GA | 1983 |
| Beta Rho* | Louisiana State University, Baton Rouge, LA | 1983 |
| Beta Sigma | Wayne State University, Detroit, MI | 1983 |
| Beta Tau* | University of Arkansas, Fayetteville, AK | 1983 |
| Beta Upsilon* | Texas A & I University, Kingsville, TX | 1983 |
| Beta Phi | University of Wisconsin, La Crosse, WI | 1983 |
| Beta Chi | University of Alabama–Birmingham, Birmingham, AL | 1984 |
| Beta Psi | State University of New York, Brockport, NY | 1984 |
| Beta Omega | New Mexico State University, Las Cruces, NM | 1984 |
| Gamma Alpha* | Western Washington University, Bellingham, WA | 1984 |
| Gamma Beta* | University of Richmond, Richmond, VA | 1984 |
| Gamma Gamma* | Virginia Tech, Blacksburg, VA | 1986 |
| Gamma Delta | Southern Illinois University, Edwardsville, IL | 1987 |
| Gamma Epsilon* | Utah State University, Logan, UT | 1987 |
| Gamma Zeta | Plymouth State University, Plymouth, NH | 1988 |
| Gamma Eta | University of Cincinnati, Cincinnati, OH | 1988 |
| Gamma Theta | Youngstown State University, Youngstown, OH | 1991 |

| | | |
|---|---|---|
| Gamma Iota | Georgia College, Milledgeville, GA | 1991 |
| Gamma Kappa | Liberty University, Lynchberg, VA | 1992 |
| Gamma Lambda | University of Texas–El Paso, El Paso, TX | 1993 |
| Gamma Mu | Western Michigan University, Kalamazoo, MI | 1993 |
| Gamma Nu* | University of Nevada–Reno, Reno, NV | 1993 |
| Gamma Xi | East Stroudsburg University, East Stroudsburg, PA | 1995 |
| Gamma Omicron* | Springfield College, Springfield, MA | 1995 |
| Gamma Pi | Hofstra University, Hempstead, NY | 1995 |
| Gamma Rho | Truman State University, Kirksville, MO | 1996 |
| Gamma Sigma* | Appalachian State University, Boone, NC | 1996 |
| Gamma Tau | University of North Texas, Denton, TX | 1996 |
| Gamma Upsilon | Georgia Southern University, Statesboro, GA | 1996 |
| Gamma Phi | North Carolina Central University, Durham, NC | 1998 |
| Gamma Chi | Clemson University, Clemson, SC | 1997 |
| Gamma Psi* | Western Oregon State University, Monmouth, OR | 1997 |
| Gamma Omega | William Paterson College, Wayne, NJ | 1997 |
| Delta Alpha* | Iowa State University, Ames, IA | 1997 |
| Delta Beta | University of Montana, Missoula, MT | 1998 |
| Delta Gamma* | Cleveland State University, Cleveland, OH | 1998 |
| Delta Delta | California State University, San Bernardino, CA | 1998 |
| Delta Epsilon | Morgan State University, Baltimore, MD | 1999 |
| Delta Zeta | Coastal Carolina University, Conway, SC | 1999 |
| Delta Eta | Ohio University, Athens, OH | 2000 |
| Delta Theta | SUNY College at Potsdam, Potsdam, NY | 2000 |
| Delta Iota | Southern Connecticut State University, New Haven, CT | 2001 |
| Delta Kappa | University of South Florida, Tampa, FL | 2002 |
| Delta Lambda | Malone College, Canton, OH | 2002 |
| Delta Mu | Morehead State University, Morehead, KY | 2002 |
| Delta Nu* | Idaho State University, Pocatello, ID | 2002 |
| Delta Xi | University of Alabama, Tuscaloosa, AL | 2003 |
| Delta Omicron | Lamar University, Beaumont, TX | 2003 |
| Delta Pi | Bridgewater State College, Bridgewater, MA | 2004 |
| Delta Rho | California State University, Fullerton, CA | 2004 |
| Delta Sigma | Keene State College, Keene, NH | 2005 |
| Delta Tau | Columbus State University, Columbus, GA | 2005 |
| Delta Upsilon | University of Wisconsin–River Falls, River Falls, WI | 2005 |
| Delta Phi | University of Michigan–Flint, Flint, MI | 2006 |
| Delta Chi | Texas State University, San Marcos, TX | 2006 |
| Delta Psi | Northern Illinois University, Dekalb, IL | 2006 |
| Delta Omega | University of Northern Iowa, Cedar Falls, IA | 2006 |
| Epsilon Alpha | Baylor University, Waco, TX | 2007 |
| Epsilon Beta | Rutgers University, New Brunswick, NJ | 2009 |
| Epsilon Gamma | Monmouth University, West Long Branch, NJ | 2009 |

*Source:* National Office of Eta Sigma Gamma, 2000 University Avenue, Muncie, IN 47306. Used with permission.

*These chapters were inactive at the time this chapter was written.

# Glossary

*A New Perspective on the Health of Canadians*
the Canadian publication that presented the
epidemiological evidence supporting the importance of lifestyle and environmental factors on
health and sickness and called for numerous national health promotion strategies to encourage
Canadians to become more responsible for their
own health.

**abstracts** short summaries of research studies that
have appeared in selected journals.

**accreditation** "the process by which a recognized
professional body evaluates an entire college or
university professional preparation program"
(Cleary, 1995, p. 39) (Chapter 6).

**action stage** a stage of the transtheoretical model
in which a person is overtly making changes.

**actual behavioral control** having the "the skills,
resources, and other prerequisites needed to
perform a given behavior" (Ajzen, 2006)
(Chapter 4).

**adjusted rate** a rate that is statistically adjusted for
a certain characteristic, such as age, expressed
for a total population.

**administrative and policy assessment** is "an
analysis of the policies, resources, and circumstances prevailing in an organizational situation
to facilitate or hinder the development of the
health program" (Green & Kreuter, 2005,
p. G-1) (Chapter 4).

**advocacy** "the actions or endeavors individuals
or groups engage in in order to alter public
opinion in favor or in opposition to a certain
policy" (Pinzon-Perez & Perez, 1999, p. 29)
(Chapter 1).

**Affordable Care Act (ACA)** the official title of
health care reform legislation that was passed
by Congress in March 2010. All of the provisions of the ACA will be fully implemented by
2020.

**American Academy of Health Behavior (AAHB)**
society of researchers and scholars in the areas
of human behavior, health education, and
health promotion.

**American Alliance for Health, Physical Education,
Recreation and Dance (AAHPERD)** a profes-
sional alliance of five national associations
(American Association for Physical Activity and
Recreations, American Association for Health
Education, National Association for Girls' and
Women's Sports, National Association for Sport
and Physical Education, National Dance
Association), six district associations (Central,
Eastern, Midwest, Northwest, Southern, and
Southwest), and a research consortium.

**American Association for Health Education
(AAHE)** a professional association within
AAHPERD.

**American College Health Association (ACHA)** a
professional association comprising mostly individuals who work in colleges and universities.

**American Public Health Association (APHA)** a
professional association for those individuals
working in the fields of public health.

**American Red Cross (ARC)** a quasi-governmental
organization.

**American School Health Association (ASHA)** a
professional association comprising
individuals interested in coordinated school
health programs.

**anonymity** exists when no one, including those
conducting the program, can relate a participant's
identity to any information pertaining to the
program.

**Asclepiads** a brotherhood of men associated with
the Asclepian temples who first began the practice of medicine based on a more rational basis.

**Asclepius** the Greek god of medicine, for whom
many temples were built.

**assessment** the estimation of the relative magnitude, importance, or value of objects observed.

**attitude toward the behavior** an attitude about a certain behavior; a construct of the theory of planned behavior.

**bacteriological period of public health** the period of 1875 to 1900, during which great advancements in the study of bacteria occurred.

**behavioral capability** the knowledge and skills necessary to perform a behavior.

**behavior change philosophy** involves a health education specialist using behavioral contracts, goal setting, and self-monitoring to help foster and motivate the modification of an unhealthy habit in an individual with whom the health education specialist is working.

**beneficence** "simply doing good" (Balog et al., 1985, p. 91) (Chapter 5).

**benevolence** see beneficence.

**browser** a software package used for exploring the World Wide Web—Internet Explorer, for example.

**caduceus** the serpent and staff symbol of medicine, which was the symbol of the Asclepian Temples.

**capacity** "refers to both individual and collective resources that can be brought to bear for health enhancement" (Gilmore & Campbell, 2005, p. 7) (Chapter 6).

**CDCynergy** a health communication planning model developed by the Office of Communication at the Centers for Disease Control and Prevention.

**certification** "a process by which a professional organization grants recognition to an individual who, upon completion of a competency-based curriculum, can demonstrate a predetermined standard of performance" (Cleary, 1995, p. 39) (Chapter 6).

**Certified Health Education Specialist (CHES)** a health education specialist who has met all necessary requirements and has been certified by the National Commission for Health Education Credentialing, Inc.

**chain of infection** a model used to help explain the spread of a communicable disease from one host to another.

**Coalition of National Health Education Organizations, USA (CNHEO)** a coalition made up of representatives from eight professional associations, of which health education specialists are members.

**code of ethics** "document that maps the dimensions of the profession's collective social responsibility and acknowledges the obligations individual practitioners share in meeting the profession's responsibilities" (Feeney & Freeman, 1999, p. 6) (Chapter 5).

**Code of Hammurabi** the earliest written record concerning public health.

**cognitive-based philosophy** a philosophy that focuses on the acquisition of content and factual information to increase knowledge so a person is better equipped to make health-related decisions.

**communicable disease model** a model used to help explain the spread of a communicable disease from one host to another via the elements of agent, host, and environment.

**communicable diseases** those diseases for which biological agents or their products are the cause and that are transmissible from one individual to another (McKenzie et al., 2012) (Chapter 1).

**community empowerment** "helping people help themselves in a way that encourages them to take ownership of their health problems and use their abilities and resources to develop solutions" (Doyle & Ward, 2001, p. 125) (Chapter 6).

**community health** "the health status of a defined group of people and the actions and conditions to protect and improve the health of the community" (Green & McKenzie, 2002, p. 247) (Chapter 1).

**community health education** health education/promotion programs conducted in departments of health, voluntary agencies, hospitals, religious organizations, and so on.

**competencies** "reflects the ability of the student to understand, know, etc." (National Commission for Health Education Credentialing, Inc., 1996, p. 12) (Chapter 6).

**Competencies Update Project (CUP)** a project to review and update both entry-level and advanced-level health education/promotion competencies.

**comprehensive school health instruction** the development, delivery, and evaluation of a planned curriculum, preschool through grade 12, with goals, objectives, content sequence, and specific classroom lessons that include, but are not limited to, the following major content areas: community health, consumer health, environmental health, family life, mental and emotional health, injury prevention and safety, nutrition, personal health, prevention and control of disease, and substance use and abuse (Joint Committee on Health Education Terminology, 1991a, p. 102) (Chapter 2).

**computerized databases** computerized storage disks containing a large compilation of references; each database is specific to a general subject area (e.g., education, medicine) and provides access to the cumulative information found in several index or abstract sources on that subject area.

**concepts** the primary elements, building blocks, or major components of theories.

**confidentiality** exists when only those responsible for conducting a program can link information about a participant with that person and have promised not to reveal such to others.

**consequentialism** see teleological theories.

**conservative** a person who generally distrusts governmental regulations and tax-supported programs for addressing social or economic problems.

**construct** a concept that has been developed, created, or adopted for use with a specific theory.

**contemplation stage** a stage of the transtheoretical model in which a person is seriously thinking about change in the next six months.

**continuum theories** those behavior change theories that identify variables that influence actions and combine them into a single equation that predicts the likelihood of action (Weinstein, Rothman, & Sutton, 1998; Weinstein, Sandman, & Blalock, 2008) (Chapter 4).

**coordinated school health program** "an organized set of policies, procedures, and activities designed to protect, promote, and improve the health and well-being of students and staff, thus improving a student's ability to learn. It includes, but is not limited to, comprehensive school health education; school health services; a healthy school environment; school counseling; psychological and social services; physical education; school nutrition services; family and community involvement in school health; and school-site health promotion for staff" (Joint Terminology Committee, 2001, p. 99) (Chapter 1).

**credentialing** a process whereby an individual or a professional preparation program meets the specified standards established by the credentialing body and is thus recognized for having done so.

**crude rate** the rate expressed for a total population.

**cue to action** a construct of the health belief model that motivates a person to act.

**culturally competent** having the ability "to understand and respect values, attitudes, beliefs, and mores that differ across cultures, and to consider and respond appropriately to these differences in planning, implementing, and evaluating health education and health promotion programs and interventions" (Joint Committee, 2001, p. 99) (Chapter 1).

**death rates** the number of deaths per 100,000 resident population, sometimes referred to as mortality or fatality rates.

**decision-making philosophy** the belief that the use of scenarios, case studies, and simulated problems is the best method to motivate persons to adopt positive health behaviors.

**demographic profile** a statistical breakdown of the population of a country, region, state, or city by age group, sex, race, and ethnicity.

**deontological theories** (or formalism or nonconsequentialism) "are those that claim that certain actions are inherently right or wrong, or good or bad, without regard for their consequences" (Reamer, 2006, p. 65) (Chapter 5).

**determinants of health** include gestational endowment (i.e., genetic makeup), social circumstances, environmental conditions, health behavior, and access to quality medical care.

**Diffusion Theory** a theory that provides an explanation for the movement of an innovation through a population.

**Directors of Health Promotion and Public Health Education (DHPE)** a professional association composed of individuals who, by position, head their state or territory public health education/promotion efforts.

**disability-adjusted life years (DALYs)** a measure of health that takes into effect the severity of the health condition, age, and impact on the future.

**disease prevention** "the process of reducing risks and alleviating disease to promote, preserve, and restore health and minimize suffering and distress" (Joint Terminology Committee, 2001, p. 99) (Chapter 1).

**distributive justice** deals with the allocation of resources (Summers, 2009) (Chapter 5).

**early adopters** a group of people who are very interested in innovation, but who do not want to be the first involved.

**early majority** a group of people who may be interested in an innovation but will need some external motivation to get involved.

**eclectic health education/promotion philosophy** a philosophical approach held by health education specialists that no one philosophy is "right" for all times and circumstances and that the best philosophy involves blending the various philosophical approaches or using different approaches depending on the setting (school, community, worksite).

**ecological approaches** those that use the various environment dimensions—physical, social, and cultural—to affect behavior.

**ecological assessment** is "a systematic assessment of factors in the social and physical environment that interact with behavior to produce health effects or quality-of-life outcomes" (Green & Kreuter, 2005, p. G-3) (Chapter 4).

**ecological perspective** see **socio-ecological approach.**

**educational assessment** is "the delineation of factors that predispose, enable, and reinforce a specific behavior, or through behavior, environmental changes" (Green & Kreuter, 2005, p. G-3) (Chapter 4).

**elaboration** the amount of cognitive processing (i.e., thought) that a person puts into receiving messages (Petty, Barden, & Wheeler) (Chapter 4).

**electronic database** see "computerized databases"

**emerging profession** an occupation that does not rank so clearly high or so clearly low on the attributes that distinguish an occupation from a profession (Barber, 1988) (Chapter 1).

**emotional-coping response** to learn, a person must be able to deal with the sources of anxiety that surround a behavior.

**empowerment** "social action process for people to gain mastery over their lives and the lives of their communities" (Minkler, Wallerstein, & Wilson, 2008, p. 294) (Chapter 1).

**enabling factor** "any characteristic of the environment that facilitates action and any skill or resource required to attain a specific behavior" (Green & Kreuter, 1999, p. 505) (Chapter 4).

**endemic** occurs regularly in a population as a matter of course.

**environment** "all those matters related to health which are external to the human body and over which the individual has little or no control" (Lalonde, 1974, p. 32) (Chapter 1).

**environmental assessment** "a systematic assessment of factors in the social and physical environment that interact with behavior to produce health effects or quality-of-life outcomes. Also referred to as **ecological assessment**" (Green & Kreuter, 1999, p. 505) (Chapter 4).

**epidemic** an unexpectedly large number of cases of an illness, specific health-related behavior, or health-related event in a population.

**epidemiological assessment** "the delineation of the extent, distribution, and causes of a health problem in a defined population" (Green & Kreuter, 2005, p. G-3) (Chapter 4).

**epidemiological data** information gathered when measuring health and ill health.

**epidemiology** "the study of the distribution and determinants of health-related states or events in specific populations, and the application of this study to control health problems" (Dictionary of Epidemiology as cited in Last, 2007, p. iii) (Chapter 1).

**epistemology** the study of knowledge (Thiroux, 1995) (Chapter 5).

**Eta Sigma Gamma (ESG)** the national health education honorary society.

**ethical** good/bad, and right/wrong.

**ethics** "the study of morality, one of the three major areas of philosophy, also referred to as moral philosophy" (Thiroux, 1995) (Chapter 5).

**evidence** a body of data that can be used to make decisions about planning.

evidence-based practice the process of systematically finding, appraising, and using evidence as the basis for decision making when planning health education/promotion programs (Cottrell & McKenzie, 2011) (Chapter 1).

expectancies values people place on expected outcomes.

expectations beliefs about the likely outcomes of certain behaviors.

formalism see deontological theories.

freeing/functioning philosophy proponents of this philosophy help the person make the best health choices possible for that person, based on the individual's needs and interests, not on societal expectations.

global health "health problems, issues, and concerns that transcend national boundaries, may be influenced by circumstances or experiences in other countries, and are best addressed by cooperative actions and solutions" (IOM, 1997, p. 2) (Chapter 1).

goodness (rightness) a state or quality of being good; one of the five principles of common moral ground.

government documents unclassified publications authored and disseminated by federal, state, or local agencies intended for public use.

governmental health agencies agencies designated as having authority for certain specific duties or tasks outlined by the governmental bodies that oversee them.

graduate research assistantship an award given a graduate student who works closely with one or more faculty members on a research project; the student is usually granted tuition assistance and a stipend in return for the work.

graduate teaching assistantship an award given a graduate student who teaches for the program and in return is usually granted tuition assistance and a stipend.

hard money funds used to support health education/promotion positions and programs that are part of the regular budget of an employer.

health "is a dynamic state or condition of the human organism that is multidimensional (i.e., physical, emotional, social, intellectual, spiritual, and occupational) in nature, a resource for living, and results from a person's interactions with and adaptations to his or her environment" (McKenzie, Pinger, & Kotecki, 2012, p. 5) (Chapter 1).

health-adjusted life expectancy (HALE) the number of years of healthy life expected, on average, in a given population.

health advocacy "the processes by which the actions of individuals or groups attempt to bring about social and/or organizational change on behalf of a particular health goal, program, interest, or population" (Joint Committee, 2001, p. 99) (Chapter 1).

health behavior see lifestyle.

Health Belief Model an intrapersonal theory that "addresses a person's perceptions of the threat of a health problem and the accompanying appraisal of a recommended behavior for preventing or managing the problem" (Glanz & Rimer, 1995, p. 17) (Chapter 4).

health care organization "consists of the quantity, quality, arrangement, nature and relationships of people and resources in the provision of health care" (Lalonde, 1974, p. 32), also referred to as the health care system.

health care settings locations for health education/ promotion programs, including public and for-profit hospitals, free-standing medical care clinics, home health agencies, and physician organizations such as health maintenance organizations (HMOs) and preferred provider organizations (PPOs).

health disparities the difference in health between different populations often caused by two health inequities—lack of access to care and lack of quality care (McKenzie et al., 2012) (Chapter 1).

health education "any combination of planned learning experiences based on sound theories that provide individuals, groups, and communities the opportunity to acquire information and the skills needed to make quality health decisions" (Joint Committee, 2001, p. 99) (Chapter 1).

health education research "a systematic investigation involving the analysis of collected information or data that ultimately is used to enhance health education knowledge or practice, and answers one or more questions about a health-related theory, behavior or phenomenon" (Cottrell & McKenzie, 2011, p. 2) (Chapter 6).

**health education specialist** "a professionally prepared individual who serves in a variety of roles and is specifically trained to use appropriate educational strategies and methods to facilitate the development of policies, procedures, interventions, and systems conducive to the health of individuals, groups, and communities" (Joint Committee, 2001, p. 99) (Chapter 1).

**health field** a term that includes all matters that affect health; far more encompassing than the health care system.

**Health Field Concept** a framework that was developed in Canada to study health; it has four elements: human biology, environment, lifestyle, and health care organization.

**health literacy** the capacity of individuals to access, interpret, and understand basic health information and services and the skills to use the information and services to promote health.

**health promotion** "any planned combination of educational, political, environmental, regulatory, or organizational mechanisms that support actions and conditions of living conducive to the health of individuals, groups, and communities" (Joint Committee, 2001, p. 101) (Chapter 1).

*Healthy People* the first major U.S. government document recognizing the importance of lifestyle in promoting health and well-being.

*Healthy People 2000: National Health Promotion and Disease Prevention Objectives* a document that contains the health objectives for the United States during the 1990s.

*Healthy People 2010: Understanding and Improving Health* a document that contains the health objectives for the United States during the 2000s.

*Healthy People 2020* the latest listing of National Health Objectives for the United States through the year 2020.

**health-related quality of life (HRQOL)** "refers to a person or group's perceived physical and mental health over time" (CDC, 2010c, ¶ 1) (Chapter 1).

**Hippocrates** a Greek physician from the Asclepian tradition who eventually became known as the father of medicine.

**holistic philosophy** the philosophy that the mind and body blend into a single unit; the person is a unified being.

**home page** analogous to a combination of a cover and table of contents in a book, a home page names a specific Web site and directs the user to options within that site.

**human biology** "all those aspects of health, both physical and mental, which are developed within the human body as a consequence of the basic biology of man [sic] and the organic make-up of an individual" (Lalonde, 1974, p. 31) (Chapter 1).

**Hygeia** the daughter of Asclepios granted the power to prevent disease.

**hypertext** a type of document that allows convenient links to other documents found on the World Wide Web; it is a simple way of cross-referencing words or phrases with additional information; words or symbols that appear in color are hypertext words, and clicking on them provides links to related documents in the field (Rivard & Olpin, 1998) (Chapter 9).

**hypertext markup language** the programming language used on the Internet.

**hypertext transfer protocol** the protocol for exchanging hypertext documents between sites on the Web.

**impact evaluation** "the assessment of program effects on intermediate objectives including changes in predisposing, enabling, and reinforcing factors, behavioral and environmental changes, and possibly health and social outcomes" (Green & Kreuter, 2005, p. G-5) (Chapter 4).

**implementation** "the act of converting program objectives into actions through policy changes, regulation and organization" (Green & Kreuter, 2005, G-5) (Chapter 4).

**indexes** reference books that provide links to articles from many refereed journals, books, and selected reports; each index is written to target specific subject headings, so one index is not all-encompassing for all subjects.

**individual freedom (equality principle, or principle of autonomy)** people, being individuals with individual differences, must have the freedom to choose their own ways and means of being moral within the framework of value of life, goodness, justice, and truth-telling (Thiroux, 1995) (Chapter 5).

**informed consent** requires: (a) disclosure of relevant information to prospective participants about the program; (b) their comprehension of the information; and (c) their voluntary agreement, free from coercion and undue influence, to participate (OHSR, 2006) (Chapter 5).

**innovators** the first people to adopt an innovation.

**intention** "is an indication of a person's readiness to perform a given behavior, and it is considered to be the immediate antecedent of behavior" (Ajzen, 2006) (Chapter 4).

**International Union for Health Promotion and Education (IUHPE)** a professional association open to individuals who are interested in health education/promotion worldwide.

**Internet** an integrated network of computers that spans the entire world; the computers can transfer data to one another via phone lines, microwaves, fiber optics, and satellites (Kittleson, 1997) (Chapter 9).

**intervention alignment** matching appropriate strategies and interventions with projected changes and outcomes.

**justice (fairness)** "human beings should treat other human beings fairly and justly in distributing goodness and badness among them" (Thiroux, 1995, p. 184) (Chapter 5); a basic principle of ethics.

**laggards** the last group of people to get involved in an innovation, if they get involved at all.

**late majority** a group of people who are skeptical and will not adopt an innovation until most people in the social system have done so.

**liberal** generally, a person who favors governmental programs to address perceived social and economic inequities between segments of society.

**licensure** "a process by which an agency or government (usually a state) grants permission to individuals to practice a given profession by certifying that those licensed have attained specific standards of competence" (Cleary, 1995, p. 39) (Chapter 6).

**life expectancy** "the average number of years of life remaining to a person at a particular age and based on a given set of age-specific death rates, generally the mortality conditions existing in the period mentioned. Life expectancy may be determined by race, sex, or other characteristics using age-specific death rates for the population with that characteristic" (NCHS, 2010, p. 525) (Chapter 1).

**lifestyle** "an aggregation of decisions by individuals which affect their health and over which they more or less have control" (Lalonde, 1974, p. 32) (Chapter 1).

**likelihood of taking action** chances that a person will behave in a particular way; a construct of the health belief model.

**local health department (LHD)** a governmental organization that is located in a city or county.

**locus of control** one's perception of the center of control over reinforcement.

**macrolevel** having health education/promotion interventions targeted to the community as a whole, instead of to individuals.

**maintenance stage** the stage of the transtheoretical model in which a person is taking steps to sustain change and resist temptation to relapse.

**Master Certified Health Education Specialist (MCHES)** an advanced level of certification available for health education specialists who health education OR a master's degree in a related field along with at least 25 semester hours of health education coursework. The MCHES exam must be taken and passed to receive this credential.

**MAPP** is the acronym for the planning model titled Mobilizing for Action through Planning and Partnerships created by the National Association of County and City Health Officials.

**MATCH** an acronym for Multilevel Approach To Community Health.

**M.A., M.Ed., M.H.S., M.P.H., M.S., M.S.P.H.** degree designations available to master's-level health education/promotion students, depending on the institution they attend and their area of emphasis.

**Medicaid** government health insurance for the poor.

**Medicare** government health insurance for the elderly and disabled.

**metaphysics** the study of the nature of reality (Thiroux, 1995) (Chapter 5).

**miasmas theory** a belief that vapors, or miasmas, rising from rotting refuse could travel through the air for great distances and result in disease when inhaled.

**microlevel** targeting health education/promotion interventions to individuals.

**model** "is a composite, a mixture of ideas or concepts taken from any number of theories and used together" (Hayden, 2009, p. 1) (Chapter 4).

**moderate** a person who acts in a more situationally specific manner in regard to using tax-supported programs to solve social problems.

**modifiable risk factors** changeable or controllable risk factors.

**moral** good/bad, and right/wrong.

**moral philosophy** see ethics.

**moral sensitivity** being aware that an ethical problem exists and having an understanding of what impact different courses of action may have on the people involved (Rest et al.,1999) (Chapter 5).

**multicausation disease model** a model that explains the onset of disease caused by more than one factor.

**multitasking** the skill of coordinating and completing multiple health education/promotion projects at the same time.

**National Commission for Health Education Credentialing, Inc.** the organization that oversees the health education certification process.

**National Task Force on the Preparation and Practice of Health Educators** the group that oversaw development of the roles and responsibilities of health education specialists and ultimately the CHES credentialing system.

**National Wellness Institute, Inc.** a professional association for those interested in wellness programs.

**needs assessment** a process that helps program planners determine what health problems might exist in any given group of people, what assets are available in the community to address the health problems, and the overall capacity of the community to address the health issues (McKenzie et al., 2009) (Chapter 6).

**networking** establishing and maintaining a wide range of contacts in the field that may be of help when looking for a job and in carrying out one's job responsibilities once hired.

**noncommunicable diseases** those that cannot be transmitted from an infected person to a susceptible, healthy one (McKenzie et al., 2012) (Chapter 1).

**nonconsequential** see deontological theories.

**nongovernmental health agencies** those that operate, for the most part, free from governmental interference as long as they comply with the Internal Revenue Service's guidelines for their tax status (McKenzie et al., 2012) (Chapter 8).

**nonmaleficence** "the non-infliction of harm to others" (Balog et al., 1985, p. 91) (Chapter 5).

**nonmodifiable risk factors** nonchangeable or noncontrollable risk factors.

**objective** statement describing specific, measurable cognitive or affective changes in the learner. An objective establishes a performance standard for the learner.

**open access journals** are journals that are available to the reader online without restriction to cost, membership, or legal barriers with the exception that the reader must be able to access the Internet.

**outcome evaluation** "assessment of the effects of a program on its ultimate objectives, including changes in health and social benefits or quality of life" (Green & Kreuter, 2005, p. G-6) (Chapter 4).

**ownership** a feeling of responsibility for program outcomes.

**Panacea** the daughter of Asclepios granted the power to treat disease.

**pandemic** an outbreak over a wide geographical area, such as a continent.

**participation** the active involvement of those in the priority population in helping identify, plan, and implement programs to address the health problems they face.

**perceived barriers** the cost of engaging in a health behavior; a construct of the health belief model.

**perceived behavioral control** a belief held by people that they have control over a behavior; a construct of the theory of planned behavior.

**perceived benefits** a belief that a particular health recommendation would be beneficial in reducing a perceived threat; a construct of the health belief model.

**perceived seriousness/severity** a belief that a health problem is serious; a construct of the health belief model.

**perceived susceptibility** a belief that one is vulnerable to a health problem; a construct of the health belief model.

**perceived threat** a belief that one is vulnerable to a serious health problem or to the sequelae of that illness or condition; a construct of the health belief model.

**philanthropic foundation** "endowed institution that donates money for the good of humankind" (McKenzie et al., 2012, p. 57) (Chapter 8).

**philodoxy** literally means "the love of opinion" but often is used in the context of letting opinion define reality.

**philosophy** a statement summarizing the attitudes, principles, beliefs, values, and concepts held by an individual or a group.

**philosophy of symmetry** a philosophy of health with physical, emotional, spiritual, and social components of health.

**popular press publications** publications ranging from weekly summary magazines (e.g., *Newsweek*) to monthly magazines (e.g., *Better Homes and Gardens*); often, articles include editorials; information from these sources should be heavily scrutinized before using.

**population-based approaches** community health methods that are used to help change behavior in groups of people. Examples include policy development, policy advocacy, organizational change, community development, empowerment of individuals, and economic supports.

**population health** "the health status of people who are not organized and have no identity as a group or locality and the actions and conditions to promote, protect, and preserve their health" (McKenzie et al., 2012, p. 7) (Chapter 1).

**portfolio** a collection of evidence that enables students to demonstrate mastery of desired course or program outcomes.

**postmodern family** any family structure that differs from a family composed of two parents and their children.

**postsecondary institution** in the United States, an institution that provides further education after high school.

**PRECEDE-PROCEED** an acronym for a theory of implementation that stands for Predisposing, Reinforcing, and Enabling Constructs in Educational/Environmental Diagnosis and Evaluation and Policy, Regulatory, and Organizational Constructs in Educational and Environmental Development.

**precontemplation stage** the stage of the transtheoretical model in which a person is not thinking about change in the next six months.

**predisposing factor** "any characteristic of a person or population that motivates behavior prior to the occurrence of the behavior" (Green & Kreuter, 2005, p. G-6) (Chapter 4).

**preparation stage** the stage of the transtheoretical model in which a person is actively planning change.

**prevention** the planning for and measures taken to forestall the onset of, limit the spread of, and rehabilitate after pathogenesis or other health problems.

**primary data** original data gathered by the health education specialist as part of a needs assessment; this includes data gathered from telephone surveys, focus groups, and interviews.

**primary prevention** preventive measures that forestall the onset of illness or injury during the prepathogenesis period.

**primary sources** published studies or eyewitness accounts written by the person(s) who actually conducted the study or observed the event.

**privacy** "the claim of individuals, groups, or institutions to determine for themselves when, how, and to what extent information about them is communicated to others" (Westin, 1968, p. 7) (Chapter 5).

**procedural justice** deals with whether or not fair procedures were in place and whether those procedures were followed (Summers, 2009) (Chapter 5).

**process evaluation** "the assessment of policies, materials, personnel, performance, quality of practice or services, and other inputs and implementation experiences" (Green & Kreuter, 2005, p. G-6) (Chapter 4).

**profession** "the sociological construct for an occupation that has special status" (Livingood, 1996, p. 421) (Chapter 1).

**professional ethics** "actions that are right and wrong in the workplace and are of public matter. Professional moral principles are not statements of taste or preference; they tell practitioners what they ought to do and what they ought not to do" (Feeney & Freeman, 1999, p. 6) (Chapter 5).

**professional health associations/organizations** organizations that promote the high standards of professional practice for their respective professions, thereby improving the health of society by improving the people in the professions (McKenzie et al., 2012) (Chapter 8).

*Promoting Health/Preventing Disease: Objectives for the Nation* a document containing 226 health objectives for the United States to be accomplished during the 1980s.

**public health** "is the science and the art of protecting and improving the health of communities through education, promotion of healthy lifestyles, and research for disease and injury prevention" (Association of Schools of Public Health, n. d., ¶ 1) (Chapter 1).

**public health agencies** also called "official governmental health agencies"; agencies usually financed through public tax monies and typically offering health promotion and education programs.

**quality assurance** "The planned and systematic activities necessary to provide adequate confidence that the product or service will meet given requirements" (Quality Assurance Solutions, 2010) (Chapter 6).

**quasi-governmental health agencies** agencies that possess some of the characteristics of a governmental health agency but also possess some of the characteristics of nongovernmental agencies.

**rate** "a measure of some event, disease, or condition in relation to a unit of population, along with some specification of time" (NCHS, 2010, p. 544) (Chapter 1).

**reciprocal determinism** "behavior changes result from an interaction between the person and the environment; change is bidirectional" (Glanz & Rimer, 1995) (Chapter 4).

**reduction of threat** a belief that a particular health recommendation would be beneficial in reducing a threat at a subjectively acceptable cost; a construct of the health belief model.

**refereed journal** a journal that publishes original manuscripts only after they have been read and critiqued by a panel of experts in the field.

**reinforcement** a response to behavior that increases the chance of recurrence.

**reinforcing factor** "any reward or punishment following or anticipated as a consequence of a behavior, serving to strengthen the motivation for the behavior after it occurs" (Green & Kreuter, 2005, G-7) (Chapter 4).

**research ethics** "comprises principles and standards that, along with underlying values, guide appropriate conduct relevant to research decisions" (Kimmel, 2007, p. 6) (Chapter 5).

**responsibilities** the seven major responsibilities of all entry-level health education specialists.

**risk factors** those inherited, environmental, and behavioral influences "which are known (or thought) to increase the likelihood of physical or mental problems" (Slee et al., 2008, p. 510) (Chapter 1).

**role delineation** the process of identifying the specific responsibilities, competencies, and subcompetencies associated with the practice of health education/promotion.

**Rule of Sufficiency** the programs, strategies, initiatives, methods implemented must be sufficiently robust, or effective enough, that the stated objectives will have a reasonable chance of being met.

**School Health Advisory Council (SHAC)** community members such as parents; medical, health, and safety professionals; and political, religious, and corporate or business leaders who assist with the planning and promotion of school health initiatives.

**school health education/promotion** health education programs that instruct school-age children about health and health-related behaviors.

**School Health Education Evaluation Study** a landmark study that examined the entire health program of selected schools in the Los Angeles area.

**School Health Education Study** a nationwide study that examined the status of health education and resulted in the development of an important curriculum.

**search engine** site on the World Wide Web specifically designed to search for all links associated with a word or phrase that the user wants information on; the search engines greatly decrease the time it takes to search for information on the Web; examples are Google, Yahoo®, and Bing.

**secondary data** preexisting data used by a health education specialist in a needs assessment.

**secondary prevention** preventive measures that lead to early diagnosis and prompt treatment of a disease or an injury to limit disability, impairment, or dependency and to prevent more severe pathogenesis.

**secondary sources** articles that often provide an overview or a summary of several related studies or that chronicle the history of several related events, written by someone who did not conduct the study or observe firsthand the event that is written about.

**self-control (self-regulation)** gaining control over one's own behavior by monitoring and adjusting it.

**self-efficacy** people's confidence in their ability to perform a certain desired task or function.

**septicemia** "the presence of bacteria in the blood (bacteremia), often associated with severe disease" (NLM & NIH, 2003, p. 1).

**service learning** course credit for students to work with a community agency to meet an identified community need.

**situational analysis** is "the combination of social and epidemiological assessments of conditions, trends, and priorities with a preliminary scan of determinants, relevant policies, resources, organizational support, and regulations that might anticipate or permit action in advance of a more complete assessment of behavioral, environmental, educational, ecological, and administrative factors" (Green & Kreuter, 2005, p. G-7 & 8) (Chapter 4).

**SMART** is an acronym for a social marketing planning model titled the Social Marketing Assessment and Response Tool.

**Smith Papyri** the oldest written document related to health, which describes various surgical techniques and dates back to 1600 B.C.

**social assessment** "the assessment in both objective and subjective terms of high-priority problems or aspirations for the common good, defined for a population by economic and social indicators and by individuals in terms of their quality of life" (Green & Kreuter, 1999, p. 509) (Chapter 4).

**social capital** "the relationships and structures within a community, such as civic participation, networks, norms of reciprocity, and trust, that promote cooperation of mutual benefit" (Putnam, 1995, p. 66) (Chapter 4).

**social change philosophy** a philosophy emphasizing the role of health education/promotion in creating social, economic, and political change that benefits the health of individuals and groups.

**social ecology** an approach to health education/promotion that goes beyond individual behavior change to examine and modify the social, political, and economic factors impacting health behavior decisions.

**social marketing** "the application of commercial marketing technologies to the analysis, planning, execution, and evaluation of programs designed to influence the voluntary behavior of target audiences in order to improve their personal welfare and that of their society" (Andreasen, 1995, p. 7) (Chapter 4).

**social network** "web of social relationships that surround people" (Heaney & Israel, 2008, p. 190) (Chapter 4).

**social networking** Using a "social structure made up of individuals (or organizations) called 'nodes,' which are tied (connected) by one or more specific types of interdependency, such as friendship, kinship, common interest, financial exchange, dislike, sexual relationships, or relationships of beliefs, knowledge or prestige" (Wikipedia, 2010). Facebook, Myspace, Cyworld, Bebo, and Twitter are examples of social networking.

**Society for Public Health Education, Inc. (SOPHE)** a professional association for health education specialists.

**Society of State Directors of Health, Physical Education, and Recreation (SSDHPER)** a professional association composed of individuals who, by position in a state/territorial department of education, represent their state/territory.

**socio-ecological approach** behavior has multiple levels of influences.

**soft money** funds to support health education/promotion positions and programs secured through grants or contracts, which may be discontinued at the end of a designated period.

**specific rate** a rate for a particular population subgroup, such as for a particular disease (i.e., disease-specific) or for a particular age of people.

**stage theories** those behavior change theories that comprise an ordered set of categories into which people can be classified, and for which factors could be identified that could induce movement from one category to the next (Weinstein & Sandman, 2002) (Chapter 4).

**sub-competencies** "reflects the ability of the student to list, describe, etc." (National Commission for Health Education Credentialing, Inc. 1996, p. 12) (Chapter 6).

**subjective norm** a belief held by people that others (individuals or groups) think they should do something and that they care about what others think; a construct of the theory of planned behavior.

**technology** any device used by society to increase access to or opportunity for people to be exposed to that device—for example, computers and television have increased educational access and opportunities for many people; thus, they are examples of technology.

**teleological theories** (or consequentialism) evaluate the moral status of an act by the goodness of the consequences (Reamer, 2006) (Chapter 5).

**termination** zero chance of relapse.

**tertiary prevention** preventive measures aimed at rehabilitation following significant pathogenesis.

**theories/models of implementation** theories and models used in planning, implementing, and evaluating health education/promotion programs.

**theory** "a set of interrelated concepts, definitions, and propositions that presents a systematic view of events or situations by specifying relations among variables in order to explain and predict the events of the situations" (Glanz et al., 2008b, p. 25) (Chapter 4).

**Theory of Planned Behavior** an intrapersonal theory that addresses individuals' intentions to perform a given behavior as a function of their attitude toward performing the behavior, their beliefs about what is relevant, what others think they should do, and their perception of the ease or difficulty in performing the behavior.

**traditional family** a family having two parents and their children.

**Transtheoretical Model** also known as the stages of change model, it is an intrapersonal theory that addresses an "individual's readiness to change or attempt to change toward healthy behaviors" (Glanz & Rimer, 1995, p. 17) (Chapter 4).

**truth telling (honesty)** to tell the truth; one of the five principles of common moral ground.

**Uniform Resource Locator (URL)** identifier for a site on the World Wide Web; specifies locations, or addresses.

**value of life** a basic principle of ethics: no life should be ended without very strong justification.

**variable** the operational (practical use) form of a construct.

**voluntary health agencies** "organizations that are created by concerned citizens to deal with health needs not met by governmental agencies" (McKenzie et al., 2012) (Chapters 7 and 8); these organizations rely heavily on volunteer help and donations to function.

**wellness** "an approach to health that focuses on balancing the many aspects, or dimensions, of a person's life through increasing the adoption of health enhancing conditions and behaviors rather than attempting to minimize conditions of illness" (Joint Committee, 2001, p. 103) (Chapter 1).

**worksite health promotion** health education/promotion programs offered by business and industry entities for their employees.

**World Wide Web** an interactive information delivery service that includes a repository of resources about most subjects; documents are related by subject area and linked together, thus creating a "web" (Madden, 2010) (Chapter 9).

**years of potential life lost (YPLL)** a measure of premature mortality calculated by subtracting a person's age at death from seventy-five years (NCHS, 2006) (Chapter 1).

# Index

Note: Page numbers followed by *f* indicate a figure or photograph, by *t* indicate a table, and by *b* indicate boxed material. Page numbers for Key Terms are in boldface.